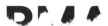

Health for all Children

Health for all Children

FIFTH EDITION

Edited by

Alan Emond

Professor of Child Health, Centre for Academic Child Health,
University of Bristol, UK

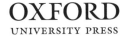

OXFORD
UNIVERSITY PRESS

OXFORD
UNIVERSITY PRESS

Great Clarendon Street, Oxford OX2 6DP,
United Kingdom

Oxford University Press is a department of the University of Oxford.
It furthers the University's objective of excellence in research, scholarship,
and education by publishing worldwide. Oxford is a registered trade mark of
Oxford University Press in the UK and in certain other countries

© Royal College of Paediatrics and Child Health 2019

Chapter 13 © Crown Copyright. Reproduced with the permission of Public Health England
under delegated authority from the Controller of HMSO.

The moral rights of the authors have been asserted

First Edition Published in 1989
Second Edition Published in 1991
Third Edition Published in 1996
Fourth Edition Published in 2003
Fourth Edition Revised Published in 2006
Fifth Edition Published in 2019

Impression: 1

Published in the United States of America by Oxford University Press
198 Madison Avenue, New York, NY 10016, United States of America

British Library Cataloguing in Publication Data
Data available

Library of Congress Control Number: 2018960020

ISBN 978–0–19–878885–0

Printed in Great Britain by
Bell & Bain Ltd., Glasgow

Preface

Health for all children—the story so far

Health services for children have been evolving in the UK since the Victorians' social reforms in the nineteenth century. After the Second World War, attention turned to early detection of disabling conditions such as cerebral palsy, learning difficulties, impaired vision or hearing, and to problems for which new treatment approaches were emerging, for example, congenital heart disease and growth disorders. Developmental and health checks of infants and children were provided by a community-based workforce which worked, and was managed, separately from hospital paediatric services or general practice.

The introduction by Guthrie in 1962 of the newborn blood spot test for phenylketonuria focused attention on screening. In 1966, Wilson and Jungner observed that the potential for screening tests in medicine was almost unlimited and they published criteria by which candidate screening procedures could be evaluated. Child health checks did not meet these criteria. The staffing levels, the target disorders and schedules of examination, and the take-up by parents varied widely. For these reasons, the term 'child health surveillance' (CHS) was preferred to 'screening'.

By the mid 1980s, many 'new' diagnoses were recognized, including autism spectrum disorders, speech and language impairments, behavioural syndromes, dyslexia, and dyspraxia. Community child health clinics were more familiar with these problems than general practitioners; however, the latter often had a more detailed knowledge of relevant family circumstances and argued that CHS was logically part of good family medicine.

In 1986, the British Paediatric Association (which became a Royal College in 1996) set up a Joint Working Party with general practitioners and health visitors, supported by the Department of Health. The brief was to review the evidence base for CHS and make recommendations for best practice. The review found that quality data were lacking, many conditions were diagnosed late, and many normal children were referred unnecessarily for specialist assessment. In 1989, the report *Health for all Children* proposed a core CHS programme—this was incorporated into a new general practice contract, backed up by an accredited training programme.

The review noted that screening programmes can do harm as well as good and stressed the ethical imperative to evaluate them, but specialists and parent organizations were often enthusiastic about screening and recommendations made by the Working Party for caution regarding unproven screening programmes were subjected to strident criticism that often went beyond academic debate. In 1996, a UK National Screening Committee was set up to develop evidence-based policy and advise Ministers. The Committee updated the Wilson and Junger criteria, recommended newborn hearing screening, and proposed expansion of the newborn blood spot programme to include many more disorders. Reviews were undertaken of growth monitoring and of screening for vision defects, language disorders, and autism.

Health promotion now has an increasingly prominent role, addressing topics such as reducing the risk of sudden infant death, immunization, nutrition, obesity, dental health, and injury prevention. There has been more investment in preschool and early intervention programmes, particularly for disadvantaged children and families.

The proposals in successive editions of *Health for all Children* were reflected in the *National Service Framework* (2004) and subsequently implemented in England in the *Healthy Child Programme* (2010). But health policy is never purely scientific—it is influenced by social attitudes and healthcare politics. Critical questions remain: for example, why do child health programmes vary so much within and between countries? Do countries with primary care paediatricians perform better?

In the UK, health visitor roles are evolving while general practitioners, who in 1989 wanted to take over CHS, now actually do less paediatrics—and there is still no obligatory paediatric training for general practice. The Quality and Outcomes Framework, an annual reward and incentive programme for all general practitioner surgeries in England, does not include any measures relevant to children. The recommendations of this fifth edition of *Health for all Children* present a challenge to professionals and politicians—I hope it will be more successful in stimulating action than its predecessors.

Professor Sir David Hall
Emeritus Professor of Community Paediatrics
University of Sheffield
Honorary Consultant
Sheffield Children's NHS Trust, UK

Acknowledgements

The section leads each made a big contribution to writing and editing the book, and deserve special thanks: Cheryll Adams, Jane Barlow, Helen Bedford, Mitch Blair, Sarah Cowley, and David Elliman

Many individuals and institutions contributed to, or commented on, early drafts of the fifth edition. Thanks to the following individuals who reviewed chapters or contributed comments: Jill Beswick, Allan Colver, Toity Deave, Diane de Bell, Gene Feder, Leon Feinstein, Amanda Hall, Munib Haroon, Alice Haynes, Lynn Kemp, Jackie Kirkham, Rachel Knowles, Simon Lenton, Jacqui Mok, Rob Moy, Robert Nettleton, Jugnoo Rahi, Robert Scott-Jupp, Tony Sirimanna, and Cathy Williams.

These stakeholders provided useful feedback: Public Health England, Public Health Wales, NHS Scotland, NHS Northern Ireland, Royal College of General Practice, Institute of Health Visiting, British Society of Paediatric Dentistry, British Association of Community Child Health, Community Practitioners and Health Visitors Association, and Royal College of Paediatrics and Child Health (General Paediatrics, Paediatric Care Online).

Special thanks to the support team at the Royal College of Paediatrics and Child Health: Lindsey Hunter, Matthew Jordan, Christopher Nelson, Raisha Sajjad and Grace Brown; and to Jamie Reeves at Imperial College London. Caroline Smith and Sylvia Warren at Oxford University Press patiently nurtured the book to publication.

Executive summary

The fifth edition of *Health for all Children* is a review of the evidence supporting preventive healthcare, health promotion, and an effective community-based response to the needs of families and children, from pregnancy to the age of 7 years. Evidence is utilized from all over the world, but referenced to UK policy and practice, taking into account different models of delivery of the child health programme in the different UK administrations.

This book summarizes evidence about 'why' and 'what works' in health promotion and health surveillance with children and families, where possible gives guidance on 'how' to implement and quality assure a programme—but does not conclude on 'who' should provide the service.

Recommendations are made for commissioners of child health services, provider organizations and Trusts, and practitioners. Each recommendation is made on the basis of evidence, and a weighting of the strength of that evidence is attached to each recommendation. The strength of recommendations is determined by the balance between the quality of evidence, variability in values and preferences, desirable and undesirable consequences of alternative strategies, and resource use. Each chapter concludes with 'Learning links': recommended e-learning courses and online materials to support evidence-based practice.

The book contains 35 chapters divided into seven sections. The first introductory section describes the scope of the book and the philosophy of improving child health by reducing inequalities with a programme based on 'proportionate universalism'. The second section on pregnancy starts with a discussion of the effects of environmental exposures and mother's diet on the fetus. The growing body of evidence of importance of parental mental health in the perinatal period and the impact of inter-personal violence in pregnancy on the developing child is reviewed in detail. Evidence-based interventions to stop smoking and avoid alcohol and substance use in pregnancy are summarized. The literature on the transition to parenthood and interventions to prepare for parenting is critically appraised.

The third section on primary prevention and health promotion is the largest in the book, with each chapter reviewing the evidence of effectiveness in a different topic area. Evidence-based recommendations are made for universal, targeted, and enhanced interventions to improve health and development of infants and children up to the age of 7 years, and examples of good practice are highlighted. Section 4 covers secondary prevention, including screening, and recommended surveillance activities. The evidence supporting 'core' reviews is summarized, and the importance of opportunistic identification of growth, developmental, and behaviour problems in primary care emphasized.

Children with additional needs are considered in Section 5, including the evidence for early identification and referral of children with atypical development. The growing literature on supporting families living in special circumstances such as migrants and gypsies/Travellers, and children who have been fostered or adopted is appraised. Good practice in safeguarding children is summarized. Interventions for medical conditions and in-hospital care of children are not included. In Section 6, the evidence for effective delivery of a child health programme is summarized, emphasizing the need for coordination between community health services, social care, and early education. The importance of school readiness as a framework and an outcome of preschool services is highlighted. Several enhancements to the child health programme in the UK are described, and the emerging evidence base for their effectiveness reviewed. The final section, Section 7, considers issues of managing and quality assuring a child health programme, the need for data to enable the reduction of inequalities in coverage and outcomes, and the importance of coordinated oversight and management of the programme.

Contents

Abbreviations

AABR	automated auditory brainstem response
ACE	adverse childhood experience
ADHD	attention deficit hyperactivity disorder
ASC	autistic spectrum conditions
ASQ-3	Ages and Stages Questionnaires
BCCEWH	British Columbia Centre of Excellence for Women's Health
BMI	body mass index
CAHMI	Child and Adolescent Health Measurement Initiative
CBT	cognitive behavioural therapy
CDSC	Caring Dads, Safer Children
CHD	congenital heart disease
CHPs	child health programmes
CHS	child health surveillance
CIRF	Comprehensive Implementation Research Framework
CM	contingency management
CO	carbon monoxide
CP	cerebral palsy
DAWBA	Development and Well-Being Assessment
DCD	developmental coordination disorder
DDH	developmental dysplasia of the hip
DfE	Department for Education
DH	Department of Health
ECD	Early Childhood Development
ED	emergency department
EU	European Union
EYFS	early years foundation stage
FASP	Fetal Anomaly Screening Programme
FNP	Family Nurse Partnership
FRAIT	Family Resilience Assessment Instrument Tool
GP	general practitioner
HCP	Healthy Child Programme
ICD-10	International Statistical Classification of Diseases, tenth edition
IDPS	Infectious Diseases in Pregnancy Screening
IDT	infant distraction test
IPV	intimate partner violence
KPI	key performance indicator

MI	motivational interviewing
NBS	newborn bloodspot screening
NCB	National Children's Bureau
NHS	National Health Service
NHSP	Newborn Hearing Screening Programme
NICE	National Institute for Health and Care Excellence
NICU	neonatal intensive care unit
NIPE	newborn and infant physical examination
OAE	otoacoustic emissions
OME	otitis media with effusion
PCB	polychlorinated biphenyl
PCHR	Personal Child Health Record
PEDS	Parents' Evaluation of Developmental Status
PHDSS	Promoting Healthy Development Survey
PND	postnatal depression
PPV	positive predictive value
PTSD	post-traumatic stress disorder
RCGP	Royal College of General Practitioners
RCPCH	Royal College of Paediatrics and Child Health
RCT	randomized controlled trial
ROI	return on investment
SACN	Scientific Advisory Committee on Nutrition
SD	standard deviation
SDQ	Strengths and Difficulties Questionnaire
SES	school entry screening
SIDS	sudden infant death syndrome
SIGN	Scottish Intercollegiate Guidelines Network
TMV	thermostatic mixing valve
TT	tongue tie
UASC	unaccompanied asylum-seeking child
UK	United Kingdom
UKNSC	United Kingdom National Screening Committee
UNS	universal newborn screening
US	United States
USS	ultrasound screening
WHO	World Health Organization

Section leads

Cheryll Adams
Executive Director, Institute of Health
Visiting, London, UK

Jane Barlow
Professor of Evidence-Based
Intervention and Policy Evaluation,
Department of Social Policy and
Intervention, University of Oxford,
Oxford, UK

Helen Bedford
Professor of Children's Health, UCL
Great Ormond Street Institute of Child
Health, London, UK

Mitch Blair
Professor of Paediatrics and Child Public
Health, Imperial College, London, UK

Sarah Cowley
Emeritus Professor, King's College
London and Trustee of the Institute of
Health Visiting, London, UK

David Elliman
Clinical Lead, National NIPE and NBS
Screening Programmes, Public Health
England; and Consultant, Great Ormond
Street Hospital, London, UK

Alan Emond
Professor of Child Health, Centre for
Academic Child Health, Bristol Medical
School, University of Bristol, Bristol, UK

Contributors

Nick Axford
Associate Professor in Health Services Research, Faculty of Medicine and Dentistry, University of Plymouth, Plymouth, UK

Peter S. Blair
Professor of Epidemiology and Statistics, Bristol Medical School, University of Bristol, UK

Alison Burton
Public Health Programme Manager, Maternity and Early Years, Public Health England, London, UK

Anna Chalkley
National Centre for Sport and Exercise Medicine—East Midlands, School of Sport, Exercise and Health Sciences, Loughborough University, Leicestershire, UK

Jane Coad
Professor in Children and Family Nursing, Coventry University, Coventry, UK

Louise Condon
Professor of Nursing, College of Human and Health Sciences, Swansea University, Swansea, UK

Vivette Glover
Institute of Reproductive and Developmental Biology, Imperial College London, London, UK

Jenny Godson
National Lead for Oral Health Improvement, Public Health England, London, UK

Alice Haynes
Development and Learning Advisor, A Better Start, London, UK

Alison M. Kemp
Professor of Child Health, Division of Population Medicine, School of Medicine, Cardiff University, Cardiff, UK

Denise Kendrick
Professor of Primary Care Research, Division of Primary Care, University of Nottingham, Nottingham, UK

Jackie Kirkham
Health Visitor, NHS Forth Valley, Stirling, UK

James Law
Professor of Speech & Language Sciences, School of Education, Communication and Language Sciences, University of Newcastle, Newcastle-upon-Tyne, UK

Mary Malone
Director of the Oxford School of Nursing and Midwifery, Oxford Brookes University, UK

Anita Schrader McMillan
Senior Research Fellow, Department of Social Policy and Intervention, University of Oxford, Oxford, UK

Julie Mytton
Associate Professor in Child Health, Centre for Academic Child Health, University of the West of England, Bristol, UK

Anna Pease
Senior Research Associate, Centre for
Academic Child Health, Bristol Medical
School, University of Bristol, Bristol, UK

Rebecca Reynolds
Professor of Metabolic Medicine,
Centre for Cardiovascular Science,
Queen's Medical Research Institute,
Edinburgh, UK

Diane Seymour
Senior Dental Public Health Manager,
Dental Public Health, Public Health
England, London, UK

Lauren Sherar
Reader in Physical Activity and
Health, National Centre for Sport and
Exercise Medicine—East Midlands,
School of Sport, Exercise and Health
Sciences, Loughborough University,
Leicestershire, UK

Douglas Simkiss
Consultant Paediatrician and Honorary
Associate Professor in Child Health,
Children and Families Division,
Birmingham Community Healthcare
NHS Foundation Trust, Birmingham, UK

Susan Soar
Early Childhood Unit, National
Children's Bureau, London, UK

Ameenat Lola Solebo
NIHR BRC Moorfields Institute
of Ophthalmology and UCL Great
Ormond Street Institute of Child Health,
London, UK

Andy Spencer
Senior Lecturer, Keele University
Medical School, Staffordshire, UK

Caroline Taylor
Research Fellow, Centre for Academic
Child Health, Bristol Medical School,
University of Bristol, Bristol, UK

Philip Wilson
Professor of Primary Care and Rural
Health, University of Aberdeen, Centre
for Rural Health, Inverness, UK

Charlotte M. Wright
Professor of Community Child
Health, School of Medicine, Dentistry
and Nursing, University of Glasgow,
Glasgow, UK

Section 1

Introduction

Chapter 1

Health for all children: philosophy and principles

Alan Emond

Summary

This chapter:

+ describes the aims of this review of the evidence supporting child health programmes

+ explains the concept of proportionate universalism

+ emphasizes that different components of a child health programme require different competencies from staff working in multidisciplinary teams

+ defines some key terms to be used throughout the book.

Life course approach

Pregnancy and the first years of life are when the foundations of future health and well-being are laid down, and this is a time when parents are particularly receptive to learning and making changes. Outcomes for both children and adults are strongly influenced by the factors that operate during pregnancy and the first years of life. Increasing strength of evidence about the sensitivity and plasticity of the developing brain, the impact of stress in pregnancy, and the importance of attachment in determining the quality of relationships throughout life, all make prevention and early intervention an imperative if the United Nations Sustainable Development Goals are to be realized.

There is an increasing body of evidence on the effects of 'toxic stress' as a result of adverse childhood experiences and harmful exposures in pregnancy (see https://developingchild.harvard.edu/). Early experiences with significant stress are critical, because they lead to physiological adaptations to the stress response (biological memories), which undermine the development of adaptive capacities and coping skills needed to deal with later challenges. A growing evidence base links childhood toxic stress to the subsequent development of unhealthy lifestyles (e.g. substance abuse and poor eating and exercise habits), persistent socioeconomic inequalities (e.g. school failure and financial hardship), and poor health (e.g. diabetes) (Shonkoff and Garner, 2011). The prevention of long-term, adverse consequences of stress is best achieved by the buffering protection afforded by stable, responsive relationships that help children develop a sense of safety.

Universal or targeted services?

In spite of declining mortality rates, there are still steep social gradients in most indicators of child health. To address these inequalities, child health programmes in the UK have been developed as a progressive universal service that offers a core programme of prevention and health promotion to all families, and a range of early intervention services for different levels of risk and assessed need. However, 'targeting' interventions may stigmatize families, and data from the US Head Start programme suggest that although early intervention programmes benefit most children, there is a risk that children in the most needy families may perform worse in some programme areas and that early intervention may actually increase inequalities.

Fair Society, Healthy Lives: The Strategic Review of Health Inequalities in England post-2010 (Marmot et al. 2010) introduced the concept of 'proportionate universalism' suggesting that 'To reduce the steepness of the social gradient in health, actions must be universal, but with a scale and intensity that is proportionate to the level of disadvantage'. There has been much debate over what 'proportionate' means (Carey 2015). A proportionate response could see direct health interventions for the most disadvantaged, or could be a dose–response approach, where those at the bottom of the gradient require more 'health action' than those higher up. Child health programmes offer universal services for all children and families, and both targeted services to certain vulnerable, disadvantaged groups, and more intensive support services to families living in socially deprived communities.

Components of child health programmes in the UK

In this review, *child health programme* is a generic term to describe proportionate universal services for children from pregnancy to the age of 7 years. The term includes the Healthy Child Programme in England, the Healthy Child Wales Programme, the child health programme in Scotland (Getting it Right for Every Child), and the Healthy Child, Healthy Future programme in Northern Ireland. All of these are coordinated programmes of activity, including health promotion and disease prevention, screening, case identification, and targeted interventions. All share the philosophy of working in partnership with families to achieve the best outcomes for children.

Working in partnership with parents

To work effectively to support families, and to help children achieve their potential, practitioners need to develop a mutually trusting relationship, allowing open exploration of the problems or difficulties facing the parent. If practitioners (in a relatively powerful position) are not trusted, parents will not talk openly. If a parent is regarded with esteem and treated with respect, he or she will feel valued, leading to increasing self-esteem and capacity to manage difficulties more effectively. See Box 1.1.

Box 1.1 Qualities needed to work in partnership with parents

- *Respect* or unconditional positive regard—valuing parents as people and assuming competence and strength, not weakness and incapacity.
- *Genuineness*—which implies attempting to be yourself, honestly and openly, and not being closed and defensive, not hiding behind a professional façade.
- *Empathy*—the attempt to understand the world from the viewpoint of the person you are trying to help, as opposed to the imposition of the helper's own views.
- *Humility* allows the person who is seeking help to contribute to the process and not to simply be in the hands of someone who is all-knowing and all-powerful.

Services that are highly rated by parents have certain characteristics in common (Box 1.2). Interventions that have these characteristics are likely to be not only effective but also acceptable and sustainable.

Competencies needed

Different components of a child health programme require different competencies from staff, supported by appropriate training. *Screening* requires the test or examination to identify the condition of interest to be applied in a structured way, following

Box 1.2 Characteristics of successful programmes and projects with families

- The staff have both the time and the skill to establish a relationship of respect and trust with families.
- The child is seen as a member of the family, and the family a part of the community.
- Services are of a broad spectrum and comprehensive, crossing traditional professional boundaries, and are coherent and easy to use.
- Both the structure and the individual staff are flexible in their ability to respond to unexpected demands.
- Projects have enthusiastic committed leadership; clearly specified, measurable aims; and focus on families with high levels of need.
- There is sustained high quality and quantity of input and, importantly, sufficient continuity of input to develop a relationship with the individual client.

a standard procedure or protocol so that true cases are not missed and false positives are kept to a minimum. Effective *case identification* requires practitioners to have an understanding of the normal, the range of variation around that norm seen in the population, and the ability to distinguish atypical patterns of child development from delay in development. *Health promotion* has to be evidence based, and delivered in a way that is appropriate to the family's educational and cultural background and economic circumstances. This needs practitioners who are both informed about the scientific evidence and culturally competent, good communicators. *Anticipatory guidance* involves giving prevention and health promotion advice in a developmental context—that is, the practitioner needs to have a 'developmental approach', to be aware of patterns of normal development, of crucial developmental windows (or 'sensitive periods'), and of the risks of injury associated with each stage of development. Finally, *assessment* of risk or of need for additional services or referral requires the highest level competencies in understanding the sources of stress to families and children; understanding how families function and how parental mental and physical health can impact children; identifying signs of neglect and maltreatment; and also recognizing a family's resources and capacity for resilience. This is a very complicated task, and tools have been created in both Scotland (Getting it Right for Every Child National Practice Model, https://www2.gov.scot/Topics/People/Young-People/gettingitright/national-practice-model) and in Wales (Family Resilience Assessment Instrument, https://www.frait.wales) to help health visitors identify protective factors within families as well as to identify additional needs and potential safeguarding concerns.

Team working

The wide range of competencies needed means that different practitioners can deliver different components of the child health programme. It is not cost-effective to have all the tasks in the universal programme undertaken by practitioners who have the level of competencies needed for assessment of risk and need, and for delivering targeted interventions. However, it is also not wise to skill-mix to the point that staff do not have the knowledge, skills, and attitudes to undertake holistic assessments, and risks are ignored, and needs are missed. Having practitioners with the capacity to undertake needs assessments is essential to the concept of proportionate universalism—to identify children and families who need an enhanced or targeted service, or who need referral to specialists.

The delivery of a child health programme therefore needs a team approach, and commissioners have a responsibility to monitor the extent to which provider organizations create functioning teams where different professionals, employed by different organizations, can communicate effectively with each other.

Health practitioners who can make up the team delivering the child health programme include nursery nurses, midwives, health visitors, general practitioners, and practice nurses. Staff working in children's centres and teachers in nurseries and schools also have important roles.

In the UK, health visitors are particularly identified with the health of mothers and preschool children, and much of the relevant research involves assessment of health visiting practice, both in the UK and overseas. In the North American literature, the term 'home visitation' is used; in some countries, the nurse is called a maternal and child health nurse.

British health visiting services are designed to offer a proportionate universal service, making use of their specific professional skills (Cowley et al., 2014) and those of team members and colleagues in, for example, children's centres. Systems that offer targeted provision from within a universal service are recommended (Daro and Dodge, 2010), ideally being organized to allow overlapping provision and encourage uptake, which will optimize preventive messages.

Definitions

Primary prevention is activity across the whole population that aims to reduce the number of new cases of a disease, disorder, or condition in a population, that is, reduction of the *incidence*.

Secondary prevention is targeted activity that aims to reduce the *prevalence* of a condition through early detection and effective intervention.

Child health surveillance is a programme of secondary prevention, and it includes *screening* and *case identification*.

Tertiary prevention is activity aimed at reducing impairments and disabilities, minimizing the impact on children and families and promoting the child's and parents' adjustment to conditions that cannot be ameliorated.

Health promotion can be defined as 'any planned and informed intervention which is designed to improve physical or mental health or prevent disease, disability and premature death'. Health in this definition is taken to mean a 'positive holistic state in which mental and social well-being are as important as physical well-being'. Successful health promotion needs both community-wide action and, at the individual level, a cooperative and respectful approach, with interpersonal skills which need to be developed to a high level.

Health education is defined as 'any activity which promotes health through learning, i.e. some relatively permanent change in an individual's capabilities or dispositions'. It can be directed at individuals, groups, or whole populations.

Health protection involves measures adopted to safeguard the health of the community as a whole; for example, clean water, good sanitation, safe roads, and playgrounds.

Healthy alliances refer to collaborations between statutory agencies and voluntary bodies in health protection, community development, and health education.

Community development is the process by which local people define their own health needs and organize themselves to make these needs known to service providers, or take action themselves in order to bring about change.

Child health programme is a generic term to describe universal services for children from pregnancy to the age of 7 years. The term includes the Healthy Child Programme in England, the Healthy Child Wales programme, the child health programme in Scotland (Getting it Right for Every Child), and the Healthy Child, Healthy Future programme in Northern Ireland.

Learning links

◆ Center on the Developing Child, Harvard University—'Resource library': https://
developingchild.harvard.edu/resources.

References

Cowley, S., Whittaker, K., Malone, M., Donetto, S., Grigulis, A., and Maben, J. (2014). Why
health visiting? Examining the potential public health benefits from health visiting practice
within a universal service: a narrative review of the literature. *International Journal of
Nursing Studies*, **52**, 465–480.

Daro, D. and Dodge, K.A. (2010). Strengthening home-visiting intervention policy: expanding
reach, building knowledge. [online] Available at: https://www.brookings.edu/wp-content/
uploads/2016/07/1013_investing_in_young_children_haskins_ch7.pdf.

Marmot, M., Allen, J., Goldblatt, P., et al. (2010). *Fair Society, Healthy Lives: The Strategic
Review of Health Inequalities in England post-2010*. London: Institute of Health Equity.
Available at: http://www.instituteofhealthequity.org/resources-reports/fair-society-healthy-
lives-the-marmot-review/fair-society-healthy-lives-full-report-pdf.

Shonkoff, J.P. and Garner, A.A. (2011). The American Academy of Pediatrics Committee on
Psychosocial Aspects of Child and Family Health. Toxic stress, brain development, and the
early childhood foundations of lifelong health. *Pediatrics*, **129**, e232–e246.

Chapter 2

The scope of the review

Alan Emond

Summary

This chapter:

◆ summarizes why a new edition of *Health for all Children* is needed

◆ explains how the quality and strength of the evidence supporting practice and commissioning have been assessed

◆ describes how the recommendations from evidence have been weighted

◆ provides an overview of the book structure.

Background

More than a decade has passed since the fourth edition of *Health for all Children*, and a new edition is overdue for several reasons:

◆ The evidence to support clinical practice in health surveillance and health promotion in the early years has expanded.

◆ The commissioning of services for children outside hospital has changed, with increasing devolution to local authorities in England.

◆ The range of professionals engaged in delivering care to young children has widened, and there are more and different types of provider.

◆ Evidence-based recommendations need to be linked to e-learning training resources.

The scope of *Health for all Children,* fifth edition

The scope of this book is to summarize evidence supporting preventive healthcare, health promotion, and an effective community-based response to the needs of families and children, from pregnancy to age seven. Each chapter will summarize evidence of effectiveness in the topic area, in health promotion, and in universal and selective interventions.

What is different about this edition of *Health for all Children* is that the review of evidence starts in pregnancy and runs until the age of 7 years. The review does not address issues of hospital or acute care, but where appropriate, links are provided to clinical management guidelines from the National Institute for Health and Care Excellence (NICE) and recommendations from the Scottish Intercollegiate Guidelines Network (SIGN) and others.

The book takes account of different government policies and different models of delivery of the child health programme in all four of the UK administrations. It utilizes evidence from all over the world, but references the evidence to UK policy and practice.

This book summarizes evidence about 'why' and 'what works' in health promotion and health surveillance with children and families, and where possible gives guidance on 'how' to implement and quality assure a programme—but does not conclude on 'who' should provide the service (this will vary according to the location, the demographic background of the families, the resources available, and many other factors).

A consistent theme throughout is that each evidence-based component of the child health programme should be linked to competencies needed to deliver that component, and the training needed to acquire and maintain those competencies. Where appropriate, recommendations are made for the skills and competencies needed by the workforce to deliver a healthy child programme, without being prescriptive about the grade or professional background of staff. Competencies do not rest exclusively with any professional group—a team is required to deliver all aspects of the child health programme. However, key messages for workforce skills and training are included. Each chapter includes 'learning links' to online training materials and e-learning for health, or to resources freely available to practitioners.

What is evidence? Definitions to be used

Quality of evidence is the degree to which bias is minimized. It concerns the extent to which a study's design, conduct, and analysis have minimized biases in selecting subjects and measuring both outcomes and differences in the study groups (other than the factors being studied) that might influence the results.

Strength of evidence is the degree to which published literature is consistent, and the quantity of evidence supporting a conclusion. Precision of results and applicability to UK settings is also considered.

Quality and strength of evidence are closely inter-related; the quality of individual studies must be graded before drawing affirmative conclusions about the strength of the aggregated evidence.

Strong evidence is based on evaluations that are sufficiently rigorous to determine whether an intervention can be causally linked to improvements in outcomes. A reliable comparison group is needed, which is why randomized controlled trials are an important method of estimating impact.

Moderately strong evidence uses evaluations based on pre–post comparisons or the use of non-experimental comparison groups.

Emerging evidence (more research is needed) uses evaluations that confirm the intervention's core assumptions and verify its primary outcome, but more research is needed to be certain about a causal relationship with improvement in outcome.

This evidence-based review builds on and draws down from several important recent reports:

- Early Intervention Foundation—'The Best Start at Home': http://www.eif.org.uk/publication/the-best-start-at-home/
- Early Intervention Foundation— 'What Works to Enhance the Effectiveness of the Healthy Child Programme: An Evidence Update': http://www.eif.org.uk/wp-content/uploads/2018/06/what-works-to-enhance-effectiveness-healthy-child_June2018.pdf
- Public Health England—'Rapid Review to Update Evidence for the Healthy Child Programme 0–5': https://www.gov.uk/government/publications/healthy-child-programme-rapid-review-to-update-evidence/.

Making recommendations

At the end of each chapter, recommendations are made for commissioners of child health services, provider organizations and trusts, and practitioners. Each recommendation is made on the basis of evidence, and a weighting of the strength of that evidence is attached to each recommendation. The strength of each recommendation is determined by the balance between the desirable and undesirable consequences of alternative strategies, quality of evidence, variability in values and preferences, and resource use.

Evidence, even when available, is rarely definitive. The level of confidence that one might have in evidence depends on the underlying robustness of the research and the analyses done to synthesize that research. It is important to remember that the 'absence of evidence' about benefits (or harms) is not the same as 'evidence of no benefit' (or harm). Many important components of a proportionate universal child health programme do not have a strong evidence base, but this is an indication that more research is needed, not that services should be cut. The final chapter of this book describes some of the policy areas where more research evidence is required.

Where there is no, uncertain, or only low-quality emerging evidence to support an activity or intervention, recommendations are made about current good practice. These are generally supported by clear statements from the National Health Service or from professional bodies.

The child health programme in different countries in the UK

This book reviews the evidence supporting a universal child health programme. The same evidence is relevant to all of the UK countries, but different countries have chosen different methods of implementation, with a different number of mandated contacts, and different tools for assessment to identify families who need an enhanced service or referral.

Further details of each country's child health programme from the age of 0 to 7 years are available from the following websites:

- England: http://www.healthychildprogramme.com
- Scotland: http://www.isdscotland.org/Health-Topics/Child-Health/Child-Health-Programme

- Wales: http://gov.wales/topics/health/publications/health/reports/healthy-child/?lang=en
- Northern Ireland: https://www.health-ni.gov.uk/publications/healthy-child-healthy-future.

Overall structure of the book

With increasing recognition of the importance of a life course approach, and a growing body of evidence about the importance of prenatal influences on child health and development, this evidence-based review starts in pregnancy. It finishes at age seven, to cover the important transition into school, and to be consistent with the early years in education.

Section 2 (Chapters 3–7) summarizes the literature on prenatal exposures affecting the fetus, the impact of parental mental health and intimate partner violence on the developing infant, and 'what works' in helping parents with smoking, drugs, and alcohol cessation. The issue of how to prepare prospective parents for parenthood is summarized.

Section 3 (Chapters 8–16) covers primary prevention, health promotion, and anticipatory guidance to be delivered as part of universal services. Although the review does not include evidence supporting health promotion with school-aged children, each topic chapter covers the issues of transition into school and the needs of children in early years educational settings.

Section 4 (Chapters 17–23) deals with secondary prevention, including screening for specific conditions and the evidence supporting different ways of case identification.

Section 5 (Chapters 24–27) reviews the evidence for early intervention and support of children identified by a child health programme and highlights the additional needs of specific groups of children living in special circumstances.

Section 6 (Chapters 28–32) summarizes what is being provided as part of child health programmes in each of the countries of the UK, and reviews the interface with early years and educational services. Some current innovations and additions to the universal child health programmes in England, Scotland, and Wales are reviewed in a chapter addressing the way in which these programmes are being enhanced.

Section 7 (Chapters 33–35) concerns the implementation of an evidence-based child health programme, including management, quality assurance, and data collection. The final chapter concludes with recommendations for future research to improve the evidence base for practice with the under sevens and their families.

Each recommendation is supported by evidence, linked to defined competencies, and the training needed to acquire and maintain those competencies.

Learning links

- Early Intervention Foundation—'The Best Start at Home': http://www.eif.org.uk/publication/the-best-start-at-home/
- E-learning for healthcare—'Healthy Child Programme': https://www.e-lfh.org.uk/programmes/healthy-child-programme/.

Recommendations

General recommendations for child health programmes

- Both universal and targeted services should be commissioned for the child health programme. Commissioners and providers should continuously monitor the coverage of the population receiving universal services. Targeted and enhanced services should focus on children with abnormal patterns of growth, development, or behaviour, or on families with recognized risk factors for abnormal child health. (*Evidence: strong.*)

- All changes or enhancements to the child health programme should be monitored and have evaluation built in. (*Evidence: strong.*)

- Formal screening should be limited to the evidence-based programmes endorsed by the National Screening Committee. Screening activities outside this framework should be treated as research, reviewed by an ethics committee, time limited, and reported for peer review. (*Evidence: strong.*)

- Commissioners can draw on the wide range of available programmes to enable early interventions in response to early signals of risk to child development. (*Evidence: moderate.*)

- Commissioners should ensure that practitioners are given the time, resources, and authority to deliver evidence-based screening, active health surveillance, and health promotion. (*Evidence: strong.*)

- Provider organizations should improve understanding among their workforces of child development and the measurement of early signals of risk, and use these indicators to better respond to risk. (*Evidence: moderate.*)

- All recommendations for interventions should be implemented in practice according to the family's situation and resources, and with sensitivity to culture and religion. (*Good practice.*)

- Practitioners need training in evidence-based practice, to maintain the specific competencies required to deliver the universal child health programme, and the skills to assess children's needs for targeted services. (*Evidence: strong.*)

- Practitioners need to be culturally competent to work effectively with the diverse population of children and their families in the UK. (*Good practice.*)

- Practitioners require regular and supportive supervision for all aspects of their work with families, not just safeguarding. (*Good practice.*)

- The principles of the child health programme, screening, case identification, and health promotion should be included in the training of all pre-registration medical and nursing students and others who will be working with children and families. (*Evidence: moderate.*)

Section 2

Pregnancy, perinatal period, and preparation for parenthood

Chapter 3

Dietary and environmental exposures in pregnancy

Caroline Taylor

Summary

This chapter:

- introduces the concept of the role of exposures during pregnancy in fetal development and programming
- summarizes the evidence for the role of diet and nutrition preconceptually and during pregnancy on key aspects of child health and development
- summarizes the evidence for the role of environmental exposures, including pollutants, medicines, and herbal remedies, preconceptually and during pregnancy on key aspects of child health and development
- provides information on relevant UK guidelines and other sources of advice
- highlights and comments on gaps in knowledge
- provides recommendations for commissioners and practitioners for improving the evidence base for screening, individual advice and management, and public health measures.

Introduction

During pregnancy, the maternal diet has to provide the nutrients to meet the needs of the growing fetus as well as those of the mother, with storage of some nutrients to ensure that requirements are met during gestation and into lactation. Maternal nutritional status at conception is an important determinant of fetal health. In addition, there is increasing recognition of the importance of both nutrition and environmental exposures in pregnancy: this is part of the theory of developmental origins of health and disease in which prenatal events are thought to have a significant impact on the emergence of later disease, as well as on many crucial aspects of child development, such as growth, cognition, and behaviour. While early interventions to prevent long-term outcomes are attractive, they require high levels of public health education and engaged public policies. This chapter provides an overview of evidence for the importance of nutrition and environmental exposures both preconceptually and in pregnancy on the long-term health and development of the child, and provides some recommendations for action points by health professionals.

Diet and nutrition

Pregnant women are advised, like the general population, to eat a healthy and varied diet (Nhs.uk, 2017a). Guidance from the National Institute for Health and Care Excellence (NICE) (2010) on healthy weight management before, during, and after pregnancy emphasizes that there is no need to 'eat for two' even for pregnancies with multiples. Details of energy requirements in pregnancy and lactation have been published by the Scientific Advisory Committee on Nutrition (2011a). The UK recommended intakes for most nutrients remain the same in pregnancy as those for women of child-bearing age, with the exception of small increments for vitamins A, C, and D, riboflavin, and folate (Committee on Medical Aspects of Food Policy, 1991). Data from the UK National Diet and Nutrition Survey (Scientific Advisory Committee on Nutrition, 2008) show that the dietary quality of young women, particularly those from deprived social backgrounds, can be poor. Specific nutrients and other food components that are of concern in pregnancy are described below.

Folic acid

Periconceptual folic acid supplementation substantially reduces the risk of neural tube defects (Scientific Advisory Committee on Nutrition, 2006) in babies. In the UK, a daily supplement (Nhs.uk, 2015) of 400 micrograms/day is recommended preconceptually until 12 weeks' gestation (5 mg per day for women who are at increased risk, such as those with a history of a neural tube defect-affected pregnancy) and folic acid is included in NHS Healthy Start vitamins (Healthy Start, 2017). Uptake of folic acid supplementation in the UK, however, is low, particularly in women with unexpected pregnancies, ethnic minorities, young women, and women with low socioeconomic status (Stockley and Lund, 2008; Peake et al., 2013). Folic acid is provided to the whole population through fortification of flour in countries such as the US and Canada, but this approach has not yet been adopted in the UK despite recommendation by advisory bodies (Walker, 2016; Scientific Advisory Committee on Nutrition, 2017). This is partly because of a fear of potential adverse effects (Scientific Advisory Committee on Nutrition, 2017), although fortification may also have protective effects (Smith et al., 2008).

Vitamin D

Vitamin D status is low (serum 25-hydroxy-vitamin D <25 nmol/L) in about 22% of UK women aged 19–64 years, particularly during winter months when synthesis through the action of sunlight on the skin is limited (Scientific Advisory Committee on Nutrition, 2016). In pregnancy, postulated adverse effects of low vitamin D status include pre-eclampsia and low birthweight, and hypocalcaemic seizures and impaired skeletal development in the baby (Royal College of Obstetricians and Gynaecologists, 2014), but evidence for these effects is inconsistent (Scientific Advisory Committee on

Nutrition, 2016). Blood markers of vitamin D status are lower in black and particularly in Asian women than in white women (McAree et al., 2013). The Scientific Advisory Committee on Nutrition (2016) has recommended that there should be national surveys focused on measurement of vitamin D status particularly in pregnant women and in minority ethnic groups. It is recommended that all pregnant women take a vitamin D supplement (Nhs.uk, 2017b); vitamin D is included in the NHS Healthy Start vitamins (Healthy Start, 2017) at 10 micrograms (400 IU) per day.

Iron

Physiological changes in pregnancy (plasma volume expansion and haemodilution) make the interpretation of markers of iron metabolism difficult (Scientific Advisory Committee on Nutrition, 2011b). Iron deficiency in pregnancy, particularly if arising early in pregnancy, may increase the risk of infection, postpartum haemorrhage, low birthweight, neonatal anaemia, preterm delivery, and small for gestational age (Allen, 2000). UK NICE guidelines (2008) recommend that women are screened at booking and at 28 weeks' gestation with treatment for haemoglobin less than 110 g/L in the first trimester and 105 g/L at 28 weeks, with follow-up checks. However, low preconception iron stores, measured by serum ferritin, are strongly predictive of anaemia in later pregnancy, and so iron deficiency anaemia should ideally be treated preconceptually (Iglesias et al., 2018). Routine iron supplementation has not been shown to have any beneficial or adverse effects on birth outcomes (Scientific Advisory Committee on Nutrition, 2011b). Maternal anaemia in the third trimester is thought not to be associated with adverse pregnancy outcomes, and may simply reflect increased plasma volume (Xiong et al., 2000).

Iodine

Iodine requirements rise in pregnancy (World Health Organization, 2007) and lactation primarily to supply an increase in thyroid hormone production in the first trimester and to enable the fetus to produce its own thyroid hormones from mid gestation onwards. Low iodine status in early pregnancy is associated with impaired measures of cognition in the offspring (Bath et al., 2013). There is increasing concern that some women of child-bearing age and pregnant women in the UK may be iodine insufficient (Kibirige et al., 2004; Bath et al., 2014). Pregnant and lactating women who avoid dairy products, eggs, and/or fish are most at risk of insufficiency and may be advised to have thyroid function tests. Iodine requirements should ideally be considered preconceptually to optimize thyroidal stores (Moleti et al., 2011). Iodine supplementation in pregnancy has been proposed as a cost-effective measure to prevent adverse effects on cognition; this would need careful tailoring to reflect local iodine status, with monitoring at a population level to prevent under/over dosing (Taylor and Vaidya, 2016).

Vitamin A

High intakes of vitamin A in pregnancy are teratogenic in animal species when given at critical periods of embryonic development (Dolk et al., 1999). The teratogenicity in humans remains unclear because clinical trials are not possible; evidence from a small number of case reports, case–control studies, and prospective studies has not provided conclusive evidence (Dolk et al., 1999). The cautious approach is therefore that periconceptually and during pregnancy, women are advised to limit vitamin A intake to a maximum of 1.5 mg/week by not taking any supplements containing vitamin A (including fish liver oil) (Nhs.uk, 2017c), as well as avoiding eating liver or any food containing liver.

Caffeine

Caffeine is rapidly absorbed and crosses the placenta freely. The concentration of caffeine that the fetus is exposed to is dependent on maternal metabolism, which varies between individuals (Sasaki et al., 2017). Caffeine interferes with intervillous blood flow in the placenta. Intakes greater than 200 mg/day (two 250 mL cups) have been associated with fetal growth restriction (CARE Study Group, 2008). The UK recommendation (Nhs.uk, 2015) in pregnancy is to limit consumption to less than 200 mg/day, but reduction preconceptually should also be considered.

Environment

Heavy metals

Lead

Recent evidence suggests that prenatal lead exposure even at low levels previously considered to be of no consequence is associated with a range of adverse outcomes including preterm birth and low birthweight, impaired cognition and school performance, and poor behaviour (Taylor et al., 2015; Shah-Kulkarni et al., 2016), with no evidence of a lower limit for effects (Taylor et al., 2016b). However, there are no national levels of concern published in the UK (Taylor et al., 2014), and there has been no population monitoring of blood lead concentrations since the mid 1990s (Primatesta et al., 1998), and no data specifically from pregnant women since the early 1990s (Taylor et al., 2014). National advice (Nhs.uk, 2017d) on reducing exposure is limited to avoidance of eating lead-shot game by children and pregnant women. Advice related to healthy living in pregnancy, such as smoking cessation, reducing alcohol intake, and restricting caffeinated tea and coffee intakes, is likely to reduce lead exposure (Taylor et al., 2013). Avoidance of home improvements in old houses where there may be exposure to lead-based paint and old dust that has accumulated lead from coal fires and industrial activities will also reduce exposure. There is also some evidence in the UK that blood lead levels are higher in pregnant women of Asian origin (Taylor et al., 2013): this may be due to the use of traditional herbal preparations that can be high in lead (Martena et al., 2010). These preparations should be avoided before and during pregnancy.

Mercury

Exposure to mercury can occur from the diet, particularly fish, as well as from dental amalgam, and from natural environmental sources. National guidance (Nhs.uk, 2017d) regarding reducing mercury exposure for pregnant women is advice on species of fish to avoid and those to limit. There is increasing evidence from observational cohort studies in the UK and in the Seychelles (where fish consumption is high) that fish consumption during pregnancy is beneficial to the development of the fetus (Davidson et al., 2011; Taylor et al., 2016a), with the adverse effects of mercury being matched or even outweighed by the beneficial effects of fish. These beneficial effects may be due to other nutrients provided by the fish, such as omega-3 fatty acids, iodine, and vitamin D, for example. It is likely that faced with the complex and confusing guidelines on eating fish in pregnancy (Nhs.uk, 2017e) in the UK and elsewhere, pregnant women reduce their fish consumption or give up eating fish altogether, as has been shown in the US (Bloomingdale et al., 2010). The UK advice to eat at least two portions of fish per week in pregnancy, with not more than two portions being oily fish, needs to be more widely promoted.

Arsenic

Diet is the main source of arsenic exposure in many countries. Although fish contains relatively large amounts of arsenic, it is present as organic arsenic, which is relatively less harmful than inorganic arsenic. In some developing countries where drinking water contains high concentrations of arsenic, prenatal exposure has been shown to be associated with low birthweight and still birth (Kippler et al., 2012b). Although such high levels of exposure are less likely in the UK, private water supplies (Drinking Water Inspectorate, 2016) can become contaminated from natural seepage from rocks and soil (Middleton et al., 2016). Regular monitoring of these supplies is advised. There has been concern recently over arsenic in rice, which is present as the more toxic inorganic arsenic. In response, the European Commission introduced maximum limits for concentrations in rice in 2016 (European Commission, 2015), but this appears to have had little impact on the arsenic content of rice-based infant foods (Signes-Pastor et al., 2017). The UK Food Standards Agency (2016) recommends that young children are not given rice-based drinks, but there is no advice specifically for pregnant women.

Cadmium

Prenatal cadmium exposure is associated with adverse effects on birth outcomes and child cognition (Kippler et al., 2012a; Johnston et al., 2014). The main route of exposure to cadmium is through smoking, with additional exposure through diet (European Food Safety Authority Panel, 2012). This reinforces public health messages on smoking cessation, and the benefits of cessation preconceptually should be emphasized.

Particulates and air pollution

Exposure to airborne particulate matter during pregnancy is associated with adverse birth outcomes (Bell et al., 2008) and with lung function deficits in childhood (Jedrychowski et al., 2010). The Department for Environment, Food and Rural Affairs (Defra) issues a daily air quality index with advice on appropriate action when air quality is poor, although the advice is not specifically for pregnant women (https://uk-air.defra.gov.uk/air-pollution/daqi).

Chemical pollutants

Pregnant women are exposed to multiple synthetic chemicals, both banned and permitted, through industrial and consumer products. Maternal exposure to individual chemicals may be associated with endocrine disruption in the both the mother and child, and adverse effects on behavioural and cognitive development in the child (Mitro et al., 2015). It is possible that adverse effects will be amplified due to interaction between the chemicals, but few studies have reported on the cumulative impacts of multi-chemical exposures in pregnancy. The Royal College of Obstetrics and Gynaecology (2013) provides some general advice on minimizing exposure to chemical pollutants.

Phthalates and phenols

Phthalates and bisphenol A are synthetic chemicals used in many products such as plastics, carpets, cosmetics, and cleaning liquids. Bisphenol A exposure during pregnancy has been associated with the risk of miscarriage and low birthweight (Huo et al., 2015). The Royal College of Obstetrics and Gynaecology (2013) advises pregnant women to avoid exposure to chemicals in plastics as a precaution until more research has been completed.

Dioxins and polychlorinated biphenyls

Levels of the persistent organic pollutants dioxins and polychlorinated biphenyls (PCBs) overall in the UK are declining (The Food and Environment Research Agency, 2012). Prenatal exposure to PCBs, which is primarily through consumption of oily fish, has been associated with adverse effects on child neurodevelopment (El Majidi et al., 2013). The risk of PCB and dioxin exposure from oily fish must be weighed against the evidence for the positive benefits due to its content of omega-3 fatty acids, iodine, vitamin D, etc. (Nhs.uk, 2017e).

Organochlorine pesticides, perfluorinated chemicals, and flame retardants

Organochlorine pesticides, perfluorinated chemicals (used to provide water and stain resistance), and some types of flame retardants persist in the environment and in human tissue. Maternal exposure may be associated with a range of adverse outcomes, including reduced fetal growth and IQ decrements in the child (Mitro et al., 2015).

Radiation

Radon

Radon is a naturally occurring radioactive gas that can accumulate in buildings (Health Protection Agency, 2009). Little is known specifically about the effects of radon exposure in pregnancy. Radon risk reports and kits for radon measurement are available through the UKradon website (http://www.ukradon.org/) and there are several recommended remediation methods available.

Electromagnetic fields

There has been extensive research into electromagnetic fields (World Health Organization, 2017) from sources such as laptops and mobile phones and there is no evidence to date of adverse effects. The World Health Organization acknowledged, however, that there are gaps in knowledge that need to be addressed before better health risk assessments can be made.

Daylight and shift work

Sleep deprivation and/or circadian rhythm disturbances, which partly arise from disrupted patterns of daylight exposure, may impair fetal growth or lead to other complications in pregnancy (Mitro et al., 2015). The Royal College of Physicians/NHS Plus provide comprehensive guidance for management of shift work in pregnancy (Royal College of Physicians, 2009).

Medicines and herbal remedies

Medicines

Most medicines are transferred freely across the placenta and can have adverse, or sometimes beneficial, effects on the fetus. There is a lack of comprehensive information on medication use in pregnancy: this has been recognized by the European Board and College of Obstetrics and Gynaecology (Van Calsteren et al., 2016).

The UK Teratology Information Service (UKTIS) provides publicly accessible information on individual medicines on its website 'bumps' (best use of medicines in pregnancy) (UK Teratology Information Service, 2017). The service also provides fuller summary documents (UK Teratology Information Service, 2015) for health professionals, with further information available from the European Medicines Agency (2017) and TOXBASE (National Poisons Information Service, 2018). UKTIS also provides information on the use of recreational drugs (e.g. cannabis, cocaine, and heroin), and on some chemicals (e.g. essential oils, hair dye, and paint) in pregnancy.

Prescription medicines

NICE advises that drugs should only be prescribed in pregnancy if the benefit to the mother is thought to be greater than the risk to the fetus, and avoided where possible in the first trimester, with a preference for drugs that have been well used in pregnancy, used in the smallest possible dose (NICE, 2017). The *British National Formulary* (*BNF*) and *BNF for Children* provide guidance on individual drugs (BNF Publications, 2017).

Over-the-counter medicines

There are insufficient data to determine the safety of many common over-the-counter medications in pregnancy conclusively. Paracetamol is recommended as being safe for use throughout pregnancy although it should be taken at as low a dose as possible and for the shortest time possible (UK Teratology Information Service, 2017). However, recent studies have suggested that use of paracetamol early in pregnancy can increase the risks of cryptorchidism (Snijder et al., 2012) and asthma (Magnus et al., 2016) in the offspring. Standard dose aspirin is not recommended after 30 weeks' gestation.

Low-dose aspirin is occasionally used beyond this date in women at high risk of pre-eclampsia. Ibuprofen is not recommended in pregnancy, especially after 30 weeks' gestation.

Herbal remedies

Herbal remedies are taken by about 25% of pregnant women in the UK (Kennedy et al., 2013). Commonly used products include ginger, raspberry, cranberry, Echinacea, peppermint, and chamomile. They are used to treat a range of conditions including nausea, anaemia, constipation, heartburn, sleeping problems, and preparation for labour. In a review of the safety of commonly used herbal products in pregnancy, none of the studies included showed any adverse effects of a range of herbal preparations, but the studies were all small and did not provide definitive evidence (Holst et al., 2011). There is also a possibility of herb–drug interactions (Holst et al., 2011). Information on the safety and efficacy of most herbal products is scant or absent and so it seems prudent to limit or eliminate exposure in pregnancy.

Learning links

- Cadmium—incident management: https://assets.publishing.service.gov.uk/government/uploads/system/uploads/attachment_data/file/527341/Cadmium_IM_PHE_120516.pdf
- Mercury—health effects incident management and toxicology: https://assets.publishing.service.gov.uk/government/uploads/system/uploads/attachment_data/file/526835/Mercury_PHE_IM_310516.pdf
- *Control of Lead at Work*, Third edition, 2002: http://www.hse.gov.uk/pUbns/priced/l132.pdf
- Working safely with lead: http://www.hse.gov.uk/lead/index.htm
- Lead—health effects, incident management, and toxicology: https://assets.publishing.service.gov.uk/government/uploads/system/uploads/attachment_data/file/522444/Lead_IM_PHE_050516.pdf
- The Royal College of Midwives, RCM i-Learn—'Nutrition in Pregnancy': http://www.ilearn.rcm.org.uk/enrol/index.php?id=13
- The Royal College of Midwives, RCM i-Learn—'Medicines Management in Maternity': http://www.ilearn.rcm.org.uk/enrol/index.php?id=247.

Recommendations

- Provide universal access to Healthy Start vitamins for all pregnant women. (*Evidence: strong.*)
- Provide health professionals with training to encourage uptake of Healthy Start vitamins in pregnant women. (*Evidence: strong.*)

- Offer a drug review, including over-the-counter medication and herbal products, as usual practice at booking (or preferably preconceptually), with appropriate advice offered. (*Good practice.*)

- Encourage pregnant and lactating women to eat iodine-containing foods (such as eggs and fish), and monitor vegans and others who avoid these foods as they are at risk of low iodine status in pregnancy. (*Evidence: strong.*)

- Promote more widely advice to pregnant women to consume at least two portions of fish per week to maximize the positive benefits of fish consumption in pregnancy. (*Evidence: strong.*)

- Assess iron status (stores) at first contact with pregnant women, correct if necessary, and start folate supplementation. (*Evidence: strong.*)

- Offer advice to pregnant women to minimize fetal exposure to heavy metals including eating a healthy diet with adequate calcium and iron, stopping smoking and alcohol, and reducing caffeine consumption to a minimum. (*Good practice.*)

- Consider offering advice to avoid paint stripping and other home improvements during pregnancy. (*Good practice.*)

- Commissioners should support local and regional initiatives on transport/environment to reduce air pollution. (*Evidence: strong.*)

References

Allen, L.H. (2000). Anemia and iron deficiency: effects on pregnancy outcome. *American Journal of Clinical Nutrition*, **71**, 1280S–1284S.

Bath, S.C., Steer, C.D., Golding, J., Emmett, P., and Rayman, M.P. (2013). Effect of inadequate iodine status in UK pregnant women on cognitive outcomes in their children: results from the Avon Longitudinal Study of Parents and Children (ALSPAC). *Lancet*, **382**, 331–337.

Bath, S.C., Walter, A., Taylor, A., Wright, J., and Rayman, M.P. (2014). Iodine deficiency in pregnant women living in the South East of the UK: the influence of diet and nutritional supplements on iodine status. *British Journal of Nutrition*, **111**, 1622–1631.

Bell, M.L., Ebisu, K., and Belanger, K. (2008). The relationship between air pollution and low birth weight: effects by mother's age, infant sex, co-pollutants, and pre-term births. *Environmental Research Letters*, **3**, 44003.

Bloomingdale, A., Guthrie, L.B., Price, S., et al. (2010). A qualitative study of fish consumption during pregnancy. *American Journal of Clinical Nutrition*, **92**, 1234–1240.

BNF Publications (2017). BNF publications. [online] Available at: https://www.bnf.org/ [Accessed 29 Sep. 2017].

CARE Study Group (2008). Maternal caffeine intake during pregnancy and risk of fetal growth restriction: a large prospective observational study. *BMJ*, **337**, a2332.

Committee on Medical Aspects of Food Policy (1991). *Dietary Reference Values for Food Energy and Nutrients for the United Kingdom*. Department of Health Report on Health and Social Subjects 41. London: Department of Health.

Davidson, P.W., Cory-Slechta, D.A., Thurston, S.W., et al. (2011). Fish consumption and prenatal methylmercury exposure: cognitive and behavioral outcomes in the main cohort at 17 years from the Seychelles child development study. *NeuroToxicology*, **32**, 711–717.

Dolk, H.M., Nau, H., Hummler, H., and Barlow, S.M. (1999). Dietary vitamin A and teratogenic risk: European Teratology Society discussion paper. *European Journal of Obstetrics, Gynecology, and Reproductive Biology*, **83**, 31–36.

Drinking Water Inspectorate (2016). Private water supplies in England and Wales. [online] Available at: http://dwi.defra.gov.uk/private-water-supply/ [Accessed 29 Sep. 2017].

El Majidi, N., Bouchard, M., and Carrier, G. (2013). Systematic analysis of the relationship between standardized prenatal exposure to polychlorinated biphenyls and mental and motor development during follow-up of nine children cohorts. *Regulatory Toxicology and Pharmacology*, **66**, 130–146.

European Commission (2015). Commission regulation (EU) 2015/1006 of 25 June 2015 amending Regulation (EC) No 1881/2006 as regards maximum levels of inorganic arsenic in foodstuffs. [online] Available at: https://eur-lex.europa.eu/legal-content/EN/TXT/?uri=OJ:JOL_2015_161_R_0006 [Accessed 27 Sep. 2017].

European Food Safety Authority Panel (2012). Cadmium dietary exposure in the European population. *EFSA Journal*, **10**, 2551.

European Medicines Agency (2017). Homepage. [online] Available at: http://www.ema.europa.eu/ema/ [Accessed 29 Sep. 2017].

Food Standards Agency (2016). *Arsenic in Rice*. London: Food Standards Agency. [online] Available at: https://www.food.gov.uk/science/arsenic-in-rice [Accessed 9 Nov. 2018].

Health Protection Agency (2009). *Radon and Public Health: Report of the Independent Advisory Group on Ionising Radiation*. London: Health Protection Agency. [online] Available at: https://assets.publishing.service.gov.uk/government/uploads/system/uploads/attachment_data/file/335102/RCE-11_for_website.pdf [Accessed 28 Sep. 2017].

Healthy Start (2017). Healthy Start vitamins. [online] Available at: https://www.healthystart.nhs.uk/healthy-start-vouchers/healthy-start-vitamins/ [Accessed 28 Sep. 2017].

Holst, L., Wright, D., Haavik, S., and Nordeng, H. (2011). Safety and efficacy of herbal remedies in obstetrics—review and clinical implications. *Midwifery*, **27**, 80–86.

Huo, W., Xia, W., Wan, Y., et al. (2015). Maternal urinary bisphenol A levels and infant low birth weight: a nested case–control study of the Health Baby Cohort in China. *Environment International*, **85**, 96–103.

Iglesias, L., Canals, J., and Arija, V. (2018). Effects of prenatal iron status on child neurodevelopment and behavior: a systematic review. *Critical Reviews in Food Science and Nutrition*, **58**, 1604–1614.

Jedrychowski, W.A., Perera, F.P., Maugeri, U., et al. (2010). Effect of prenatal exposure to fine particulate matter on ventilatory lung function of preschool children of nonsmoking mothers. Krakow inner city birth cohort prospective study. *Paediatric and Perinatal Epidemiology*, **24**, 492–501.

Johnston, J.E., Valentiner, E., Maxson, P., Miranda, M.L., and Fry, R.C. (2014). Maternal cadmium levels during pregnancy associated with lower birth weight in infants in a North Carolina cohort. *PLoS One*, **9**, e109661.

Kennedy, D.A., Lupattelli, A., Koren, G., and Nordeng, H. (2013). Herbal medicine use in pregnancy: results of a multinational study. *BMC Complementary and Alternative Medicine*, **13**, 355.

Kibirige, M.S., Hutchison, S., Owen, C.J., and Delves, H.T. (2004). Prevalence of maternal dietary iodine insufficiency in the north east of England: implications for the fetus. *Archives of Disease in Childhood. Fetal and Neonatal Edition*, **89**, F436–F439.

Kippler, M., Tofail, F., Gardner, R., et al. (2012a). Maternal cadmium exposure during pregnancy and size at birth: a prospective cohort study. *Environmental Health Perspectives*, **120**, 284–289.

Kippler, M., Wagatsuma, Y., Rahman, A., et al. (2012b). Environmental exposure to arsenic and cadmium during pregnancy and fetal size: a longitudinal study in rural Bangladesh. *Reproductive Toxicology*, **34**, 504–511.

Magnus, M.C., Karlstad, O., Haberg, S.E., Nafstad, P., Davey Smith, G., and Nystad, W. (2016). Prenatal and infant paracetamol exposure and development of asthma: the Norwegian Mother and Child Cohort Study. *International Journal of Epidemiology*, **45**, 512–522.

Martena, M.J., Van Der Wielen, J.C., Rietjens, I.M., Klerx, W.N., De Groot, H.N., and Konings, E.J. (2010). Monitoring of mercury, arsenic, and lead in traditional Asian herbal preparations on the Dutch market and estimation of associated risks. *Food Additives & Contaminants. Part A, Chemistry, Analysis, Control, Exposure & Risk Assessment*, **27**, 190–205.

McAree, T., Jacobs, B., Manickavasagar, T., et al. (2013). Vitamin D deficiency in pregnancy – still a public health issue. *Maternal & Child Nutrition*, **9**, 23–30.

Middleton, D.R., Watts, M.J., Hamilton, E.M., et al. (2016). Urinary arsenic profiles reveal exposures to inorganic arsenic from private drinking water supplies in Cornwall, UK. *Scientific Reports*, **6**, 25656.

Mitro, S.D., Johnson, T., and Zota, A.R. (2015). Cumulative chemical exposures during pregnancy and early development. *Current Environmental Health Reports*, **2**, 367–378.

Moleti, M., Di Bella, B., Giorgianni, G., et al. (2011). Maternal thyroid function in different conditions of iodine nutrition in pregnant women exposed to mild–moderate iodine deficiency: an observational study. *Clinical Endocrinology*, **74**, 762–768.

National Institute for Health and Care Excellence (2008). Antenatal care for uncomplicated pregnancies. [online] Available at: https://www.nice.org.uk/guidance/cg62/chapter/introduction [Accessed 28 Sep. 2017].

National Institute for Health and Care Excellence (2010). Weight management before, during and after pregnancy. [online] Available at: https://www.nice.org.uk/guidance/ph27 [Accessed 28 Sep. 2017].

National Institute for Health and Care Excellence (2017). Prescribing in pregnancy. [online] Available at: https://bnf.nice.org.uk/guidance/prescribing-in-pregnancy.html [Accessed 29 Sep. 2017].

National Poisons Information Service (2018). TOXBASE. [online] Available at: https://www.toxbase.org/.

Nhs.uk. (2015). Should I limit caffeine during pregnancy? [online] Available at: https://www.nhs.uk/common-health-questions/pregnancy/should-i-limit-caffeine-during-pregnancy/ [Accessed 29 Sep. 2017].

Nhs.uk. (2017a). Have a healthy diet in pregnancy. [online] Available at: https://www.nhs.uk/conditions/pregnancy-and-baby/healthy-pregnancy-diet/ [Accessed 28 Sep. 2017].

Nhs.uk. (2017b). Vitamins, supplements and nutrition in pregnancy. [online] Available at: https://www.nhs.uk/conditions/pregnancy-and-baby/vitamins-minerals-supplements-pregnant/ [Accessed 28 Sep. 2017].

Nhs.uk. (2017c). Vitamin A. [online] Available at: http://www.nhs.uk/conditions/vitamins-minerals/pages/vitamin-a.aspx [Accessed 29 Sep. 2017].

Nhs.uk. (2017d). Foods to avoid in pregnancy. [online] Available at: https://www.nhs.uk/conditions/pregnancy-and-baby/foods-to-avoid-pregnant/ [Accessed 29 Sep. 2017].

Nhs.uk. (2017e). Should pregnant and breastfeeding women avoid some types of fish? [online] Available at: https://www.nhs.uk/common-health-questions/pregnancy/should-pregnant-and-breastfeeding-women-avoid-some-types-of-fish/ [Accessed 2 Oct. 2017].

Peake, J.N., **Copp, A.J.**, and **Shawe, J.** (2013). Knowledge and periconceptional use of folic acid for the prevention of neural tube defects in ethnic communities in the United Kingdom: systematic review and meta-analysis. *Birth Defects Research Part A. Clinical and Molecular Teratology*, **97**, 444–451.

Primatesta, P., **Dong, W.**, **Bost, L.**, **Poulter, N.R.**, and **Delves, H.T.** (1998). Survey of blood lead levels in the population in England, 1995. In: Gompertz, D. (Ed.) *IEH Report on Recent UK Blood Lead Surveys, Report R9*, pp. 9–52. Norwich: Medical Research Council, Institute for Environmental Health.

Royal College of Obstetricians and Gynaecologists (2013). *Chemical Exposures During Pregnancy: Dealing with Potential, but Unproven, Risks to Child Health*. Scientific Impact Paper No 37. London: Royal College of Obstetricians and Gynaecologists . [online] Available at: https://www.rcog.org.uk/globalassets/documents/guidelines/scientific-impact-papers/sip_37.pdf [Accessed 28 Sep. 2017].

Royal College of Obstetricians and Gynaecologists (2014). *Vitamin D in Pregnancy*. Scientific Impact Paper No 43. London: Royal College of Obstetricians and Gynaecologists. [online] Available at: https://www.rcog.org.uk/globalassets/documents/guidelines/scientific-impact-papers/vitamin_d_sip43_june14.pdf [Accessed 9 Nov. 2018].

Royal College of Physicians (2009). *Physical and Shift Work in Pregnancy: Occupational Aspects of Management*. London: Royal College of Physicians. Available at: https://www.rcplondon.ac.uk/guidelines-policy/physical-and-shift-work-pregnancy-occupational-aspects-management-2009 [Accessed 29 Sep. 2017].

Sasaki, S., **Limpar, M.**, **Sata, F.**, **Kobayashi, S.**, and **Kishi, R.** (2017). Interaction of maternal caffeine intake during pregnancy and CYP1A2 C164A polymorphism affects infant birth size in the Hokkaido Study. *Pediatric Research*, **82**, 19–28.

Scientific Advisory Committee on Nutrition (2006). *Folate and Disease Prevention*. London: The Stationery Office. [online] Available at: https://www.gov.uk/government/uploads/system/uploads/attachment_data/file/338892/SACN_Folate_and_Disease_Prevention_Report.pdf [Accessed 28 Sep. 2017].

Scientific Advisory Committee on Nutrition (2008). *The Nutritional Wellbeing of the British Population*. London: The Stationery Office. [online] Available at: http://webarchive.nationalarchives.gov.uk/20131102012210/http://www.sacn.gov.uk/reports_position_statements/reports/the_nutritional_wellbeing_of_the_british_population.html [Accessed 28 Sep. 2017].

Scientific Advisory Committee on Nutrition (2011a). *Dietary Reference Values for Energy*. London: The Stationery Office.

Scientific Advisory Committee on Nutrition (2011b). *Iron and Health*. London: The Stationery Office.

Scientific Advisory Committee on Nutrition (2016). *Vitamin D and Health*. London: The Stationery Office.

Scientific Advisory Committee on Nutrition (2017). *Update on Folic Acid*. London: The Stationery Office.

Shah-Kulkarni, S., Ha, M., Kim, B.M., et al. (2016). Neurodevelopment in early childhood affected by prenatal lead exposure and iron intake. *Medicine (Baltimore)*, **95**, e2508.

Signes-Pastor, A.J., Woodside, J.V., McMullan, P., et al. (2017). Levels of infants' urinary arsenic metabolites related to formula feeding and weaning with rice products exceeding the EU inorganic arsenic standard. *PLoS One*, **12**, e0176923.

Smith, A.D., Kim, Y.I., and Refsum, H. (2008). Is folic acid good for everyone? *American Journal of Clinical Nutrition*, **87**, 517–533.

Snijder, C.A., Kortenkamp, A., Steegers, E.A., et al. (2012). Intrauterine exposure to mild analgesics during pregnancy and the occurrence of cryptorchidism and hypospadia in the offspring: the Generation R Study. *Human Reproduction*, **27**, 1191–1201.

Stockley, L. and Lund, V. (2008). Use of folic acid supplements, particularly by low-income and young women: a series of systematic reviews to inform public health policy in the UK. *Public Health Nutrition*, **11**, 807–821.

Taylor, C.M., Golding, J., and Emond, A.M. (2014). Lead, cadmium and mercury levels in pregnancy: the need for international consensus on levels of concern. *Journal of Developmental Origins of Health and Disease*, **5**, 16–30.

Taylor, C.M., Golding, J., and Emond, A.M. (2015). Adverse effects of maternal lead levels on birth outcomes in the ALSPAC study: a prospective birth cohort study. *BJOG: An International Journal of Obstetrics and Gynaecology*, **122**, 322–328.

Taylor, C.M., Golding, J., and Emond, A.M. (2016a). Blood mercury levels and fish consumption in pregnancy: risks and benefits for birth outcomes in a prospective observational birth cohort. *International Journal of Hygiene and Environmental Health*, **219**, 513–520.

Taylor, C.M., Golding, J., Hibbeln, J., and Emond, A.M. (2013). Environmental factors in relation to blood lead levels in pregnant women in the UK: the ALSPAC study. *PLoS One*, **8**, e72371.

Taylor, C.M., Tilling, K., Golding, J., and Emond, A.M. (2016b). Low level lead exposure and pregnancy outcomes in an observational birth cohort study: dose–response relationships. *BMC Research Notes*, **9**, 291.

Taylor, P.N. and Vaidya, B. (2016). Iodine supplementation in pregnancy – is it time? *Clinical Endocrinology*, **85**, 10–14.

The Food and Environment Research Agency (2012). *Organic Environmental Contaminants in the 2012 Total Diet Study Samples: Report to the Food Standards Agency*. York: The Food and Environment Research Agency. [online] Available at: https://www.food.gov.uk/sites/default/files/media/document/research-report-total-diet-study.pdf [Accessed 29 Sep. 2017]

UK Teratology Information Service (2015). Maternal exposure. [online] Available at: http://www.uktis.org/html/maternal_exposure.html [Accessed 29 Sep. 2017].

UK Teratology Information Service (2017). Bumps: best use of medicine in pregnancy. [online] Available at: http://www.medicinesinpregnancy.org/ [Accessed 29 Sep. 2017].

Van Calsteren, K., Gersak, K., Sundseth, H., et al. (2016). Position Statement from the European Board and College of Obstetrics & Gynaecology (EBCOG): the use of medicines during pregnancy: call for action. *European Journal of Obstetrics & Gynecology and Reproductive Biology*, **201**, 211–214.

Walker, D. (2016). Fortification of flour with folic acid is an overdue public health measure in the UK. *Archives of Disease in Childhood*, **101**, 593.

World Health Organization (2007). *Assessment of Iodine Deficiency Disorders and Monitoring their Elimination: A Guide for Programme Managers*, 3rd edn. Geneva: World Health Organization.

World Health Organization (2017). Electromagnetic fields (EMF): research. [online] Available at: http://www.who.int/peh-emf/research/en/ [Accessed 29 Sep. 2017].

Xiong, X., Buekens, P., Alexander, S., Demianczuk, N., and **Wollast, E.** (2000). Anemia during pregnancy and birth outcome: a meta-analysis. *American Journal of Perinatology*, **17**, 137–146.

Chapter 4

Perinatal parental mental health problems

Vivette Glover, Rebecca Reynolds,
Nick Axford, and Jane Barlow

Summary

This chapter contains:

- a description of the nature and prevalence of mental health problems in men and women during the perinatal period
- a summary of the evidence regarding the impact of such problems on young children
- a summary of the evidence regarding the effectiveness of primary and secondary interventions aimed at promoting parental mental health
- some suggestions regarding the implications of the findings for workforce development
- recommendations for practice.

Introduction

Mental health problems such as stress, anxiety, and depression are common in the perinatal period. For example, the evidence suggests that depression (both minor and major) affects around 11% of pregnant women and 13% in the first 3 months postnatally (Gavin et al., 2005), with continuity across the postnatal period (Markus et al., 2003). The prevalence of perinatal anxiety of any type in the last trimester is also in the region of 13% (Vesga-Lopez et al., 2008). Two recent reviews suggest that perinatal anxiety and depression in men are also common, with between 5% and 10% of men experiencing clinical depression (with higher rates being experienced in the 3–6-month postnatal period) (Paulson and Bazemore, 2010), and between 5% and 15% of men being affected by anxiety disorders (Leach et al., 2016). A positive moderate correlation with maternal postnatal depression has also been identified (Paulson and Bazemore, 2010).

There are different pathways leading to mental health problems in the pre- and postnatal periods. This chapter examines these pathways and will describe the effects of antenatal and postnatal parental mood (stress, anxiety, and depression) on child outcomes, and what is known about the use of interventions to prevent or treat parent mental health problems. The chapter does not address more severe mental health problems such as personality or psychotic disorders (for a discussion of these, see National Institute for Health and Care Excellence (NICE) (2014) guidelines) due to the focus of the book on primary and secondary prevention.

Impact of maternal *antenatal* anxiety/stress and/or depression

The antenatal period has been identified as being a key period in terms of promoting the long-term wellbeing of the child, with maternal antental anxiety/stress and/or depression being potentially important factors in terms of all aspects of the development of the foetus. Stein et al. (2014) reviewed the evidence on antenatal anxiety and depression, finding effects of antenatal depression on premature delivery and low birthweight, the latter especially in lower-income countries but no association with pre-eclampsia, Apgar scores, or admission to neonatal intensive care units. Antenatal stress has, however, been found to be associated with an increased risk of asthma (Khashan et al., 2012) and neurodevelopmental problems for the child, including an increased risk of emotional and behavioural problems such as symptoms of anxiety and depression, attention deficit hyperactivity disorder, conduct disorder (O'Connor et al., 2002), autism spectrum disorder (Hecht et al., 2016), schizophrenia (Khashan et al., 2008), and cognitive difficulties (Laplante et al., 2008). These problems can last until adolescence and early adulthood (Pearson et al., 2013).

Impact of *postnatal* maternal mental health problems

*The postnatal period has been identified as being of particular importance in terms of the infant's need for sensitive parenting (De Wolff and van Ijzendoorn, 1997) and for parental reflective functioning (Fonagy and Target, 1997), both of which are now thought to be central to the infant's capacity to develop a secure attachment to the primary caregiver. Parental psychosocial functioning can impact on the parent's capacity to provide this type of parenting. For example, one study found that depressed mothers were less sensitively attuned to their infants, less affirming, and more negating of infant experience compared with parents not experiencing postnatal depression (Murray, 1992), while a review found that maternal postpartum depression reduces children's cognitive performance (Mirhosseini et al., 2015). There is also evidence of an impact on the long-term emotional and cognitive development of the child (Murray et al., 2009), including a fourfold increase in risk of psychiatric diagnosis at age 11 years (Pawlby et al., 2008), and a five-fold increase in the risk of being depressed by 16 years of age (Murray et al., 2011). Neurodevelopmental research suggests that postnatal depression can also impact on the child's developing neurological system (Schore, 2005).

---

* Section reproduced with permission from Barlow J. et al. 'Group-based parent training programmes for improving parental psychosocial health.' *Cochrane Database of Systematic Reviews*, Issue 5, Copyright © 2014 The Cochrane Collaboration. Published by John Wiley & Sons, Ltd. Art. No.: CD002020.

For example, one study found that infants of depressed mothers exhibited reduced left frontal electroencephalogram activity (Dawson et al., 1997).

The impact of *paternal* mental health problems pre- and postnatally

A small number of studies have examined the impact of paternal stress/distress and/or depression on the interaction and involvement of fathers with the infant. Most (for an exception, see McElwain and Volling, 1999) show an adverse impact on inter-action, including an increase in infant-directed negativity in verbal comments to and regarding the infant (Sethna et al., 2009), less involvement (Roggman et al., 2002), including less reading, singing, and storytime (Paulson et al., 2006), and lower attach-ment to the infant (Buist et al., 2003). Better psychological well-being in fathers has also been found to be associated with an increased sensitivity in interaction with in-fants and toddlers (Broom, 1994).

There is also increasing evidence regarding the impact of perinatal mental health problems in fathers on the later development of children, with the available find-ings suggesting a similar and independent impact on the child's well-being to that of mental health problems in women (i.e. this occurs irrespective of whether the mother is depressed). One study showed that boys of fathers who were depressed during the postnatal period had an increased risk of conduct problems at age 3.5 years, and that boys of fathers who were depressed during both the prenatal and postnatal periods had the highest risks of subsequent psychopathology at 3.5 years and psychiatric diagnosis at 7 years of age (Ramchandani et al., 2005, 2008), with the most significant effects occurring when the father was depressed during both the pre- and postnatal periods.

What should we be doing?

The following sections examine what the evidence tells us regarding the identification, prevention, and treatment of depression and anxiety in the antenatal period. This evi-dence draws on the NICE (2014) guidance on antenatal and postnatal mental health which is summarized in the update of the evidence supporting the Healthy Child Programme (Axford et al., 2015, pp. 49–54). We also summarize more recent evidence where this is available.

Identification

#NICE (2014) guidance recommends that at a woman's first contact with primary care or her booking visit, and during the early postnatal period, the practitioner should consider asking the two Whooley questions (Whooleyquestions.ucsf.edu, 2015) as

---

Section adapted under the Open Government Licence v3.0 from Axford N. et al. '*Rapid Review to Update Evidence for the Healthy Child Programme 0–5*'. Public Health England, London, UK, © Crown Copyright 2015, https://assets.publishing.service.gov.uk/government/uploads/system/uploads/attachment_data/file/429740/150520RapidReviewHealthyChildProg_UPDATE_poisons_final.pdf.

part of a general discussion about a woman's mental health and well-being. The guidance recommends that practitioners should also consider asking about anxiety using the two-item Generalized Anxiety Disorder scale (GAD-2) (ACP Depression Care Guide, 2016).

These questions should be used as a preliminary means of assessing whether the practitioner should then conduct further assessment using standardized screening tools for either anxiety, depression, or both. NICE (2014) recommends, for example, that if a woman responds positively to either of the depression identification questions or is at risk of developing a mental health problem, or if there is clinical concern, practitioners should consider using the Edinburgh Postnatal Depression Scale (EPDS) (Psychology Tools, 2017) or the Patient Health Questionnaire (PHQ-9) (Patient Health Questionnaire-9, 2017) as part of a full assessment.

In the case of anxiety, if a woman scores 3 or more on the GAD-2 scale, practitioners should consider using the seven-item GAD-7 scale (Patient.info, 2017) for further assessment. If a woman scores less than 3 on the GAD-2 scale, but the practitioner is still concerned that she may have an anxiety disorder, they should ask the following question: 'Do you find yourself avoiding places or activities and does this cause you problems?' and if she responds positively, practitioners should consider using the GAD-7 scale for further assessment. In either case, the practitioner should consider referring the woman to her general practitioner or, if a severe mental health problem is suspected, to a mental health professional.

The evidence that maternal mental health problems such as anxiety and depression can impact on mother–infant interaction (e.g. Murray et al., 1996; Murray and Cooper, 1997) suggests that where there are concerns about the mother's mental health, the practitioner should also assess whether this is affecting her interaction with the baby, and the assessment should cover verbal interaction, emotional sensitivity, and physical care (NICE, 2014). This assessment may also be done using simple assessment tools, such as the Parent–Infant Interaction Observation Scale (PIIOS) (Svanberg et al., 2013) or the Keys to Parenting Interaction Scale (KIPS) (Comfort et al., 2011).

Prevention of perinatal depression/anxiety

#There are a number of opportunities for practitioners working with pregnant women to prevent antenatal depression and anxiety (see Department of Health, 2009), but there is currently limited evidence available regarding effective methods of working (see Howard et al., 2014; NICE, 2014).

There is currently limited evidence concerning the benefits of cognitive behavioural therapy (CBT) for preventing antenatal anxiety (summarized in Howard et al., 2014), or providing feedback during the ultrasound scan in reducing anxiety and depression (Nabhan and Faris, 2010), or the effectiveness of mind–body interventions such as psychoeducation, relaxation, and meditation during pregnancy on perceived

---

Section adapted under the Open Government Licence v3.0 from Axford N. et al. '*Rapid Review to Update Evidence for the Healthy Child Programme 0–5*'. Public Health England, London, UK, © Crown Copyright 2015, https://assets.publishing.service.gov.uk/government/uploads/system/uploads/attachment_data/file/429740/150520RapidReviewHealthyChildProg_UPDATE_poisons_final.pdf.

stress or mood (Beddoe and Lee, 2008). The evidence concerning the effectiveness of hypnotherapy, imagery, and autogenic training during pregnancy and the immediate postnatal period in preventing or treating anxiety is also inconclusive (Marc et al., 2011). Although these reviews found no benefits in terms of the use of yoga during pregnancy to reduce state anxiety, later reviews (Kawanishi et al., 2015; Sheffield and Woods-Giscombé, 2016) are more positive, suggesting that prenatal yoga can improve the mental health (stress, depression, and anxiety) of healthy and at-risk pregnant women. There is insufficient evidence to suggest that exercise-based interventions could prevent antenatal depression (Daley et al., 2015) and poor quality evidence concerning the effectiveness of mindfulness training during pregnancy in terms of stress, depression, and anxiety (Hall et al., 2016).

Women who receive a psychosocial or psychological intervention are significantly less likely to develop postpartum depression compared with those who received standard care (Dennis and Dowswell, 2013). This review focused on women in pregnancy and up to 6 weeks postpartum. Promising interventions include (i) intensive, professionally-based postpartum home visits provided by public health nurses or midwives; (ii) flexible, individualized midwifery-based postpartum care that incorporates postpartum depression screening tools; (iii) telephone-based peer support; and (iv) interpersonal psychotherapy (which is well placed to address two of the strongest risk factors for postpartum depression: marital conflict and lack of support). Antenatal classes addressing postpartum depression and in-hospital psychological debriefing are less promising, and it is not clear whether home visits conducted by laypeople are effective (Dennis and Dowswell, 2013).

A review of omega-3 supplementation during pregnancy found no association with the prevention of postpartum depression (Saccone et al., 2016).

Little is known about whether there are particular interventions to address obesity in pregnancy with the aim of reducing the risk of anxiety and depression. To date, most trials have only considered short-term outcomes such as gestational weight gain and birthweight of the baby (Dodd et al., 2014; Chiswick et al., 2015). The assessment of maternal mood should therefore be included in the design of future intervention studies in obese pregnant women, and long-term evaluation of the effect on infants is also needed.

Treatment of perinatal depression/anxiety

The NICE (2014) guidance on ante- and postnatal mental health provides clear recommendations regarding the treatment of antenatal depression and anxiety.

Depression

[#]This guidance recommends that women with persistent *subthreshold* depressive symptoms, or *mild to moderate* depression in pregnancy or the postnatal period, should be

----

[#] Section adapted under the Open Government Licence v3.0 from Axford N. et al. '*Rapid Review to Update Evidence for the Healthy Child Programme 0–5*'. Public Health England, London, UK, © Crown Copyright 2015, https://assets.publishing.service.gov.uk/government/uploads/system/uploads/attachment_data/file/429740/150520RapidReviewHealthyChildProg_UPDATE_poisons_final.pdf.

offered facilitated self-help (delivered as described in recommendation 1.4.2.2 of the guideline on depression in adults (NICE guideline CG90)). However, for a woman with a history of *severe* depression but who initially presents with mild depression in pregnancy or the postnatal period, tricyclic antidepressants (TCA), selective serotonin reuptake inhibitors (SSRI), or (serotonin and) norepinephrine reuptake inhibitors (S) NRI antidepressants should be considered.

A number of options have been identified as being effective for women experiencing *moderate or severe* depression in pregnancy, including the following:

◆ A high-intensity psychological intervention (e.g. CBT).

◆ A TCA, SSRI, or (S)NRI antidepressant if the woman understands the risks associated with the medication and the mental health problem in pregnancy and the postnatal period and:

  • she has expressed a preference for medication; or

  • she declines psychological interventions; or

  • her symptoms have not responded to psychological interventions.

◆ A high-intensity psychological intervention in combination with medication if the woman understands the risks associated with the medication and the mental health problem in pregnancy, and there is no response, or a limited response, to a high-intensity psychological intervention or medication alone.

Anxiety

[#]NICE (2014) recommends that a woman with persistent *subthreshold* symptoms of anxiety in pregnancy or the postnatal period should be offered facilitated self-help. This should consist of the use of CBT-based self-help materials over 2–3 months with support (either face-to-face or by telephone) for a total of 2–3 hours over six sessions.

For a woman with an anxiety disorder in pregnancy or the postnatal period, the guideline recommends that she be offered a low-intensity psychological intervention (e.g. facilitated self-help) or a high-intensity psychological intervention (e.g. CBT) as initial treatment in line with the recommendations set out in the NICE guideline for the specific mental health problem. The guidelines note that it is important to be aware that:

◆ only high-intensity psychological interventions are recommended for post-traumatic stress disorder

◆ high-intensity psychological interventions are recommended for the initial treatment of social anxiety disorder

◆ progress should be closely monitored and a high-intensity psychological intervention offered within 2 weeks if symptoms have not improved.

[#] Section adapted under the Open Government Licence v3.0 from Axford N. et al. '*Rapid Review to Update Evidence for the Healthy Child Programme 0–5*'. Public Health England, London, UK, © Crown Copyright 2015, https://assets.publishing.service.gov.uk/government/uploads/system/uploads/attachment_data/file/429740/150520RapidReviewHealthyChildProg_UPDATE_poisons_final.pdf.

More recent evidence

Support for these recommendations are supported by a review which found that psychosocial interventions, such as peer support and non-directive counselling, and psychological interventions, such as CBT and interpersonal psychotherapy, are effective in reducing depressive symptoms in the first year postpartum (Dennis and Hodnett, 2007) but also by more recent reviews: one (Sockol, 2015) found strong evidence that CBT interventions are effective for treating depression in the perinatal period, noting that those initiated in the postpartum period are more effective than those delivered antenatally; and the other, on interpersonal psychotherapy, showed overall clinical improvement in depression measures in postpartum depressed women and often full recovery in several cases of treated patients (Miniati et al., 2014). The inconclusive evidence for the effectiveness of a number of alternative therapies, including maternal massage, bright light therapy, acupuncture, and omega-3 fatty acids, for treating antenatal depression has been covered by the NICE 2014 guidelines.

Another recent review suggests that there is insufficient evidence to make recommendations about the effectiveness of mindfulness training during pregnancy in reducing perinatal mental health problems generally (Hall et al., 2016). In contrast, there is significant evidence that exercise-based interventions can reduce symptoms of depression during pregnancy (Daley et al., 2015), although there is no clear difference in terms of benefit between aerobic exercise (running, walking, swimming, and aerobic classes) and non-aerobic exercise (strength-based training, yoga, and tai chi). It is, however, uncertain whether exercise interventions reduce symptoms of postnatal depression (Daley et al., 2009).

Computer- or web-based interventions for perinatal mental health are also promising. They entail various therapeutic approaches (e.g. CBT, relaxation, biofeedback, mindfulness, and stress management) and often involve therapist contact. The majority of the interventions in the two relevant reviews identified were targeted rather than universal. Ashford et al. (2016) found mainly positive effects in terms of reducing depression symptoms, but predominantly no significant outcomes for anxiety (although anxiety was rarely a target for intervention). Preventive interventions appeared to be less effective than those targeting an existing mental health issue. Lee et al. (2016) concluded that web-based interventions for perinatal depression delivered in the postpartum period may play a role in improving maternal mood. This is a developing field and more studies are needed, particularly on antenatal interventions.

Non-pharmacological treatment is particularly important in the perinatal period because of maternal treatment preferences and potential concerns about fetal and infant health outcomes (Howard et al., 2014). There are few high-quality studies on the effectiveness or safety of pharmacological treatments in the perinatal period, but general principles of prescribing drugs in the perinatal period have been described (see Howard et al., 2014, pp. 1781–1784).

Addressing mother–child interaction

Where there are concerns about the mother–infant interaction as a result of maternal mental health problems such as anxiety and depression and that do not resolve, further support targeting the dyad (mother and infant) should be provided (NICE, 2014). A range of evidence-based interventions can be used, ranging from infant massage through to more intensive models of work such as video feedback and parent–infant psychotherapy (Barlow et al., 2016) (see Chapter 10).

Supporting fathers in the perinatal period

Although research has shown that participation in a fathers' group can help fathers to cope with their partner's depression (Davey et al., 2006), and that partner support in the provision of treatment for women with postnatal depression can reduce maternal depressive symptoms (Misri et al., 2000), there is very little research that explicitly examines the effectiveness of interventions for fathers experiencing mental health problems. Furthermore, while many types of intervention that are provided in the perinatal period explicitly target the couple (e.g. preparation for parenthood programmes—see Chapter 7), most services that are aimed at addressing perinatal mental health problems target the mother only (see the Fatherhood Institute (2010) for an overview of some of innovative methods that are being tried).

Although the implications for practice are currently unclear, good practice would appear to include practitioners ensuring that services are clearly targeted at, and welcoming to, both parents (The Dad Project, 2017). Furthermore, groups that are provided especially for fathers, without necessarily focusing explicitly on mental health issues, may be a way of enabling fathers to begin to discuss openly the problems that they are experiencing.

Workforce skills and training

[#]NICE (2014) recommends that all healthcare professionals providing assessment and interventions for mental health problems in pregnancy and the postnatal period should understand the variations in their presentation and course at these times, how these variations affect treatment, and the context in which they are assessed and treated (e.g. maternity services, health visiting, and mental health services).

The recommended techniques for identifying women who may be in need of further comprehensive assessment requires training for health professionals in the skilful interpersonal process for psychosocial assessment (Howard et al., 2014, p. 1780).

[#] Section adapted under the Open Government Licence v3.0 from Axford N. et al. '*Rapid Review to Update Evidence for the Healthy Child Programme 0–5*'. Public Health England, London, UK, © Crown Copyright 2015, https://assets.publishing.service.gov.uk/government/uploads/system/uploads/attachment_data/file/429740/150520RapidReviewHealthyChildP rog_UPDATE_poisons_final.pdf.

NICE (2014) recommends that all interventions for mental health problems in pregnancy and the postnatal period should be delivered by competent practitioners. Psychological and psychosocial interventions should be based on the relevant treatment manual(s), which should guide the structure and duration of the intervention. Practitioners should consider using competence frameworks developed from the relevant treatment manual(s) and for all interventions practitioners should:

- receive regular high-quality supervision
- use routine outcome measures and ensure that the woman is involved in reviewing the efficacy of the treatment
- engage in the monitoring and evaluation of treatment adherence and practitioner competence—for example, by using video and audio tapes, and external audit and scrutiny where appropriate.

A review of qualitative evidence suggests that 'women's experience of accessing and engaging with care for mental health problems could be improved if they are given the opportunity to develop trusting relationships with healthcare professionals who acknowledge and reinforce the woman's role in caring for her baby in a non-judgemental and compassionate manner, and foster hope and optimism about treatment' (Megnin-Viggars et al., 2015, p. 745).

Learning links

The Institute of Health Visiting have developed three e-learning modules:

- Module 1—'Perinatal depression and other maternal mental health disorders': https://ihv.org.uk/for-health-visitors/resources-for-members/resource/ e-learning/perinatal-depression-and-other-maternal-mental-health-disorders-module-1/
- Module 2—'How to recognise perinatal anxiety and depression': https:// ihv.org.uk/for-health-visitors/resources-for-members/resource/e-learning/ perinatal-depression-and-other-maternal-mental-health-disorders-module-2/
- Module 3—'Interventions for perinatal anxiety, depression and related disorders': https://ihv.org.uk/for-health-visitors/resources-for-members/resource/ e-learning/perinatal-depression-and-other-maternal-mental-health-disorders-module-3/.

Recommendations

- Commission and deliver a structured child health programme to provide key opportunities to work with families and address common problems. (*Evidence: strong.*)
- Provide early intervention in perinatal mental health services to promote the well-being of both the parent and the child. (*Evidence: strong.*)

- ◆ Key health professionals (such as midwives and health visitors) should be alert to the possibility of anxiety and depression at all meetings with pregnant women and their partners. (*Evidence: strong.*)
- ◆ Follow NICE (2014) guidance for prevention and treatment of common mental health problems. (*Evidence: strong.*)
- ◆ Target services at both mothers and fathers to support both parents experiencing mental health problems. (*Good practice.*)

References

ACP Depression Care Guide. (2016). GAD-2. [online] American College of Physicians. Available at: https://integrationacademy.ahrq.gov/sites/default/files/GAD-2_0.pdf [Accessed 29 Sep. 2017].

Ashford, M.T., Olander, E.K., and **Ayers, S.** (2016). Computer- or web-based interventions for perinatal mental health: a systematic review. *Journal of Affective Disorders*, **197**, 134–146.

Axford, N., Barlow, J., Coad, J., et al. (2015). *Rapid Review to Update Evidence for the Healthy Child Programme 0–5*. London: Public Health England.

Barlow, J., Schrader-McMillan, A., Axford, N., et al. (2016). Attachment and attachment-related outcomes in pre-school children: a review of recent evidence. *Child and Adolescent Mental Health*, **21**, 11–20.

Beddoe, A. and **Lee, K.** (2008). Mind-body interventions during pregnancy. *Journal of Obstetric, Gynecologic and Neonatal Nursing*, **37**, 165–175.

Broom, B.L. (1994). Impact of marital quality and psychological well-being on parental sensitivity. *Nursing Research*, **43**, 138–143.

Buist, A., Morse, C.A., Durkin, S. (2003). Men's adjustment to fatherhood: implications for obstetric health care. *Journal of Obstetrics, Gynecology and Neonatal Nursing*, **32**, 172–180.

Chiswick, C., Reynolds, R.M., Denison, F., et al. (2015). Effect of metformin on maternal and fetal outcomes in obese pregnant women (EMPOWaR): a randomised, double-blind, placebo-controlled trial. *Lancet Diabetes Endocrinology*, **10**, 778–786.

Comfort, M., Gordon, P.R., and **Naples, D.** (2011). KIPS: an evidence-based tool for assessing parenting strengths and needs in diverse families. *Infants and Young Children: An Interdisciplinary Journal of Early Childhood Intervention*, **24**, 56–74.

Daley, A., Jolly, K., and **MacArthur, C.** (2009). The effectiveness of exercise in the management of post-natal depression: systematic review and meta-analysis. *Family Practice*, **26**, 154–162.

Daley, A.J., Foster, L., Long, G., et al. (2015). The effectiveness of exercise for the prevention and treatment of antenatal depression: systematic review with meta-analysis. *British Journal of Obstetrics and Gynaecology*, **122**, 57–63.

Davey, S.J., Dziurawiec, S., and **O'Brien-Malone, A.** (2006). Men's voices: postnatal depression from the perspective of male partners. *Qualitative Health Research*, **16**, 206–220.

Dawson, G., Frey, K., Panagiotides, H., Osterling, J., and Hessl, D. (1997). Infants of depressed mothers exhibit atypical frontal brain activity: a replication and extension of previous findings. *Journal of Child Psychology and Psychiatry*, **38**, 179–186.

De Wolff, M.S. and van Ijzendoorn, M.H. (1997). Sensitivity and attachment: a meta-analysis on parental antecedents of infant attachment security. *Child Development*, **68**, 604–609.

Dennis, C.L. and Dowswell, T. (2013). Psychosocial and psychological interventions for preventing postpartum depression. *Cochrane Database of Systematic Reviews*, **2**, CD001134.

Dennis, C.L. and Hodnett, E. (2007). Psychosocial and psychological interventions for treating postpartum depression. *Cochrane Database of Systematic Reviews*, **4**, CD006116.

Department of Health (2009). Healthy Child Programme: pregnancy and the first five years. [online] https://www.gov.uk/government/publications/healthy-child-programme-pregnancy-and-the-first-5-years-of-life [Accessed 1 June 2017].

Dodd, J.M., Turnbull, D., McPhee, A., et al. (2014). Antenatal lifestyle advice for women who are overweight or obese: LIMIT Randomised Trial. *BMJ*, **348**, G1285.

Fatherhood Institute (2010). Fatherhood Institute Research Summary: Fathers and Postnatal Depression. [online] Fatherhood Institute. Available at: http://www.fatherhoodinstitute.org/2010/fatherhood-institute-research-summary-fathers-and-postnatal-depression/ [Accessed 29 Sep. 2017].

Fonagy, P. and Target, M. (1997). Attachment and reflective function: their role in self-organization. *Development and Psychopathology*, **9**, 679–700.

Gavin, N.I., Gaynes, B.N., Lohr, K.N., Meltzer-Brody, S., Gartlehner, G., and Swinson, T. (2005). Perinatal depression: a systematic review of prevalence and incidence. *Obstetrics and Gynaecology*, **106**, 1071–1083.

Hall, H.G., Beattie, J., East, C., and Biro, M.A. (2016). Mindfulness and perinatal mental health: a systematic review. *Women and Birth*, **29**, 62–71.

Howard, L.M., Molyneaux, E., Dennis, C.-L., Rochat, T., Stein, A., and Milgrom, J. (2014). Perinatal mental health 1: non-psychotic mental disorders in the perinatal period. *The Lancet*, **384**, 1775–1788.

Kawanishi, Y., Hanley, S.J., Tabat, K., et al. (2015). Effects of prenatal yoga: a systematic review of randomized controlled trials. *Nihon Koshu Eisei Zasshi*, **62**, 221–231.

Khashan, A.S., Abel, K.M., Mcnamee, R., Pedersen, M.G., Webb, R.T., and Baker, P.N. (2008). Higher risk of offspring schizophrenia following antenatal maternal exposure to severe adverse life events. *Archives of General Psychiatry*, **65**, 146–152.

Khashan, A.S., Wicks, S., Dalman, C., et al. (2012). Prenatal stress and risk of asthma hospitalization in the offspring: a Swedish population-based study. *Psychosomatic Medicine*, **74**, 635–641.

Laplante, D.P., Brunet, A., Schmitz, N., Ciampi, A., and King, S. (2008). Project Ice Storm: prenatal maternal stress affects cognitive and linguistic functioning in 5 1/2-year-old children. *Journal of the American Academy of Child and Adolescent Psychiatry*, **47**, 1063–1072.

Leach, L.S., Poyser, C., Cooklin, A.R., and Giallo, R. (2016). Prevalence and course of anxiety disorders (and symptom levels) in men across the perinatal period: a systematic review. *Journal of Affective Disorders*, **190**, 675–686.

Lee, E.W., Denison, F.C., Hor, K., and Reynolds, R.M. (2016). Web-based interventions for prevention and treatment of perinatal mood disorders: a systematic review. *BMC Pregnancy and Childbirth*, **16**, 38.

Marc, I., Toureche, N., Ernst, E., et al. (2011). Mind-body interventions during pregnancy for preventing or treating women's anxiety. *Cochrane Database of Systematic Reviews*, 7, CD007559.

McElwain, N.L. and Volling, B.L. (1999). Depressed mood and marital conflict: relations to maternal and paternal intrusiveness with one-year-old infants. *Journal of Applied Developmental Psychology*, **20**, 63–83.

Megnin-Viggars, O., Symington, I., Howard, L.M., and Pilling, S. (2015). Experience of care for mental health problems in the antenatal or postnatal period for women in the UK: a systematic review and meta-synthesis of qualitative research. *Archive of Women's Mental Health*, **18**, 745–759.

Miniati, M., Callari, A., Calugi, S., et al. (2014). Interpersonal psychotherapy for postpartum depression: a systematic review. *Archives of Womens Mental Health*, **17**, 257–268.

Mirhosseini, H., Moosavipoor, S. A., Nazari, M. A., Dehghan, A., Mirhosseini, S., Bidaki, R., & Yazdian-Anari, P. (2015). Cognitive Behavioral Development in Children Following Maternal Postpartum Depression: A Review Article. Electronic physician, 7(8), 1673–1679.

Misri, S., Kostaras, X., Fox, D., and Kostaras, D. (2000). The impact of partner support in the treatment of postpartum depression. *Canadian Journal of Psychiatry*, **45**, 554–558.

Murray, L. (1992). The impact of postnatal depression on infant development. *Journal of Child Psychology and Psychiatry*, **33**, 543–561.

Murray, L., Arteche, A., Fearon, P., Halligan, S., Goddyer, I., Cooper, P. Maternal postnatal depression and the development of depression in offspring up to 16 years of age. *Journal of the American Academy of Child and Adolescent Psychiatry*, 50(5), 460–470.

Murray, L. and Cooper, P.J. (1997). The effects of postnatal depression on infant development. *Archives of Disease in Childhood*, **77**, 99–101.

Murray, L., Fiori-Cowley, A., Hooper, R., and Cooper, P. (1996). The impact of postnatal depression and associated adversity on early mother-infant interactions and later infant outcome. *Child Development*, **67**, 2512–2526.

Murray, L., Halligan, S.L, Cooper, P.J., Wachs, T., Bremner, G. (2009). Effects of postnatal depression on mother-infant interactions, and child development. *Handbook of Infant Development*. Oxford: Wiley-Blackwell.

Nabhan, A.F. and Faris, M.A. (2010). High feedback versus low feedback of prenatal ultrasound for reducing maternal anxiety and improving maternal health behaviour in pregnancy. *Cochrane Database of Systematic Reviews*, **4**, CD007208.

National Institute for Health and Care Excellence (2014). *Antenatal and Postnatal Mental Health: Clinical Management and Service Guidance*. Clinical guideline [CG192]. London: NICE. Available at: https://www.nice.org.uk/guidance/cg192 [Accessed 29 Sep. 2017].

O'Connor, T.G., Heron, J., Golding, J., Beveridge, M., and Glover, V. (2002). Maternal antenatal anxiety and children's behavioural/emotional problems at 4 years. report from the Avon Longitudinal Study of Parents and Children. *British Journal of Psychiatry*, **180**, 502–508.

Patient Health Questionnaire-9 (PHQ-9) (2017). Patient Health Questionnaire-9 (PHQ-9). [online] Patient Platform Limited. Available at: http://www.phqscreeners.com/sites/g/files/g10016261/f/201412/PHQ-9_English.pdf [Accessed 29 Sep. 2017].

Patient.info (2017). GAD7 Anxiety Test Questionnaire. [online] Available at: https://patient.info/doctor/generalised-anxiety-disorder-assessment-gad-7 [Accessed 29 Sep. 2017].

Paulson, J.F. and **Bazemore, S.D.** (2010). Prenatal and postpartum depression in fathers and its association with maternal depression: a meta-analysis. *Journal of the American Medical Association*, **303**, 1961–1969.

Paulson, J.F., **Dauber, S.**, and **Leiferman, J.A.** (2006). Individual and combined effects of postpartum depression in mothers and fathers on parenting behavior. *Pediatrics*, **118**, 659–668.

Pawlby, S., **Sharpe, D., Hay, D.**, and **O'Keane, V.** (2008). Postnatal depression and child outcome at 11 years: the importance of clinical diagnosis. *Journal of Affective Disorders*, **107**, 241–245.

Pearson, R.M., **Evans, J., Kounali, D., Lewis, G., Heron, J.**, and **Ramchandani, P.G.** (2013). Maternal depression during pregnancy and the postnatal period: risks and possible mechanisms for offspring depression at age 18 years. *JAMA Psychiatry*, **70**, 1312–1319.

Psychology Tools (2017). Edinburgh Postnatal Depression Scale. [online] Psychology Tools. Available at: https://psychology-tools.com/epds/ [Accessed 29 Sep. 2017].

Ramchandani, P., **O'Connor, T.G., Evans, J., Heron, J., Murray, L.**, and **Stein, A.** (2008). The effects of pre- and postnatal depression in fathers: a natural experiment comparing the effects of exposure to depression on offspring. *Journal of Child Psychology and Psychiatry*, **49**, 1069–1078.

Ramchandani, P., **Stein, A., Evans, J., O'Connor, T.G.**, and **ALSPAC study team.** (2005). Paternal depression in the postnatal period and child development: a prospective population study. *The Lancet*, **365**, 2201–2205.

Roggman, L.A., **Boyce, L.K., Cook, G.A.**, and **Cook, J.** (2002). Getting dads involved: predictors of father involvement in early head start and with their children. *Infant Mental Health Journal*, **23**, 62–78.

Saccone, G., **Saccone, I.**, and **Berghella, V.** (2016). Omega-3 long-chain polyunsaturated fatty acids and fish oil supplementation during pregnancy: which evidence? *Journal of Maternal and Fetal Neonatal Medicine*, **29**, 2389–2397.

Schore, A.N. (2005). Back to basics: attachment, affect regulation, and the developing right brain: linking developmental neuroscience to pediatrics. *Pediatrics in Review*, **26**, 204–217.

Sethna, V., **Murray, L., Psychogiou, L.**, and **Ramchandani, P.** (2009). The impact of paternal depression in infancy: a mechanism for the intergenerational transmission of risk. *European Psychiatry*, **24**, 236.

Sheffield, K.M. and **Woods-Giscombé, C.L.** (2016). Efficacy, feasibility and acceptability of perinatal yoga on women's mental health and well-being: a systematic literature review. *Journal of Holistic Nursing*, **34**, 64–79.

Sockol, L.E. (2015). A systematic review of the efficacy of cognitive behavioral therapy for treating and preventing perinatal depression. *Journal of Affective Disorders*, **177**, 7–21.

Stein, A., **Pearson, R.M., Goodman, S.H., Rapa, E., Rahman, A.**, and **Mccallum, M.** (2014). Effects of perinatal mental disorders on the fetus and child. *The Lancet*, **384**, 1800–1819.

Svanberg, P.O., **Barlow, J.**, and **Tigbe, W.W.** (2013). The parent–infant interaction observation scale: reliability and validity of a screening tool. *Journal of Reproductive and Infant Psychology*, **31**, 5–14.

The Dad Project. (2017). [ebook] NSPCC. Available at: https://www.nspcc.org.uk/globalassets/documents/research-reports/all-babies-count-dad-project.pdf [Accessed 29 Sep. 2017].

Vesga-Lopex, O., **Blanco, C.**, **Keyes, K.**, **Olfson, M.**, **Grant, B.F.**, and **Hasin, D.S.** (2008). Psychiatric disorders in pregnant and postpartum women in the United States. *Archives of General Psychiatry*, **65**, 830–836.

Whooleyquestions.ucsf.edu (2015). Whooley Questions for Depression Screening. [online] Available at: http://whooleyquestions.ucsf.edu/ [Accessed 29 Sep. 2017].

Chapter 5

Intimate partner violence

Anita Schrader McMillan and Nick Axford

Summary

This chapter:

+ outlines the prevalence of intimate partner violence (IPV) in the UK
+ describes the adverse effects of IPV for adult and child survivor-victims
+ synthesizes evidence on the effectiveness of interventions to (i) prevent IPV, (ii) identify IPV, (iii) support adults and children affected by IPV, and (iv) treat perpetrators
+ makes recommendations for practice.

Introduction

Intimate partner violence (IPV) includes acts of physical, emotional, psychological, and financial abuse by those who are or have been intimate partners or family members, as well as sexual abuse and stalking (Home Office, 2013). The first part of this chapter presents recent evidence about the prevalence of IPV in the UK and its impact on survivor-victims and children. The remainder of the chapter summarizes the evidence about effective prevention and identification/screening for IPV, effective methods of supporting adults and children affected by IPV, and methods for treating perpetrators.

Prevalence, impact, and modalities of intimate partner violence

Prevalence and impact on victim-survivors

A recent study estimated that in the UK 1.3 million women/girls (8.2% of the population) and 600,000 men/boys (4%) were victims of IPV in 2014/2015 (Office for National Statistics, 2016). Both men and women perpetrate violence in heterosexual and same-sex relationships but women are more likely to be exposed to coercive control and severe or sexual violence and to die at the hands of a partner or ex-partner (Donovan et al., 2006).

IPV is not a homogeneous phenomenon. Although all typologies are contested, they do signal the need for different approaches to intervention and treatment—and in particular, that no 'one-size-fits-all' approach is likely to be suitable in work with perpetrators. For example, Johnson (1995) distinguishes between coercive controlling violence, violence that is used in self-defence, and 'situational' violence that can be initiated by either partner in the context of escalating fights. Although the latter is the most common form of IPV, it is least likely to attract outside help (Stith et al., 2011). A different typology identifies broad three types of perpetrators: (i) 'family-only' types, who are rarely violent, only violent within the family, and do not have co-occurring addiction or psychopathology; (ii) dysphoric/borderline perpetrators with moderate to high levels of violence, psychological and sexual abuse, and high levels of depression and anger; and, at the most extreme end, (iii) generally violent or antisocial perpetrators who demonstrate antisocial/psychopath personality disorders and engage in high levels of violence in a range of settings.

In victims of both sexes, IPV is associated with an increased risk of poor health, depressive symptoms, substance use, chronic disease, chronic mental illness, and injury (Lawrence et al., 2012). Its impact on women is compounded by generally higher levels of fear, an important dynamic in abuse. The consequences of both psychological and physical abuse are significantly worse for victims who are unemployed and/or on a low income and from minority ethnic groups (Lawrence et al., 2012). Both men and women with a long-term illness or disability are at increased risk of IPV (Office for National Statistics, 2016).

Infants and young children in the context of IPV

IPV features in over half of the serious case reviews in the UK (Sidebotham et al., 2016) and there are no reliable figures about those exposed to low-level violence that does not reach the attention of police or welfare services. There is, however, robust evidence about the adverse impact of IPV on children's emotional, social, and cognitive development and their physical health (MacDonell, 2013). Antenatal IPV is associated with an increased risk of miscarriage, preterm birth, low birthweight, and neonatal death (Jasinksy, 2004). In infants and toddlers, exposure to IPV can affect developmental milestones, including language learning and toilet training, and lead to sleep disturbances, emotional distress, and fear of being alone (Osofsky, 2003). Under-fives are especially vulnerable because of the plasticity of the infant brain and because IPV undermines the conditions necessary for infants to create secure attachment (Sturge-Appel et al., 2012). Unlike older children, for whom school may offer a refuge, infants cannot escape from violence at home and nor do they have the capacity to verbalize or make sense of their experience. Longitudinal studies show that adverse effects are linked to children's age when first exposed to IPV, chronicity, and whether IPV is compounded—as it often is—by other threats to the child (Chan and Yeung, 2009). Children who appear to cope better tend to have strong attachments to a non-violent parent or other significant adult, and to have had the opportunity to engage in therapeutic work sooner rather than later (Devaney, 2014). IPV is the crime most likely to reoccur, and often co-occurs with alcohol and drug abuse, so children are rarely exposed to just a single distressing event (Finkelhor et al., 2007; Stanley, 2011). Early intervention is essential both to prevent or end IPV and to mitigate its effects on children (Heise, 1998; Hibel et al., 2011).

Preventing violence

Preventing 'dating violence' in adolescence

School-based dating violence prevention programmes (usually universal) comprise a curriculum delivered by teachers in group settings over the course of several sessions. Overall, they are promising; there is reasonably strong evidence of positive effects in terms of improvement in participants' attitudes and increased knowledge around dating violence, and weaker evidence that they can reduce perpetration and victimization (Whitaker et al., 2006, 2013; British Columbia Centre of Excellence for Women's Health (BCCEWH), 2013; Fellmeth et al., 2013; DeGue et al., 2014; De Koker et al., 2014; De La Rue et al., 2014; Petering et al., 2014; Stanley et al., 2015a, 2015b). The same evidence base shows that mostly targeted community-based interventions can also reduce dating violence victimization or perpetration. However, most trials of dating violence prevention programmes have involved adolescents in North America, often from minority ethnic groups, so there is a need to develop and rigorously test such interventions in the UK (Stanley et al., 2015a).

Notwithstanding these concerns about their transferability, dating violence prevention programmes are considered likely to be most effective at reducing victimization and perpetration if they:

> focus on a broader range of risk factors and behaviour change theories; involve repeated exposure in multiple settings (school and community); train participants in emotional intelligence and effective communication and conflict resolution skills; focus on influencing key people in the adolescent's environment (as well as the adolescent themselves); promote equal gender roles; build links with support services that can respond to disclosures and support high-risk children; provide teachers with more and better training from people with specialist knowledge and skills in domestic abuse; are sensitive to the local cultural context; and, in the case of school-based interventions, are delivered in schools that are properly ready for implementation. (Axford et al., 2018, p. 69.)

Prevention of IPV in adults

Several authors propose developing awareness campaigns that operate concurrently at both the societal and individual level to create a supportive context for violence prevention (BCCEHW, 2013). Interventions for adults that are designed to prevent IPV tend to involve media and educational campaigns and there are few effectiveness studies (BCCEHW, 2013). There is inconsistent evidence that media campaigns addressing IPV can help improve recall, raise awareness of available resources, increase calls to hotlines, and improve knowledge of IPV among target audiences. Some studies have demonstrated positive effects, while others have not because the intended audience had limited awareness of the campaign.

Perinatal home visiting programmes that screen for IPV find high rates of IPV and that IPV limits the ability of the intervention to improve maternal and child outcomes (Sharps et al., 2008). Home visiting interventions that include specific content on IPV and support women who are abused can reduce women's exposure in the short term, although their effect in the long term is not known (Prosman et al., 2015). The most effective home visiting programmes for reducing violence last 12–24 months and are delivered by trained nurses rather than paraprofessionals (Van Parys et al., 2014).

Screening and assessment

The early identification of IPV through routine questioning has been the focus of numerous studies, primarily in emergency department, antenatal care, and primary care settings (Rabin et al., 2009; O'Reilly et al., 2010; O'Campo et al., 2011; Todahl and Walters, 2011; Taft et al., 2013). There is much less research examining the identification of IPV in social care environments, or evaluating integrated approaches to identification across various health and social care settings. Assessment for IPV can be built into home visiting programmes, although those involved in delivery need appropriate training, including on how to make referrals to local specialist agencies (Sharps et al., 2008; Van Parys et al., 2014).

Although not universally accepted as 'screening', the evidence shows that standardized enquiry leads to increased disclosure and identification of IPV, particularly when it is built into the routine care of women during pregnancy and the postnatal period (Taft et al., 2013). However, there is no evidence that such assessment results in an actual reduction of exposure to violence for women identified as at risk, or that it leads to better outcomes than routine or opportunistic enquiry. Standardized assessment isn't necessarily part of a care pathway, so those identified may not be referred to appropriate services or offered support for their health, social, and safety needs (O'Campo et al., 2011). Even where services are offered, there has been little measurement of the relationship between provision and take-up rates.

Health service users—including victims of violence—are generally supportive of universal questioning for IPV, provided that a rationale is given and that it is done in private and with a non-judgemental attitude (Todahl and Walters, 2011). In contrast, the degree to which clinicians agree with routine assessment varies greatly, from 15% to 95% across studies (Feder et al., 2009).

Studies of organizations that have implemented routine screening have identified four elements that increase provider efficacy (these are also true for any form of identification): (i) the organization's expectation that practitioners will undertake this assessment, and support for them to do so; (ii) effective protocols; (iii) ongoing skills development training; and (iv) on-site access to help with referrals to support services (Todahl and Walters, 2011; Sprague et al., 2012; Taft et al., 2013). A critical element of success is practitioners being able to communicate with sensitivity in order to encourage clients to speak about IPV when necessary (O'Reilly et al., 2010). There is some evidence for the benefits of services having on-site support and a manager or coordinator who can quickly access the support in terms of improving screening and disclosure rates and provider confidence and self-efficacy (O'Reilly et al., 2010; O'Campo et al., 2011).

Although the National Institute for Health and Care Excellence (NICE) (2014) finds insufficient evidence to recommend screening or routine enquiry in healthcare settings, it recommends that health and social care practitioners should be able to: recognize indicators of domestic violence and ask relevant questions to help people disclose; know about and have access to relevant services; understand the effects of violence on children and how to refer to child protection services; and respond with empathy and understanding.

Treatment

Work with victim-survivors of IPV

Most studies of interventions for victims of IPV have been conducted with women in shelter populations, and in health or criminal justice settings (which tend to involve perpetrators/victims of IPV). This is despite most commissioned services being delivered in the community by domestic violence services and agencies working together across the range of children's and early years provision. Unless otherwise specified, the evidence in Box 5.1 draws from BCCEWH (2013), the comprehensive review that underpins the NICE (2014) guidelines.

Work with perpetrators of IPV

This section also draws on the BCCEWH (2013) review but more recent individual studies are included too. Although several studies in the review included women who perpetrate IPV, the majority concerned interventions for heterosexual males. Studies varied in whether participants were court-mandated, non-mandated, or both.

♦ Short group approaches (16 weeks or less) included 'family of origin group therapy, a solution- and goal-focused group treatment programme, CBT, unstructured supportive group therapy, group counselling and group sessions based on the Duluth model' (BCCEWH, 2013, p. 211). On the whole, the evidence is stronger for improvements in attitudinal, psychological, and interpersonal outcomes than it is for reductions in recidivism.

♦ Long approaches (over 16 weeks) included 'CBT programs, psycho-educational components, abuser schema therapy and Duluth-based group therapy' (BCCEWH 2013, p. 212). As with short-term interventions, most studies demonstrate 'improvements on measures such as communication, motivation to change and attitudes towards violence and conflict management skills' (p. 15) but limited effectiveness with respect to actual behavioural change (BCCEWH, 2013). Dropout is a problem in most treatment studies for perpetrators but may be reduced by the use of motivational interviewing techniques.

♦ Batterer Intervention Programmes based on psychoeducational/Duluth models have consistently produced low effect sizes for perpetrator behaviour change. Effects are stronger for changes in beliefs and attitudes associated with violence.

Box 5.1 Evidence underpinning the NICE (2014) guidelines on working with victim-survivors of IPV

Advocacy interventions involve helping victims of IPV to access a range of services and supports, and ensuring that their rights and entitlements are upheld. BCCEWH (2013) finds moderate evidence that such services can improve women's access to community resources, reduce rates of IPV, improve safety, decrease depression, reduce various stressors and improve parenting stress and children's well-being. However, cumulative evidence on their *long-term* effects finds very high levels of recidivism (i.e. re-exposure to partner violence). A more recent Cochrane review concluded that intensive advocacy may improve short-term quality of life and reduce physical abuse one to two years after the intervention for women recruited from domestic violence shelters and refuges (Rivas et al., 2015). It also found that brief advocacy may provide small short-term mental health benefits and reduce abuse, particularly in pregnant women and for less severe abuse.

- ◆ *Practical skill-building* (such as groups, or training sessions) for victim-survivors of IPV is associated with improvements in well-being, decision-making abilities and safety (BCCEWH, 2013). The skills taught (e.g. coping skills, conflict resolution, safety planning, decision-making, economic education, and sleep training) vary between interventions.

- ◆ '*Counselling interventions* may improve PTSD symptoms, depression, anxiety, self-esteem, stress management, independence, support, re-occurrence of violence, birth outcomes for pregnant women, motivational level, readiness to change, and/or forgiveness' (BCCEWH, 2013, p. 188). These interventions tend to be based on brief educational, cognitive behavioural, and motivational interviewing approaches. While the majority of interventions reported improvements on the various outcomes measured, some reported only modest improvements or improvements on some but not all measures.

- ◆ *Therapy* may be effective in improving PTSD symptoms, depression, parenting, and family-related outcomes (BCCEWH, 2013), and in some cases may reduce the likelihood of future IPV or re-abuse (although findings relating to re-victimization are mixed). Interventions included cognitive processing and written account therapies, cognitive behavioural therapy (CBT), emotion- and goal-focused group therapy, psychosocial group therapy, dialectical behavioural therapy, and holistic group therapy. Most studies involved low-income women, and the strength of effectiveness varied (BCCEWH, 2013). A more recent review (Arroyo et al., 2017) found that short-term psychotherapy interventions for survivors of IPV are particularly effective in reducing PTSD symptoms and symptoms of depression and general distress, and increasing self-esteem and life functioning. They also generate moderate effects for outcomes such as substance abuse, emotional well-being, a sense of safety, and instances of subsequent IPV. CBT and interpersonal therapies that are specifically tailored to individuals who had experienced IPV were most effective, with other interventions (exposure therapy, yoga, dialectical behaviour therapy, and education about feminism or grief) showing moderate effects. Individually delivered interventions produced stronger outcomes than those delivered in a group format, and a higher dosage is linked to stronger outcomes. Short-term psychotherapy interventions are therefore an important component of a coordinated community response to IPV, although systematic institutional, financial, and cultural barriers also need to be addressed.

- ◆ *Group-based interventions* such as the Freedom Programme, often show good user satisfaction, but evidence on their outcomes is limited (Williamson and Abrahams, 2010).

Source: data from *Review of Interventions to Identify, Prevent, Reduce and Respond to Domestic Violence*, prepared by the British Columbia Centre of Excellence for Women's Health, 2013, available from https://www.nice.org.uk/guidance/ph50/resources/review-of-interventions-to-identify-prevent-reduce-and-respond-to-domestic-violence3.

◆ Individual (one-to-one) interventions include 'case management, an individual level intervention combined with community outreach services, solution-focused therapy, educational interventions and motivational interviewing' (BCCEWH 2013, p. 211). As with group work, the BCCEWH (2013) review found that individual 'interventions appeared to have a greater effect on attitudinal outcomes than recidivism/ violence outcomes (which, when measured improved in some but not all studies)' (p. 211). There is also evidence to support motivational interviewing in terms of increased adherence to treatment.

◆ A significant subset of men with histories of IPV are concerned about the impact of their violence on their children (Rothman et al., 2007). Some new interventions have been designed to combine a focus on IPV cessation with improved parenting for men, using the man's role as a father to motivate change. A quasi-experimental study of the Caring Dads, Safer Children (CDSC) programme for men who perpetrated violence towards their partners found evidence of reduced incidence of IPV reported by men and their partners among a proportion of men who completed the programme (McConnell et al., 2016). IPV reduction was sustained and generated greater subjective feelings of security within in children. However, CDSC had high levels of attrition (at 49%), and even among some fathers who completed the programme, change was insufficient to cease monitoring their contact families; in such circumstances, feedback to referrers from CDSC workers informed decision-making about the father's access to his children.

◆ Fathers for Change is an intervention for fathers with co-occurring IPV and substance abuse problems. A randomized controlled trial (RCT) found statistically significant improvements for men involved in Fathers for Change in terms of reduced IPV, improved parenting, and reduced substance abuse relative to the control group (Stover, 2015). The programme also has a high level of user satisfaction.

These findings are based on work with small samples and further, larger-scale longitudinal research is needed. Overall, the evidence points to the need to integrate evidence-based treatment for substance abuse and trauma-focused interventions into IPV treatments (BCCEWH, 2013).

Other reviews have also found little evidence of the effectiveness of perpetrator-focused interventions. Smedsund et al. (2011) concluded that there was insufficient evidence to draw conclusions about the effectiveness of CBT interventions (with or without additional components) for physically abusive men in reducing violence against women. Akoensi et al. (2013) found that group-based interventions for perpetrators reduced abuse but weaknesses in the study designs mean that the effects could not be attributed to the programmes alone. Gilchrist et al. (2015) found insufficient evidence to draw conclusions about the effectiveness of group-based CBT (with anger management components) targeted at alcohol-abusing males. NICE (2014) therefore recommends commissioning and evaluating new forms of treatment for IPV perpetration. One area for exploration concerns emerging insights from neurobiology and attachment research, which point to the need to develop programmes that integrate emotional/affect regulation, the development of reflective functioning, communication, and safety planning (Hamel, 2008, 2014; Sieger, 2014).

Couples work with and without treatment for substance abuse

The evidence to support other types of intervention, including couples groups and conjoint interventions, is still fairly limited, but this is due to the smaller number of studies on newer approaches to intervention for IPV (Heru, 2007). The BCCEWH (2013) review found preliminary evidence to support the efficacy of behavioural couples therapy adapted to couples in situations where IPV is compounded by alcohol and/or drug abuse. Although the quality of studies is weak, the findings indicate reduced aggression and conflict and improved relationship skills and satisfaction. Effects were modest for conjoint work among couples who did not need treatment for substance abuse. All forms of couples work in the context of IPV require careful screening for risk.

A further review focused on interventions aimed at improving inter-parental relationships, sometimes but not always in the context of IPV (Harold et al., 2016). Interventions were categorized as CBT, skills training, psychoeducation, and conflict reappraisal. Some were group based, some for couples, and some for individuals. They varied in terms of whether they were preventive or targeted and for intact or separated couples, and whether they were primarily concerned about the couple relationship itself or the children.

In general, they were shown to have the potential to improve the couple relationship, parental well-being, parenting behaviour, and child outcomes. Positive outcomes for children are seen in couples interventions that focus on conflict management and communication for couples. This can happen at key transition points (e.g. becoming a parent) and especially difficult points (e.g. divorce). Even when parenting skills are not targeted directly, interventions that target couple communication and conflict resolution skills demonstrate improvements in parenting and child outcomes. However, there are risks inherent in work with couples and it is appropriate only in the context of reactive (situational) violence that has never reached a critical threshold. Specifically, it requires careful screening by trained practitioners (see Stith et al.'s (2011) work on couples therapy in the context of IPV for examples of screening tools and procedures).

Children exposed to IPV

There is limited published work on the effectiveness of interventions designed for pre-school children exposed to IPV. A comprehensive recent review on improving outcomes for children exposed to domestic violence (Howarth et al., 2016) identified three studies involving children aged 5 years or less, of which only one (Lieberman et al., 2005) included infants. All three approaches involved conjoint work with mothers and children but varied in location, duration, and outcomes measured in the respective studies. No study measured changes in maternal sensitivity or infant attachment security.

One of these studies concerned a group-based psychoeducation programme, the Moms' Empowerment Program, which works with both mothers and children and has been tailored for children aged 4–6 years (Graham-Bermann et al., 2015). It involves educating women about the effects of IPV on themselves and their children, building parenting competence and managing child behaviour, and helping parents to understand and correctly attribute children's emotions. Intent-to-treat analyses in an efficacy trial indicated that the programme reduced internalizing problems for girls at follow-up (8 months post intervention), and per-protocol analyses indicated that the programme reduced internalizing problems for both boys and girls post intervention.

There is also some evidence to support mother–child play therapy in terms of improved parent–child interaction. One model, Family Interaction for Improving Occupational Performance (FI-OP), engages mothers and children aged 1–5 years once or twice per week for 8 weeks. A small trial in a women's refuge found that mother–child interaction was significantly better in the FI-OP group compared with the playroom group (Waldman-Levi and Weintraub, 2015).

The most robust evidence supports child–parent psychotherapy (in which the non-victimized parent–child relationship is focused on as the means of therapeutic change) combined with advocacy and advice. Children in the study, an RCT, were aged 3–5 years, and the intervention was delivered to non-abusive parent and child dyads weekly for 50 weeks. The findings provide evidence of the efficacy of child–parent psychotherapy in reducing children's total behaviour problems, traumatic stress symptoms, and diagnostic status, and mothers' avoidance symptoms, with positive trends on post-traumatic stress disorder (PTSD) symptoms and general distress (Liebermann et al., 2005). As noted above, this appears to be most effective in combination with advocacy and adjunctive support for the specific challenges faced by the family.

Other approaches to work with women and children

The CEDAR programme involves parallel groups for mothers who are victim-survivors and their children over a 12-week period. One of the core objectives of the programme, which was developed in the UK, is to strengthen women's support for their children's recovery and their parenting. A qualitative study of CEDAR reports improvements in the mother–child relationship and children's emotional well-being (Sharps and Jones, 2011). Most (94%) of the children in the CEDAR study were aged 7 years or older, and further, robust research is needed. However, these findings are congruent with research elsewhere which suggests that supporting victimized parents (primarily but not always mothers) and children to rebuild their relationship can enable both to recover and move on from their experiences (Humphreys et al., 2006).

Further work is also needed on interventions such as Fathers for Change (Stover, 2013) that work with male perpetrators of IPV and incorporate a focus on emotional regulation combined with a parenting component. Findings from one RCT show improvements in terms of violence reduction/cessation and other measures (Stover, 2015). The direct and long-term effect on children has not been studied.

Learning links

- E-learning for health have developed three modules on 'Domestic Violence and Abuse': https://www.e-lfh.org.uk/programmes/domestic-violence-and-abuse/
- The Royal College of General Practitioners' Violence Against Women and Children e-learning course enables general practitioners and other primary care professionals to improve their recognition of and response to patients suffering from violence: http://elearning.rcgp.org.uk/course/info.php?id=88.

Recommendations

Prevention

- Home visiting interventions need to include specific content on IPV, support women who are abused and be delivered by trained nurses over at least 12 months (Evidence: moderate)
- School-based (usually universal) and community-based (usually targeted) dating violence prevention programmes for adolescents deserve to be further evaluated in a UK context. (*Evidence: moderate.*)
- All health and social care practitioners involved in assessing, caring for, and supporting people experiencing or perpetrating IPV and abuse should have sufficient and appropriate training and competencies in IPV. (*Evidence: strong.*)
- Practitioners must be aware of local referral pathways for domestic violence and be able to offer referrals to specialist support services targeted to the level of risk, patterns of perpetration, and specific needs of individuals and families. (*Evidence: strong.*)

Interventions for victim/survivors of IPV

- Treatment needs to be tailored to the needs of victim/survivors. Evidence supports therapy combined with advocacy services and skill building interventions including a focus on parenting where necessary. (*Evidence: moderate.*)
- National guidelines recommend integrating trauma-focused work, substance abuse, and couples-focused interventions into IPV treatments. (*Evidence: strong.*)

Interventions for preschool children exposed to IPV

- Therapeutic/psychoeducational work that strengthens the parent–child relationship is recommended. This should include an advocacy component. (*Evidence: moderate.*)

Interventions for perpetrators

- NICE (2014) guidelines recommend commissioning and evaluating new forms of treatment for IPV perpetration. (*Evidence: strong.*)

Acknowledgements

This chapter contains public sector information licensed under the Open Government Licence v3.0, including Axford et al. (2015, 2018) and Schrader-McMillan and Barlow (2017).

References and further reading

Akoensi, T., Koehler, J., Lösel, F., and Humphreys, D. (2013). Domestic violence perpetrator programs in Europe, Part II: a systematic review of the state of evidence. *International Journal of Offender Therapy and Comparative Criminology*, **57**, 1206–1225.

Arroyo, K., Lundahl, B., Butters, R., Vanderloo, M., and Wood, D.S. (2017). Short-term interventions for survivors of intimate partner violence: a systematic review and meta-analysis. *Trauma, Violence and Abuse*, **18**, 155–171.

Axford, N., Barlow, J., Coad, J., et al. (2015). *Rapid Review to Update Evidence for the Healthy Child Programme 0–5*. London: Public Health England.

Axford, N., Lowther, K., Timmons, L., Brook, L., Webb, L., and Sonthalia, S. (2018). *Rapid Review on Safeguarding to Inform the Healthy Child Programme 5–19*. London: Public Health England.

British Columbia Centre of Excellence for Women's Health (BCCEWH) (2013). Review of Interventions to Identify, Prevent, Reduce and Respond to Domestic Violence. [online] https://www.nice.org.uk/guidance/ph50/resources/review-of-interventions-to-identify-prevent-reduce-and-respond-to-domestic-violence2 [Accessed 22 Feb. 2016].

Chan, Y. and Yeung, J.W. (2009). Children living with violence within the family and its sequel: a meta-analysis from 1995–2006. *Aggression and Violent Behaviour*, **14**, 313–322.

DeGue, S., Valle, L.A., Holt, M.K., Massetti, G.M., Matjasko, J.L, and Tharp, A.T. (2014). A systematic review of primary prevention strategies for sexual violence perpetration. *Aggression and Violent Behavior*, **19**, 346–362.

De Koker, P., Mathews, C., Zuch, M., Bastien, S., and Mason-Jones, A.J. (2014). A systematic review of interventions for preventing adolescent intimate partner violence. *Journal of Adolescent Health*, **54**, 3–13.

De La Rue, L., Polanin, J., Espelage, D., and Pigott, T. (2014). School-based interventions to reduce dating and sexual violence: a systematic review. *Campbell Systematic Reviews*, 7.

Devaney, J. (2015). Research review: the impact of domestic violence on children. *Irish Probation Journal*, **12**, 79–94.

Donovan, C., Hester, M., Holmes, J., and McCarry, M. (2006). Comparing Domestic Abuse in Same Sex and Heterosexual Relationships. [online] Available at: https://www.researchgate.net/publication/228537060_Comparing_Domestic_Abuse_in_Same_Sex_and_Heterosexual_Relationships.

Feder, G., Ramsay, J., Dunne, D., et al. (2009). How far does screening women for domestic (partner) violence in different health-care settings meet criteria for a screening programme? Systematic reviews of nine UK National Screening Committee criteria. *Health Technology Assessment*, **13**, iii–iv, xi–xiii, 1–113, 137–347.

Fellmeth, G., Heffernan, C., Nurse, J., Habibula, S., and Sethi, D. (2013). Educational and skills-based interventions for preventing relationship and dating violence in adolescents and young adults. *Cochrane Database of Systematic Reviews*, **6**, CD004534.

Finkelhor, D., Ormrod, R.K., and Turner, H.A. (2007). Poly-victimization: a neglected component in child victimization. *Child Abuse and Neglect*, **31**, 7–26.

Gilchrist, G., Tirado Munoz, J., and Easton, C.J. (2015). Should we reconsider anger management when addressing physical intimate partner violence perpetration by alcohol abusing males? A systematic review. *Aggression and Violent Behavior*, **25**, 124–132.

Graham-Bermann, S.A., Miller-Graff, L.E., Howell, K.H., and Grogan-Kaylor, A. (2015). An efficacy trial of an intervention program for children exposed to intimate partner violence. *Child Psychiatry and Human Development*, **46**, 928–939.

Hamel, J. (2008). *Intimate Partner and Family Abuse: A Casebook of Gender Inclusive Therapy*. New York: Springer.

Hamel, J. (2014). *Gender-Inclusive Treatment of Intimate Partner Abuse: Evidence-Based Approaches* (2nd edn). New York: Springer.

Harold, G., Acquah, D., Sellers, R., and Chowdry, H. (2016). *What Works to Enhance Inter-Parental Relationships and Improve Outcomes for Children*. DWP ad hoc research report no. 32. London: DWP/Early Intervention Foundation.

Heise, L.L. (1998). Violence against women: an integrated, ecological framework. *Violence Against Women*, **4**, 262–290.

Heru, A.M. (2007). Intimate partner violence: treating abuser and abused. *Advances in Psychiatric Treatment*, **13**, 376–383.

Hibel, L., Granger, D.A., Blair, C., Cox, M.J., and Family Life Project Key Investigators. (2011). Maternal sensitivity buffers the adrenocortical implications of intimate partner violence exposure during early childhood. *Development and Psychopathology*, **23**, 689–701.

Home Office (2013). *Information for Local Areas on the Change to the Definition of Domestic Violence and Abuse*. London: Home Office.

Howarth, E., Moore, T.H.M., Welton, N.J., et al. (2016). *IMPRoving Outcomes for children exposed to domestic ViolencE (IMPROVE): An Evidence Synthesis*. Southampton: NIHR Journals Library.

Humphreys, C., Mullender, A., Thiara, R., and Skamballis, A. (2006). 'Talking to my mum': developing communication between mothers and children in the aftermath of domestic violence. *Journal of Social Work*, **6**, 53–63.

Johnson, M. (1995). Patriarchal terrorism and common couple violence: two forms of violence against women. *Journal of Marriage and the Family*, **57**, 283–294.

Lawrence, E., Orengo-Aguayo, R., Langer, A., and Brock, R. (2012). The impact and consequences of partner abuse on partners. *Partner Abuse*, **3**, 406–428.

Lieberman, A.F., Van Horn, P., and Ghosh Ippen, C. (2005). Toward evidence-based treatment: child-parent psychotherapy with preschoolers exposed to marital violence. *Journal of the American Academy of Child and Adolescent Psychiatry*, **44**, 1241–1248.

MacDonell, K. (2013). The combined and independent impact of witnessed intimate partner violence and child maltreatment. *Partner Abuse*, **3**, 358–378.

McConnell, N., Holdsworth, T., Barnard, M., and Taylor, J. (2016). *Caring Dads: Safer Children: Learning from Delivering the Programme*. London: NSPCC.

National Institute for Health and Care Excellence (NICE) (2014). *Domestic Violence and Abuse: How Health Services, Social Care and the Organisations They Work With Can Respond Effectively*. PH50. London: NICE.

O'Campo, P., Kirst, M., Tsamis, C., Chambers, C., and Ahmad, F. (2011). Implementing successful intimate partner violence screening programs in health care settings: evidence generated from a realist-informed systematic review. *Social Science & Medicine*, **72**, 855–866.

Office for National Statistics (2016). March 2015 Crime Survey for England and Wales (CSEW). Available at: http://www.safelives.org.uk/policy-evidence/about-domestic-abuse#top 10.

O'Reilly, R., Beale, B., and **Gillies, D.** (2010). Screening and intervention for domestic during pregnancy care: a systematic review. *Trauma Violence Abuse,* **11,** 190–201.

Osofsky, J.D. (2003). Prevalence of children's exposure to marital violence and child maltreatment: implications for prevention and intervention. *Clinical Child and Family Psychology Review,* **6,** 161–170.

Petering, R., Wenzel, S., and **Winetrobe, H.** (2014). Systematic review of current intimate partner violence prevention programs and applicability to homeless youth. *Journal of the Society for Social Work and Research,* **5,** 107–135.

Prosman, G., Lo Fo Wong, S.H., van der Wouden, J.C., and **Lagro-Janssen, A.L.** (2015). Effectiveness of home visiting in reducing partner violence for families experiencing abuse: a systematic review. *Family Practice,* **32,** 247–256.

Rabin, R.F., Jennings, J.M., Campbell, J.C., and **Bair-Merritt, M.H.** (2009). Intimate partner violence screening tools: a systematic review. *American Journal of Preventive Medicine,* **36,** 439–445.

Rivas, C., Ramsay, J., Sadowski, L., et al. (2015). Advocacy interventions to reduce or eliminate violence and promote the physical and psychosocial well-being of women who experience intimate partner abuse. *Cochrane Database of Systematic Reviews,* **12,** CD005043.

Rothman, E.F., Mandel, D.G., and **Silverman, J.G.** (2007). Abusers' perceptions of the effect of their intimate partner violence on children. *Violence Against Women,* **13,** 1179–1191.

Schrader McMillan, A. and **Barlow, J.** (2017). *Improving the Effectiveness of the Child Protection System.* London: Early Intervention Foundation.

Sharps, C. and **Jones, J.** (2011). *We Thought They Didn't See: Cedar in Scotland – Children and Mothers Experiencing Domestic Abuse Recovery.* Edinburgh: Scottish Women's Aid and Research for Real. Available at: https://www.cedarnetwork.org.uk/wp-content/uploads/2011/03/Evaluation-Report-DOWNLOAD1.pdf [Accessed 12 Aug. 2017].

Sharps, P.W., Campbell, J., Baty, M.L., Walker, K.S., and **Bair-Merritt, M.H.** (2008). Current evidence on perinatal home visiting and intimate partner violence. *Journal of Obstetric, Gynecologic and Neonatal Nursing,* **37,** 480–490.

Sidebotham, P., Brandon, M., Bailey, S., et al. (2016). *Pathways to Harm, Pathways to Protection: A Triennial Analysis of Serious Case Reviews 2011 to 2014: Final Report.* London: Department for Education.

Sieger, B. (2014). The clinical practice of harm reduction psychotherapy. In: Straussner, S.L.A. (Ed.), *Clinical Work with Substance-Abusing Clients* (3rd edn), pp. 165–178. New York, NY: Guilford Press.

Smedslund, G., Dalsbø, T.K., Steiro, A., Winsvold, A., and **Clench-Aas, J.** (2011). Cognitive behavioural therapy for men who physically abuse their female partner. *Cochrane Database of Systematic Reviews,* **2,** CD006048.

Sprague, S., Madden, K., Simunovic, N., et al. (2012). Barriers to screening for intimate partner violence. *Women and Health,* **52,** 587–605.

Stanley, N. (2011). *Children Experiencing Domestic Violence: A Research Review.* Dartington: Research in Practice.

Stanley, N., Ellis, J., Farrelly, N., Hollinghurst, S., Bailey, S., and **Downe, S.** (2015a). Preventing domestic abuse for children and young people (PEACH): a mixed knowledge scoping review. *Public Health Research,* **3,** 1–230.

Stanley, N., Ellis, J., Farrelly, N., Hollinghurst, S., and Downe, S. (2015b). Preventing domestic abuse for children and young people: a review of school-based interventions. *Children and Youth Services Review*, **59**, 120–131.

Stith S., McCollum E., and Rosen K. (2011). *Couples Therapy for Domestic Violence: Finding Safe Solutions*. Washington, DC: American Psychological Association.

Stover, C. (2015). Fathers for Change for substance use and intimate partner violence: initial community pilot. *Family Process*, **54**, 600–609.

Stover, C.S. (2013). Fathers for change: a new approach to working with fathers who perpetrate intimate partner violence. *Journal of the American Academy of Psychiatry and the Law*, **41**(1), 65–71.

Stover, C., Meadows, A.L., and Kaufman, J. (2009). Interventions for intimate partner violence: review and implications for evidence-based practice. *Professional Psychology, Research and Practice*, **40**, 223–233.

Sturge-Appel M., Skibo, M.A., and Oavies, P.T. (2012). Impact of parental conflict and emotional abuse on children and families. *Partner Abuse*, **3**, 379–400.

Taft, A., O'Doherty, L., Hegarty, K., Ramsay, J., Davidson, L., and Feder, G. (2013). Screening women for intimate partner violence in healthcare settings. *Cochrane Database of Systematic Reviews*, **4**, CD007007.

Todahl, J. and Walters, E. (2011). Universal screening for intimate partner violence: a systematic review. *Journal of Marital and Therapy*, **37**, 355–369.

Van Parys, A., Verhamme, A., Temmerman, M., and Verstraelen, H. (2014). Intimate partner violence and pregnancy: a systematic review of interventions. *PLoS One*, **9**, e85084.

Waldman-Levi, A. and Weintraub, N. (2015). Efficacy of a crisis intervention in improving mother-child interaction and children's play functioning. *American Journal of Occupational Therapy*, **69**, 1–11.

Whitaker, D.J., Morrison, S., Lindquist, C., et al. (2006). A critical review of interventions for the primary prevention of perpetration of partner violence. *Aggression and Violent Behavior*, **11**, 151–166.

Whitaker, D.J., Murphy, C.M., Eckhardt, C.I., Hodges, A.E., and Cowart, M. (2013). Effectiveness of primary prevention efforts for intimate partner violence. *Partner Abuse*, **4**, 175–195.

Williamson, E. and Abrahams, H. (2010). *Evaluation of the Bristol Freedom Programme*. Bristol: University of Bristol. Available at: http://www.bristol.ac.uk/media-library/sites/sps/migrated/documents/rj4997finalreport.pdf.

Chapter 6

Tobacco, alcohol, and substance use in the perinatal period

Jane Barlow and Nick Axford

Summary

This chapter:

- demonstrates that exposure to teratogenic substances such as tobacco, alcohol, or substances during pregnancy can affect the unborn and newborn infant, with long-term consequences in terms of the later development of the child

- presents evidence regarding what works during the perinatal period in terms of both universal and targeted interventions for smoking cessation, and preventing and treating alcohol and drug misuse

- makes recommendations for practice, drawing on the evidence presented and best practice guidance, and focusing on strategies for identification and intervention.

Introduction

Exposure to teratogens (i.e. substances that may cause birth defects) such as tobacco, alcohol, and illicit substances during pregnancy and the postnatal period is still common, and there is now comprehensive evidence regarding the consequences of this for the developing fetus and infant. The first part of the chapter presents the evidence regarding the prevalence of exposure to teratogenic substances in pregnancy, in addition to the consequences for the developing fetus and child. The remainder of the chapter examines strategies for effectively preventing or addressing smoking, alcohol use, and drug use by women during pregnancy and after birth. It also summarizes best practice in identifying families in need of additional support.

Exposure to teratogenic substances during the perinatal period

Internationally, the evidence suggests that significant numbers of women consume alcohol, tobacco, or illicit substances in pregnancy. For example, a US survey showed 5.9% of pregnant women use illicit drugs, 8.5% drink alcohol, and 15.9% smoke cigarettes (United States Department of Human Services et al., 2013), with a similar prevalence in Europe (European Monitoring Centre for Drugs and Drug Addiction, 2011) and Australia (Passey et al., 2014).

In the UK, the Infant Feeding Survey (2010) found that around one-quarter (26%) of women smoked in the 12 months before or during their pregnancy, of whom over half (54%) gave up at some point before the birth (McAndrew et al., 2012). Twelve per cent of mothers continued to smoke throughout their pregnancy, a reduction of 5% from 17% in 2005. This survey showed that age and social class are strongly associated with smoking in pregnancy, with younger women (i.e. mothers aged under 20) (57%) and mothers in routine and manual occupations (40%) having the highest prevalence. They were also the least likely to have given up smoking before or during pregnancy (Health and Social Care Information Centre, 2013).

Smoking and environmental tobacco exposure during pregnancy affect fetal nutrition, increasing the risk of negative birth outcomes (World Health Organization, 2011) including miscarriage, stillbirth, preterm birth, risk of low birth weight or reduced birth length and head circumference, risk of birth defects (cleft palate), risk of sudden infant death syndrome, pulmonary growth neurobehavioural abnormalities, lower IQ, and childhood cancer.

Exposure to environmental tobacco smoke during infancy and childhood can similarly impact negatively on child health outcomes, including: asthma in children who have not previously exhibited symptoms; increased risk for sudden infant death syndrome; lower respiratory tract infections, such as pneumonia and bronchitis; middle ear infections; neurobehavioural and neurodevelopmental deficits; and childhood cancer (World Health Organization, 2011).

A survey (Office for National Statistics, 2015) of drinking habits in pregnancy showed that around one-third (28%) of pregnant women in Britain had had a drink in pregnancy, although fewer than one in ten pregnant women drank in the week before the interview compared with more than five in ten of those who were not pregnant or unsure. While low levels of alcohol consumption (one or two drinks per week) does not appear to be associated with an impact on the developing fetus, the evidence is not strong enough to conclude that there is no risk, and public health bodies in many countries (e.g. the UK, Canada, the US, Ireland, and New Zealand) recommend that no alcohol should be consumed in pregnancy. This reflects both areas of continuing concern (e.g. brain imaging results showing that low/moderate levels can produce functional damage to the brain, and in particular the corpus callosum, leading to adverse cognitive and neurological development that may affect speech and language development (Gray et al., 2009; Lebel et al., 2011), and the fact that alcohol crosses the placental barrier, meaning that the fetus is exposed to alcohol at sensitive developmental periods for key organs such as the brain and liver, irrespective of its impact. Higher levels of alcohol consumption including binge drinking have been shown to have a highly deleterious impact on the fetus, including being one of the main causes of intellectual deficiencies in childhood (Riley et al., 2011). The impact of such alcohol dependency is discussed in later sections with substance dependency because most epidemiological studies do not distinguish between the two.

Around one-third of drug users in the UK are women, of whom as many as 90% are of childbearing age (Day and George, 2005). Estimates show that around 2–3% of children under 16 years have a parent who is a problematic drug user and around 1% of births are to drug users and a similar number to problem drinkers (Advisory Council on the Misuse of Drugs, 2003). Of children less than 1 year old in England, it has been estimated that 19,500 live with a parent who has used Class A drugs in the last year and 93,500 live with a parent who is a problem drinker (McManus et al., 2009).

Substance misuse (e.g. cocaine, amphetamines, opioids, and marijuana) during pregnancy has been found to be associated with a number of adverse neonatal outcomes, depending on the nature and frequency of the drug use. For example, cannabis use in pregnancy, particularly where usage is heavy, and co-morbid substance use, is associated with an increased preterm labour, low birthweight, small for gestational age infants, and an adverse impact on fetal and adolescent brains (e.g. reduced attention and executive functioning, poorer academic achievement, and more behavioural problems); cocaine use has been associated with premature rupture of membranes, placental abruption, preterm birth, low birthweight, and small for gestational age infants, although the evidence about language, motor, and cognitive impact is inconclusive (Forray, 2016). Opioid use is associated with a greater risk of low birthweight, respiratory problems, third-trimester bleeding, toxaemia, and mortality; it is also associated with neonatal abstinence syndrome, which is itself associated with significant neonatal morbidity (Forray, 2016). The latter is, as such, a significant concern for maternity services and neonatologists compared with recreational drug use. These problems are exacerbated by the problems that typically co-occur with substance use, including poor diet, co-morbid psychiatric illness, chronic medical problems, poverty, and domestic abuse (Forray, 2016).

In the postnatal period, parental substance use can adversely impact on the parent–child relationship, further affecting children's socio-emotional development. Drug-dependent parents are at high risk for maltreatment of their children. Around 25% of all children subject to a child protection plan are cared for by a parent with a substance misuse problem (Advisory Council on the Misuse of Drugs, 2004) and one study found a significantly higher risk of child protection proceedings among infants of substance-misusing parents compared with infants of non-drug users (32.4% vs 7.1%) (Street et al., 2004). Substance-dependent parents demonstrate a range of parenting difficulties and deficits (Dawe et al., 2007), and a recent review of the evidence found a reduced capacity for sensitivity and attunement in the postnatal period (Hatzis et al., 2017). The poor quality of caregiving is influenced by the problems that co-occur with drug dependence, such as psychiatric disorders and psychopathology (Suchman et al., 2005; Forray, 2016), particularly disorders of affect regulation (Taylor, 1997).

Illicit drug use has changed considerably over the past 10 years, with an increase in the use of novel psychoactive substances known as 'legal highs', but there is currently little evidence concerning the prevalence of this in pregnancy, or the longer-term consequences in terms of fetal and infant outcomes.

Smoking

Identification

Best practice guidance recommends that health visitors and other health professionals (e.g. general practitioners, family nurses) use any meeting to ask women who are pregnant if they smoke and, if they do, to advise them to stop, explain how the NHS Stop Smoking service can help and make a referral to the service (with consent) (National Institute of Health and Care Excellence (NICE), 2010a). Those with specialist training should give pregnant women who smoke information about the risks to the unborn child of smoking when pregnant, the hazards of exposure to second-hand smoke for both mother and baby, and the benefits of stopping (not just cutting down) smoking.

Given good evidence that women in the UK under-report smoking during pregnancy and that carbon monoxide (CO) monitoring in antenatal clinics can help to identify pregnant smokers, best practice guidance recommends that in pregnancy clinics midwives implement routine CO testing to help identify women who smoke (NICE, 2010a). Current smokers and those who stopped in the previous 2 weeks should be referred to NHS Stop Smoking services, as should those with a CO reading of 7 ppm or above, and light or infrequent smokers even if they register a lower reading.[1] They should also be given the NHS Pregnancy Smoking Helpline number and local helpline numbers.

Interventions

Psychosocial interventions refer to non-pharmacological strategies that use cognitive behavioural, motivational, and supportive therapies to help women to quit. A recent major review concluded that such interventions can increase the proportion of women who stop smoking in late pregnancy and reduce the proportion of infants born with low birthweight (Chamberlain et al., 2017). While counselling, feedback, and incentives were found to be effective, the effect of health education and social support was less clear.

Contingency management (CM) with financial incentives is arguably the most effective approach for smoking cessation in pregnancy (Forray and Foster, 2015). A number of reviews have examined the use of financial incentives for maternal non-smoking during pregnancy (Higgins et al., 2012), incentives and CM programmes (Cahill et al., 2015), and incentives for smoking and other health behaviours (Giles et al., 2014; Mantzari et al., 2015). Incentives typically include financial rewards, lottery tickets or prize draws, and vouchers for goods and groceries. These reviews suggest that overall incentives are highly effective up to the 6-month follow-up and that the effect does not necessarily fade once they have finished. These schemes may meet the specific needs of socio-economically disadvantaged

---

[1] If mothers have a high CO reading (more than 10 ppm) but say they do not smoke, it is recommended that midwives advise them about possible CO poisoning and ask them to call the free Health and Safety Executive gas safety advice line (NICE, 2010a).

women and heavy smokers, and there is some evidence that *financial* incentives— especially higher value ones—are the most beneficial, although there are political considerations around their roll-out.

Another review found that self-help smoking cessation interventions for pregnant smokers nearly doubled the odds of quitting compared with standard care (Naughton et al., 2008). Further analysis found no evidence that more intensive input was significantly more effective than less intensive interventions. The effects were less clear when provided as part of broader health interventions rather than targeted smoking cessation programmes. Counselling interventions show a clear effect on stopping smoking compared with usual care and a smaller effect when compared with less intensive interventions (Chamberlain et al., 2017). Another review concluded that proactive telephone counselling can result in higher quit rates in both pregnant and non-pregnant women (Stead et al., 2013). Telephone quitlines provide an important route of access to support for smokers, and call-back counselling enhances their usefulness. There is limited evidence about the optimal number of calls, although low-intensity interventions (one to two calls) appear to be less beneficial.

Other non-pharmacological interventions with some evidence of effectiveness as regards smoking cessation in pregnancy include nurse home visiting, social marketing campaigns, brief feedback of urinary cotinine results, and text messaging or smartphone interventions (Forray and Foster, 2015). Interventions to establish smoke-free homes in pregnancy and the neonatal period include counselling, education, plans for smoke-free homes, and motivational interviewing (MI), although evidence for their effectiveness is inconclusive (Baxter et al., 2011).

Internet-based youth smoking prevention and cessation programmes, which are potentially relevant for young mothers, have also been found to be effective, at least in the short term (up to 3 months post intervention) (Park and Drake, 2015). Mindfulness-based interventions are promising in terms of smoking cessation, relapse prevention, and number of cigarettes smoked (De Souza et al., 2015).

Women who quit smoking during pregnancy may demonstrate high rates of relapse in pregnancy and the postpartum period. Preventing relapse is therefore an important means of preventing environmental tobacco smoke exposure for their children (Priest et al., 2008). Although one review found no evidence overall to support the use of brief counselling sessions, telephone contact, psychotherapy, or MI for relapse prevention (Hajek et al., 2013), a more recent review—not specific to pregnancy—concluded that text-messaging support programmes, alone or in combination with face-to-face assessments or online programmes, increase the likelihood of staying quit (6-month cessation outcomes) compared with smokers who did not receive such messages (Whittaker et al., 2016).

The safety and efficacy of pharmacological interventions for pregnant and postpartum women is still to be established. Nicotine replacement therapy has limited efficacy in increasing abstinence rates in pregnant women (Forray and Foster, 2015), with a major review recommending that it should be combined with behavioural support (Coleman et al., 2015). Electronic cigarettes have not been tested with pregnant women. However, a review of e-cigarettes in adults found that the odds of quitting were improved by 28% (Kalkhoran and Glantz, 2016). Similarly, Orr et al. (2014) reviewed data demonstrating effective smoking cessation with e-cigarettes. Most studies showed a significant decrease in cigarette use acutely, although there is limited evidence for their long-term effectiveness.

Alcohol

Identification

If *alcohol* misuse is suspected, best practice guidance recommends that the Alcohol Use Disorders Identification Test (AUDIT) be used to help decide whether to offer a brief intervention (and if so what) or to make a referral to specialist services in the case of dependency (NICE, 2010b, 2011, 2014).

Interventions

A review of reviews concluded that brief interventions delivered in primary healthcare are effective in reducing hazardous and harmful drinking (O'Donnell et al., 2014). There is a lack of research on the effectiveness of CM for perinatal alcohol use specifically (Forray and Foster, 2015). However, reviews have shown that brief psychological and educational interventions, especially those using MI, can increase abstinence and reduce perinatal alcohol use, although mixed results, methodological limitations, and the paucity of studies urge caution (Stade et al., 2009; Gilinsky et al., 2011). Effects may be stronger where women participate with a partner (in the case of heavier drinking) and choose abstinence as their drinking goal. There is also a case for making interventions during pregnancy more intensive (Gilinsky et al., 2011).

An alternative to brief interventions delivered by health professionals is computer-tailored advice delivered via the internet, whereby messages are adapted according to each respondent's situation (e.g. their alcohol use and coping plans). This has been shown in one study to be effective in reducing alcohol use during pregnancy (van der Wulp et al., 2014). Another study showed that telephone-based brief intervention may be as effective as in-person brief interventions in reducing the risk of an alcohol-exposed pregnancy (Wilton et al., 2013).

There is insufficient evidence to support the use of home visiting (Turnbull and Osborn, 2012), telephone support (Lavender et al., 2013), or public health interventions such as media campaigns (Crawford-Williams et al., 2015) for women who engage in heavy drinking in pregnancy, and no evidence regarding the impact of using pharmacological interventions with pregnant women enrolled in alcohol treatment programmes (Smith et al., 2009).

Other drugs

Identification

Best practice guidance on the identification of drug misuse in the antenatal and postnatal period advises asking questions about drug misuse (e.g. type, quantity, and frequency), making an assessment and agreeing a care plan, and (for health professionals) using biological testing as part of a comprehensive assessment of drug misuse (but not relying on it as the sole method of diagnosis and assessment) (NICE, 2007a, 2014).

Interventions

Cannabis

Although there is a lack of interventions aimed specifically at antenatal cannabis use, several psychosocial interventions not tested with pregnant users have nonetheless been shown to be somewhat effective in reducing cannabis use in women, including MI, cognitive behavioural therapy (CBT), and CM therapies (Forray and Foster, 2015). A recent major review of psychosocial interventions for cannabis disorder concluded that, compared with minimal treatment controls, they reduce the frequency of use and severity of dependence, at least in the short term, although abstinence rates are low (Gates et al., 2016). The most consistent support was for an intensive intervention provided over more than four sessions based on the combination of motivational enhancement therapy and CBT with abstinence-based incentives.

There is currently no approved pharmacotherapy for cannabis-use disorders, but some approaches appear promising and clinical trials are continuing (Copeland and Pokorski, 2016).

Cocaine

Evidence-based treatments for cocaine use in pregnancy are behavioural and include CBT, MI, and CM, with the latter showing the most potential, including a longer duration of abstinence (Forray and Foster, 2015). However, a major review focusing on pregnant women in outpatient illicit drug treatment programmes found no difference in retention or abstinence between CM or MI-based techniques and usual care, which included pharmacological treatment such as methadone maintenance, counselling, prenatal care, and child care (Terplan et al., 2015).

Although there are no evidence-based pharmacological interventions for antenatal cocaine use, early tests of progesterone in the postpartum period show promise (Forray and Foster, 2015).

Treatments for other stimulant use, such as methamphetamine, are limited; reinforcement-based therapy is deemed to have potential, particularly in increasing treatment retention in pregnant women, but needs more research as studies to date have shown no effect on actual use with this group (Jones et al., 2011; Forray and Foster, 2015).

Opiates

The standard treatment for pregnant women using opiates is methadone maintenance, although buprenorphine has also emerged as a potential therapy for opioid use in pregnancy (Forray and Foster, 2015). CM has also been found to increase abstinence and treatment attendance compared to controls (Jones et al., 2001), and is regarded as an important addition to methadone or buprenorphine in pregnant women.

Learning links

- Alcohol and pregnancy e-learning modules: https://alcoholpregnancy. telethonkids.org.au/alcohol-pregnancy-and-breastfeeding/diagnosing-fasd/ e-learning-modules/
- Institute of Health Visiting—'Fetal Alcohol Syndrome' e-learning module: https://ihv.org.uk/for-health-visitors/resources-for-members/resource/ e-learning/foetal- alcohol-syndrome-e-learning/
- Module 10 (Health Promotion) of the Healthy Child Programme outlines vital areas of interest in promoting health from the start in pregnancy through to the first 5 years of life, with a focus on smoking, obesity, mental health and substance misuse: https://www.e-lfh.org.uk/programmes/healthy-child-programme/.

Recommendations

- Advise pregnant women to stop smoking and explain that the NHS Stop Smoking service can help and make a referral if appropriate. (*Evidence: strong.*)
- Healthcare professionals with specialist training in smoking cessation should provide advice about risk to the unborn child, the hazards of exposure to second-hand smoke for both mother and baby, and the benefits of stopping smoking. CO monitoring should be used for monitoring purposes and motivation. (*Evidence: strong.*)
- Use the AUDIT followed by a brief intervention or referral to specialist clinic for suspected alcohol misuse. Ask questions (e.g. type, quantity, and frequency) when drug misuse is suspected, make an assessment, and agree a care plan. Biological testing may also be needed. (*Evidence: strong.*)
- Use psychosocial interventions to help pregnant smokers cut down or, as much as possible, quit; these include self-help, counselling, nurse home visiting, feedback, text messaging, and smartphone interventions. (*Evidence: strong.*)
- Use text messaging to help recent smokers who have quit to maintain their non-smoking behaviour. (*Evidence: strong.*)
- Consider combination therapy (i.e. more than one form of nicotine replacement therapy, e.g. patch plus gum, or patch plus nasal spray) for smokers in pregnancy when psychosocial interventions for smoking cessation are not effective. E-cigarettes should only be used after nicotine replacement therapy has been tried and found not to work. (*Evidence: moderate.*).
- Use brief (psychosocial) interventions for hazardous drug or alcohol misuse (e.g. information and advice to motivate patients to change their behaviour, covering potential harms of their behaviour, reasons to change, barriers to change, strategies, and setting goals). (*Evidence: strong.*)

- Refer women if harmful or dependent drug or alcohol misuse is identified in pregnancy or the postnatal period to a specialist substance misuse service for advice and treatment (e.g. for psychosocial or psychological interventions or other forms of treatment). (*Evidence: strong.*)
- Refer pregnant women if they do not wish to reduce their harmful alcohol or substance misuse to children's social care. (*Good practice.*)

References

Advisory Council on the Misuse of Drugs (2003). Hidden Harm: *Responding to the Needs of Children of Problem Drug Users*. London: Home Office.

Advisory Council on the Misuse of Drugs (2004). *Annual Report Accounting Year 2003–2004*. London: Home Office.

Baxter, S., Blank, L., and **Everson-Hock, E.S.** (2011). The effectiveness of interventions to establish smoke-free homes in pregnancy and in the neonatal period: a systematic review. *Health Education Research*, **26**, 265–282.

Cahill, K., Hartmann-Boyce, J., and **Perera, R.** (2015). Incentives for smoking cessation. *Cochrane Database of Systematic Reviews*, **5**, CD004307.

Chamberlain, C., O'Mara-Eves, A., Porter, J., et al. (2017). Psychosocial interventions for supporting women to stop smoking in pregnancy. *Cochrane Database of Systematic Reviews*, **2**, CD001055.

Coleman, T., Chamberlain, C., Davey, M., Cooper, S.E., and **Leonardi-Bee, J.** (2015). Pharmacological interventions for promoting smoking cessation during pregnancy. *Cochrane Database of Systematic Reviews*, **12**, CD010078.

Copeland, J. and **Pokorski, I.** (2016). Progress toward pharmacotherapies for cannabis-use disorder: an evidence-based review. *Substance Abuse Rehabilitation*, **7**, 41–53.

Crawford-Williams, F., Fielder, A., Mikocka-Walus, A., and **Esterman, A.** (2015). A critical review of public health interventions aimed at reducing alcohol consumption and/or increasing knowledge among pregnant women. *Drug and Alcohol Review*, **34**, 154–161.

Day, E. and **George, S.** (2005). Management of drug misuse in pregnancy. *Advances in Psychiatric Treatment*, **11**, 253–261.

Dawe, S., Frye, S., Best, D., et al. (2007). *Drug Use in the Family: Impacts and Implications for Children*. ANCD Research Paper 13. Canberra: Australian National Council on Drugs. Available at: http://www.doryanthes.info/Portable%20documents/rp13_drug_use_in_family.pdf [Accessed 29 Sep. 2017].

de Souza, I., de Barros, V.V., Gomide, HP., et al. (2015). Mindfulness-based interventions for the treatment of smoking: a systematic literature review. *Journal of Alternative and Complementary Medicine*, **21**, 129–140.

European Monitoring Centre for Drugs and Drug Addition (EMCDDA). (2011). *The State of the Drugs Problem in Europe*. Luxembourg: EMCDDA.

Forray, A. (2016). Substance use during pregnancy. *F1000Research*, **5**, F1000 Faculty Rev-887.

Forray, A. and **Foster, D.** (2015). Substance use in the perinatal period. *Current Psychiatry Reports*, **17**, 91.

Gates, P.J., Sabioni, P., Copeland, J., Le Foll, B., and **Gowing, L.** (2016). Psychosocial interventions for cannabis use disorder. *Cochrane Database of Systematic Reviews*, **5**, CD005336.

Giles, E.L., Robalino, S., McColl, E., Sniehotta, F., and Adams, J. (2014). The effectiveness of financial incentives for health behaviour change: systematic review and meta-analysis. *PLoS One*, **9**, e90347.

Gilinsky, A., Swanson, V., and Power, K.G. (2011). Interventions delivered during antenatal care to reduce alcohol consumption during pregnancy: a systematic review, *Addiction Research and Theory*, **19**, 235–250.

Gray, R., Mukherjee, R.A.S., and Rutter, M. (2009). Alcohol consumption during pregnancy and its effects on neurodevelopment: what is known and what remains uncertain. *Addiction*, **104**, 1270–1273.

Hajek, P., Stead, L.F., West, R., Jarvis, M., Hartmann-Boyce, J., and Lancaster, T. (2013). Relapse prevention interventions for smoking cessation. *Cochrane Database of Systematic Reviews*, **8**, CD003999.

Hatzis, D.M., Dawe, S., Harnett, P., and Barlow, J. (2017). Quality of caregiving in substance misusing mothers: a meta-analysis. *Substance Abuse, Research and Treatment*, **11**, 1178221817694038.

Health and Social Care Information Centre (2013). *Statistics on Smoking: England, 2013*. London: Health and Social Care Information Centre. Available at: http://content.digital. nhs.uk/catalogue/PUB11454/smok-eng-2013-rep.pdf [Accessed 29 Sep. 2017].

Higgins, S.T., Washio, Y., Heil, S.H., et al. (2012). Financial incentives for smoking cessation among pregnant and newly postpartum women. *Preventive Medicine*, **55**, S33–S40.

Jones, H.E., Haug, N., Silverman, K., et al. (2001). The effectiveness of incentives in enhancing treatment attendance and drug abstinence in methadone-maintained pregnant women. *Drug and Alcohol Dependency*, **61**, 297–306.

Jones, H.E., O'Grady, K.E., and Tuten, M. (2011). Reinforcement-based treatment improves the maternal treatment and neonatal outcomes of pregnant patients enrolled in comprehensive care treatment. *American Journal of Addiction*, **20**, 196–204.

Kalkhoran, S. and Glantz, S.A. (2016). E-cigarettes and smoking cessation in real-world and clinical settings: a systematic review and meta-analysis. *The Lancet Respiratory Medicine*, **4**, 116–128.

Lavender, T., Richens, Y., Milan, S.J., Smyth, R., and Dowswell, T. (2013). Telephone support for women during pregnancy and the first six weeks postpartum. *Cochrane Database of Systematic Reviews*, **7**, CD009338.

Lebel, C., Roussotte, F., and Sowell, E.R. (2011). Imaging the impact of prenatal alcohol exposure on the structure of the developing human brain. *Neuropsychological Review*, **21**, 102–118.

Mantzari, E., Vogt, F., Shemilt, I., Wei, Y., Higgins, J.P.T., and Marteau, T.M. (2015). Personal financial incentives for changing habitual health-related behaviors: a systematic review and meta-analysis. *Preventive Medicine*, **75**, 75–85.

McAndrew, F., Thompson, J., Fellow, L., Large, A., Speed, M., and Renfrew, M.J. (2012). *Infant Feeding Survey 2010*. Dundee: Health and Social Care Information Centre. Available at: http://content.digital.nhs.uk/catalogue/PUB08694/Infant-Feeding-Survey-2010-Consolidated-Report.pdf [Accessed 11 Sep. 2017].

McManus, S., Meltzer, H., Brugha, T.S., Bebbington, P.E., and Jenkins, R. (2009). *Adult Psychiatric Morbidity in England, 2007: Results of a Household Survey*. London: NHS Information Centre for Health and Social Care. Available at: http://content.digital.nhs. uk/catalogue/PUB02931/adul-psyc-morb-res-hou-sur-eng-2007-rep.pdf [Accessed 29 Sep. 2017].

National Institute of Health and Care Excellence (NICE) (2007a). *Drug Misuse: Psychosocial Interventions*. CG51. [Reviewed 2011.] London: NICE.

National Institute of Health and Care Excellence (NICE) (2007b). *Drug Misuse in Over 16s: Opioid Detoxification*. CG52. [Reviewed February 2014.] London: NICE.

National Institute of Health and Care Excellence (NICE) (2010a). *Quitting Smoking in Pregnancy and Following Childbirth*. PH26. London: NICE.

National Institute of Health and Care Excellence (NICE) (2010b). *Alcohol-use Disorders: Preventing Harmful Drinking*. PH24. London: NICE.

National Institute of Health and Care Excellence (NICE) (2011). *Alcohol-use Disorders: Diagnosis, Assessment and Management of Harmful Drinking and Alcohol Dependence*. CG115. London: NICE.

National Institute of Health and Care Excellence (NICE) (2014). *Antenatal and Postnatal Mental Health: Clinical Management and Service Guidance*. CG192. London: NICE.

Naughton, F., Prevost, A.T., and Sutton, S. (2008). Self-help smoking cessation interventions in pregnancy: systematic review and meta-analysis. *Addiction*, **103**, 566–579.

O'Donnell, A., Anderson, P., Newbury-Birch, D., Schulte, B., Schmidt, C., Reimer, J., and Kaner, E. (2014). The impact of brief alcohol interventions in primary healthcare: a systematic review of reviews. *Alcohol and Alcoholism*, **49**, 66–78.

Office for National Statistics (2015). Adult Drinking Habits in Great Britain, 2013. [online] Available at: https://www.ons.gov.uk/peoplepopulationandcommunity/healthandsocialcare/ healthandlifeexpectancies/compendium/opinionsandlifestylesurvey/2015-03-19/adultdrink inghabitsingreatbritain2013 [Accessed 29 Sep. 2017].

Orr, K. (2014). Efficacy of electronic cigarettes for smoking cessation. *Annals of Pharmacotherapy*, **48**, 1502–1506.

Park, E. and Drake, E. (2015). Systematic review: internet-based program for youth smoking prevention and cessation. *Journal of Nursing Scholarship*, **47**, 43–50.

Passey, M.E., Sanson-Fisher, R.W., D'Este, C.A., et al. (2014). Tobacco, alcohol and cannabis use during pregnancy: clustering of risks. *Drug and Alcohol Dependency*, **134**, 44–50.

Priest, N., Roseby, R., Waters, E., et al. (2008). Family and carer smoking control programmes for reducing children's exposure to environmental tobacco smoke. *Cochrane Database Systematic Reviews*, **3**, CD001746.

Riley, E.P., Infante, M.A., and Warren, K.R. (2011). Fetal alcohol spectrum disorders: an overview. *Neuropsychology Review*, **21**, 73–80.

Smith, E.J., Lui, S., and Terplan, M. (2009). Pharmacologic interventions for pregnant women enrolled in alcohol treatment. *Cochrane Database of Systematic Reviews*, **3**, CD007361.

Stade, B.C., Bailey, C., Dzendoletas, D., Sgro, M., Dowswell, T., and Bennett, D. (2009). Psychological and/or educational interventions for reducing alcohol consumption in pregnant women and women planning pregnancy. *Cochrane Database of Systematic Reviews*, **2**, CD004228.

Stead, L.F., Hartmann-Boyce, J., Perera, R., and Lancaster, T. (2013). Telephone counselling for smoking cessation. *Cochrane Database of Systematic Reviews*, **8**, CD002850.

Street, K., Harrington, J., Chiang, W., Cairns, P., and Ellis, M. (2004). How great is the risk of abuse in infants born to drug using mothers? *Child: Care Health and Development*, **30**, 325–330.

Suchman, N.E., McMahon, T.J., Slade, A., and Luthar, S.S. (2005). How early bonding, depression, illicit drug use, and perceived support work together to influence drug-dependent mothers' caregiving. *American Journal of Orthopsychiatry*, **75**, 431–445.

Taylor, G.J. (1997). Substance use disorders. In: Taylor, G.J., Bagby, R.M., and Parker, J.D.A. (Eds.), *Disorders of Affect Regulation: Alexithymia in Medical and Psychiatric Illness*, pp. 166–189. Cambridge: Cambridge University Press.

Terplan, M., Ramanadhan, S., Locke, A., Longinaker, N., and Lui, S. (2015). Psychosocial interventions for pregnant women in outpatient illicit drug treatment programs compared to other interventions. *Cochrane Database of Systematic Reviews*, **4**, CD006037.

Turnbull, C. and Osborn, D.A. (2012). Home visits during pregnancy and after birth for women with an alcohol or drug problem. *Cochrane Database of Systematic Reviews*, **1**, CD004456.

United States Department of Human Services, Substance Abuse and Mental Health Services Administration, Center for Behavioral Health Statistics and Quality (2013). *National Survey on Drug Use and Health, 2012*. Ann Arbor, MI: Inter-university Consortium for Political and Social Research.

van der Wulp, N.Y., Hoving, C., Eijmael, K., et al. (2014). Reducing alcohol use during pregnancy via health counselling by midwives and internet-based computer-tailored feedback: a cluster randomized trial. *Journal of Medical Internet Research*, **16**, e274.

Whittaker, R., McRobbie, H., Bullen, C., Rodgers, A., and Gu, Y. (2016). Mobile phone-based interventions for smoking cessation. *Cochrane Database of Systematic Reviews*, **4**, CD006611.

Wilton, G., Moberg, D.P., Va Stelle, K.R., Dold, L.L., Obmascher, K., and Goodrich, J.A (2013). Randomized trial comparing telephone versus in-person brief intervention to reduce the risk of an alcohol-exposed pregnancy. *Journal of Substance Abuse Treatment*, **45**, 389–394.

World Health Organization (2011). Second hand tobacco smoke and children. [online] World Health Organization. Available at: http://who.int/ceh/capacity/tobacco1.pdf [Accessed 29 Sep. 2017].

Chapter 7

Transition to parenthood programmes

Jane Barlow

Summary

This chapter:

♦ describes the transition to parenthood, and the nature and prevalence of problems encountered during this time

♦ summarizes the needs of unborn and newborn babies

♦ reviews the evidence regarding the effectiveness of transition to parenthood programmes

♦ makes recommendations for practice.

Introduction

The 'transition to parenthood' has been identified as being a significant period in the lives of men and women who are expecting their first or subsequent child and following delivery a in terms of the changes for the parents and the related stress that such changes may involve. Furthermore, the perinatal period is now recognized to be a 'sensitive' developmental period. These factors mean that the perinatal period is a significant window of opportunity to equalize the life chances of all children (Marmot et al., 2010).

This chapter examines what is meant by the 'transition to parenthood' and why this period is important in terms of the long-term well-being of the infant and child. It goes on to describe some of the innovative methods of working that have been developed over the course of the last decade to support the couple in the transition to parenthood, and concludes by examining what the evidence tells us about the effectiveness of such programmes in terms of both parental and infant well-being.

The transition to parenthood

$The transition to parenthood refers to the period during which the pregnant couple moves towards becoming parents, and spans the period from conception to the first

$ Section adapted with permission from AIMH UK Best Practice Guidance (BPG) No. 1. Improving Relationships in the Perinatal Period: What Works? *International Journal of Birth and Parent Education*. Volume 3, Issue 3 (Supplement). Copyright © Birth and Parent Education Ltd 2016. Available from https://ijbpe.com/.

2–4 months following the birth of the baby. It has long been recognized that pregnancy involves significant physical and psychological changes for pregnant women, but there is now recognition that this period involves emotional changes that affect the father as well as the mother, as a result of the significant changes to lifestyle and roles that occur during this period (Boyce et al., 2007).

The transition to parenthood has been identified as a time of potential stress for the pregnant woman and her partner, due largely to the impact that a pregnancy and newborn baby has on the couple's relationship, but also possibly as a result of the impact of the father's psychological stress/distress on the couple relationship (Raphael-Leff, 1992) (for a comprehensive discussion, see http://www.encyclopedia.com/topic/Transition_to_Parenthood.aspx). Feelings of stress/distress have been linked to higher levels of anxiety and irritability in expectant fathers (Fletcher et al., 2006). Perhaps most importantly, it is the time during which couple relationship satisfaction can become diminished, and relationship breakdown can occur. For example, there is evidence to suggest that marital satisfaction is stable during pregnancy but very often declines significantly during the postnatal period for both parents, with higher levels of variability post birth (Lawrence et al., 2008). Factors affecting such satisfaction include depression, aggression, and the reasons developed to explain their partner's behaviours, in addition to more specific factors such as whether the pregnancy was planned, infant temperament and sex, and division of childcare labour (Lawrence et al., 2008). For example, one study found that in the post-birth period, women experiencing more depression and an infant with a difficult temperament had higher levels of relationship dissatisfaction, while for men, the tendency to find less benign reasons for partner behaviour predicted less satisfaction (Lawrence et al., 2008).

Although such relationship dissatisfaction does not necessarily lead to divorce or separation (i.e. there is no difference in divorce rates for couples with children compared to those without (Office for National Statistics, 2012), the high levels of family discord that are accompanied by such relationship dissatisfaction can cause problems in terms of the long-term adjustment of the children. For example, research suggests that destructive parental conflict is associated with higher levels of emotional insecurity in young children including reports of fear, avoidance, and reduced involvement with people (Davies et al., 2002).

There is also evidence that relationship problems before the birth of the baby can affect the well-being of the mother, with consequences for the fetus/unborn baby. For example, the Norwegian Mother and Child Cohort Study found that dissatisfaction with the partner relationship is a significant predictor of maternal emotional distress in pregnancy, and that a positive relationship has a protective effect against some stressors (Røsand et al., 2011). Stress, anxiety, and depression in pregnancy have been found to be associated with compromised outcomes for both the fetus and child (e.g. Stein et al., 2014), and there is also evidence to suggest that stress/depression in fathers during both the pre- and postnatal periods is linked with later child psychopathology (Ramchandani et al., 2005, 2008).

Around 30% of domestic abuse begins during pregnancy (Lewis and Drife, 2005), and around 9% of women experience such abuse during pregnancy or after giving birth (Taft, 2002). Domestic abuse in the perinatal period is associated with a wide range of compromised outcomes both physically (e.g. miscarriage, low birthweight, placental abruption, and preterm birth) and psychologically (e.g. postnatal depression (Flach et al., 2011) and post-traumatic stress disorder (PTSD) (Loring et al., 2001)). There is also evidence to suggest that babies who witness such violence can develop symptoms of PTSD, manifested in terms of an increase in feeding problems, sleep disturbances, lack of typical responses to adults, loss of previously acquired developmental skills, reduced capacity for emotional regulation, and increased occurrence of later behavioural problems, although the extent to which this happens depends on the mother's capacity to maintain her sensitivity, in addition to her mental health and stress levels (Carpenter and Stacks, 2009).

Preparation for parenthood programmes

While traditional antenatal education has been aimed at preparing parents-to-be for pregnancy and labour, recent research about the psychological and biologically driven processes that both men and women face as part of the transition to parenthood, has raised questions about the focus of 'traditional' antenatal programmes, and their adequacy in supporting parents (Deave and Johnson, 2008; Deave et al., 2008; Barlow and Schrader-MacMillan, 2009). This has led to the emergence of preparation for parenthood programmes that are aimed explicitly at addressing issues that have been highlighted as being key for parents-to-be and new parents. While these programmes were initially designed to be run alongside traditional antenatal classes, more recently developed programmes frequently incorporate the standard material on preparation for childbirth alongside the new material.

Preparation for parenthood programmes can be provided on a universal basis to all parents who are expecting their first or subsequent baby, or on a targeted basis to parents who may be experiencing socio-economic disadvantage, low social support, or other such difficulties. Like the traditional antenatal/parentcraft classes, preparation for parenthood classes are group-based with a maximum group size being around eight couples. They typically begin in the second or third trimester of pregnancy and many continue into the postnatal period for between 4 and 8 weeks. Some of the targeted programmes can also provide a home visit at the beginning of the programme or following the birth of the baby.

Most of these programmes focus primarily on issues related to the transition to parenthood including preparation for new roles, the couple and parent relationship, and the parent and fetal/infant relationship.

A number of UK-based perinatal preparation for parenthood programmes have been developed for use with both universal populations (e.g. Solihull Approach—'Journey to Parenthood: Understanding pregnancy, labour, birth and your baby'; Family Links—'Welcome to the World') and targeted populations (e.g. National Society for the Prevention of Cruelty to Children—'Baby Steps'; Mellow Parenting—'Mellow Bumps' and 'Dads-To-Be'), but most have not so far been subject to rigorous evaluation.

What does the evidence tell us about the effectiveness of preparation for parenthood programmes in terms of outcomes for parents and babies in the perinatal period?

[$]Two systematic reviews have explicitly examined the effectiveness of interventions delivered during the perinatal period with the aim of improving the transition to parenthood (Petch and Halford, 2008; Pinquart and Teubert, 2010). Pinquart and Teubert (2010) examined the effectiveness of interventions that began in pregnancy and that had an explicit component aimed at improving the couple relationship. The review included 21 controlled studies (16 of which were randomized controlled trials (RCTs)) of couple-focused interventions that had targeted heterosexual expectant and new parents. Eighteen interventions were universal in terms of their focus on the prevention of couple adjustment problems, and three studies were delivered on a selective basis to parents at risk of poor outcomes. Seven interventions were delivered before birth, seven after birth, and eight included both before and after-birth components. The mean number of sessions attended was 11.4 (range 1–82). The results of the meta-analysis showed small effects on couple communication, psychological well-being, and couple adjustment. This review found that the more successful interventions included more than five sessions, had an antenatal and postnatal component, and were led by professionals rather than semi-professionals. One of the main limitations of this review is that it focuses only on programmes that uniquely address the couple relationship during the transition to parenthood. This means that it does not include studies of interventions that may have focused on other aspects of the transition to parenthood.

Petch and Halford (2008) examined the effectiveness of universal interventions (e.g. couple or parenting programmes, the latter of which are not reported further here), and selective interventions for high-risk couples (e.g. home-visiting programmes—not reported further here; and other non-home-visiting interventions). They identified eight RCTs that had evaluated the effectiveness of universal psychoeducation programmes aimed at improving the transition to parenthood, three of which were delivered exclusively during the antenatal period, the remainder being provided both ante- and postnatally. The intensity of the interventions ranged from minimal additional support (e.g. an extra antenatal class offering information and group discussion on couple adjustment) through to 24 weekly group sessions. The focus of these programmes included couple communication and relationship skills ($n = 5$ studies), and parenting adjustment/competence/interaction ($n = 3$ studies), or mental health ($n = 3$ studies).

The findings show that couple relationship satisfaction was improved in three of five studies, and one further study that compared two interventions found that the mother-focused parenting programme prevented declining relationship satisfaction in women but not men. Couple communication was assessed and found to be improved in two studies. Mental health was improved in two out of three studies in which it was assessed, but only one study comparing a mother-focused and couple-relationship

---

[$] Section adapted with permission from AIMH UK Best Practice Guidance (BPG) No. 1. *Improving Relationships in the Perinatal Period: What Works? International Journal of Birth and Parent Education.* Volume 3, Issue 3 (Supplement). Copyright © Birth and Parent Education Ltd 2016. Available from https://ijbpe.com/.

focused intervention examined the effects on co-parenting practices, and this found high parenting adjustment in both conditions.

The limitations of this review are that the data from the included studies were not combined to produce an overall estimate of the effectiveness of this group of programmes. In addition, the authors draw attention to the fact that most of the included parents were highly educated, there were no effects for the lowest dose couple programme (e.g. one additional hourly session per week), and that long-term effectiveness was only assessed in one study, which showed sustained effects over 5 years following an intensive programme of 24 weekly sessions that involved approximately 50 hours of professional contact per couple.

The effectiveness of a number of other preparation for parenthood programmes have been examined using RCTs that have been published since the above-mentioned reviews. Family Foundations is a group-based programme that can be delivered both on a universal or targeted basis (i.e. it has modified versions for high-risk couples and for teenage parents). The programme involves a 16-hour intervention that is delivered in eight, 2-hour sessions (four in the ante- and four in the postnatal periods). A RCT that included 169 heterosexual, first-time pregnant couples found significant programme effects on co-parental support, maternal depression and anxiety, distress in the parent–child relationship, and infant self-regulation. The programme showed more impact for lower-educated parents (Feinberg and Kan, 2008). Evidence of continued effectiveness at 1 year post intervention was found for all domains (i.e. couple relations, parent well-being, parenting quality, and child outcomes). Intervention effects on mothers' parenting were mediated by co-parenting quality, and effects on child self-regulation were mediated by the combination of co-parenting quality and parenting quality (Feinberg et al., 2009). At 3-year follow-up, the results showed an impact on parental stress and depression, co-parenting, and harsh parenting for all families. Among families of boys, programme effects were found for child behaviour problems and couple relationship quality (Feinberg et al., 2010).

A further study of the effectiveness of brief (i.e. 6-hour) psychoeducational transition to parenthood groups, targeting high-risk pregnant couples, examined two interventions that both involved four 90-minute sessions, two of which were delivered before birth and two after. One intervention focused on relationship quality and the second on the co-parenting relationship. These two brief interventions were compared with an information-only control arm (Doss et al., 2014). The results of an RCT involving 90 heterosexual couples showed that women and high-risk men in both the couple and co-parenting interventions showed less decline in relationship satisfaction and other areas of relationship functioning than the control group. Women also reported improved co-parenting in both intervention groups and perceived themselves to have experienced less stress during the first year after birth.

In the UK, the effectiveness of a 2-hour, universal psychoeducational adjunct to existing antenatal classes has been evaluated (Daley-McCoy et al., 2015). The intervention focused on promoting realistic expectations about becoming a parent, and the development of communication skills to optimize effective problem-solving. The course was midwife led and consisted of five weekly evening sessions that lasted for 2 hours, one of which involved a group exercise in which the participating couples explored what a day in the life of a new parent might involve and in particular, common areas of disagreement among new parent couples. It also included discussions within couples about their individual expectations of new parenthood, which were used to help them to develop communication and problem-solving skills. The results of a feasibility cluster RCT (i.e. antenatal *classes* were randomized rather than *individuals*) involving 83 couples showed that the intervention was feasible in terms of delivery, acceptable to parents, and that there was evidence of less deterioration in relationship quality for women, less deterioration in couple communication for men, and a significant improvement in psychological distress for both.

Some programmes, however, have not been found to be effective. The Danish Prevention and Relationship Enhancement Program (PREP) Denmark (Trillingsgaard et al., 2012), targeted first-time couples and involved the delivery of communication skills training. However, the results of an RCT comparing this programme with (a) an information-based control group and (b) care as usual, found no differences between any of the groups, and the authors concluded that none of the interventions prevented the decline in relationship satisfaction during the transition to parenthood.

Promising approaches that have not yet been tested using rigorous research designs include the Mindfulness-Based Childbirth and Parenting (MBCP) programme (Duncan and Bardacke, 2010), which comprises a formal adaptation of the Mindfulness-Based Stress Reduction programme. This programme is designed to promote family health and well-being through the practice of mindfulness during pregnancy, childbirth, and early parenting. The results of a small, one-group evaluation showed statistically significant increases in mindfulness and positive affect, and decreases in pregnancy anxiety, depression, and negative affect in mothers-to-be from pre to post test (Duncan and Bardacke, 2010).

Workforce delivery and skills

[$]The evidence suggests the four key areas on which antenatal education should focus are preparation for new roles, the couple relationship, the parent–fetal/infant relationship, and co-parenting. Practitioners and commissioners should ensure that whatever programme is implemented addresses all of these issues. The evidence also points to the importance of ensuring that both parents attend the programme. Many men have felt excluded or marginalized in traditional antenatal classes, and many existing programmes continue to target the pregnant woman (Deave and Johnson, 2008; Fenwick et al., 2012).

The evidence also suggests that preparation for parenthood programmes should be provided by a professional although this does not necessarily need to be a midwife. Many of the UK-based programmes that target high-risk groups (e.g. 'Baby Steps') are very often provided by two professionals, one of whom is from health (e.g. midwife or health visitor) and the other from social care (e.g. family centre worker, social worker, etc.). Key skills needed include experience of working with parents during the perinatal period, and skills in working with groups.

....

[$] Section adapted with permission from AIMH UK Best Practice Guidance (BPG) No. 1. Improving Relationships in the Perinatal Period: What Works? *International Journal of Birth and Parent Education.* Volume 3, Issue 3 (Supplement). Copyright © Birth and Parent Education Ltd 2016. Available from https://ijbpe.com/.

Although it is currently unclear whether it is better for the traditional antenatal class to be supplemented by adjunctive sessions that address the transition to parenthood (see, e.g. Daley-McCoy et al., 2015) or for them to be replaced with transition to parenthood programmes, the evidence strongly suggests that at least five sessions should be provided, although there is some evidence of effectiveness with a smaller number of sessions when provided on a universal basis. Key issues for parents include the amount of time required to attend the course, in addition to how convenient it is in terms of timing and location.

Learning links

- Future Learn course—'Babies in Mind: Why the Parent's Mind Matters': https://www.futurelearn.com/courses/babies-in-mind
- Key findings from a selection of research studies examining factors that affect couple relationships when partners become parents, and that are particularly relevant to practice: https://aifs.gov.au/cfca/publications/supporting-couples-across-transition-parenthood/key-factors-affecting-relationship.

Recommendations

- Consider commissioning transition to parenthood programmes as part of the child health programme (Department of Health, 2009). (*Evidence: strong.*)
- Deliver targeted transition to parenthood programmes with two skilled health professionals and consisting of at least five group-based sessions (*Evidence: strong.*)

References

Carpenter, G.L. and Stacks, S.M. (2009). Developmental effects of exposure to intimate partner violence in early childhood: a review of the literature. *Children and Youth Services Review*, **31**, 831–839.

Boyce, P., Condon, J., Barton, J., and Corkingdale, C. (2007). First-time fathers study: psychological distress in expectant fathers during pregnancy. *Australian and New Zealand Journal of Psychiatry*, **41**, 718–725.

Daley-McCoy, C., Rogers, M., and Slade, P. (2015). Enhancing relationship functioning during the transition to parenthood: a cluster-randomised controlled trial. *Archives of Women's Mental Health*, **18**, 681–692.

Davies, P.T., Harold, G.T., Goeke-Morey, M.C., et al. (2002). Child emotional security and interparental conflict. *Monographs of the Society for Research in Child Development*, **67**, i–v, vii–viii, 1–115.

Deave, T. and Johnson, D. (2008). The transition to parenthood: what does it mean for fathers? *Journal of Advanced Nursing*, **63**, 626–633.

Deave, T., Johnson, D., and Ingram, J. (2008). Transition to parenthood: the needs of parents in pregnancy and early parenthood. *BMC Pregnancy and Childbirth*, **8**, 30.

Department of Health (2009). *Healthy Child Programme: Pregnancy and the First Five Years of Life*. London: Department of Health.

Doss, B.D., Cicila, L.N., Hsueh, A.C., Morrison, K.R., and Carhart, K. (2014). A randomized controlled trial of brief co-parenting and relationship interventions during the transition to parenthood. *Journal of Family Psychology*, **28**, 4483–4494.

Duncan, L.G. and Bardacke, N. (2010). Mindfulness-based childbirth and parenting education: promoting family mindfulness during the perinatal period. *Journal of Child and Family Studies*, **19**, 190–202.

Feinberg, M.E. and Kan, M.L. (2008). Establishing family foundations: impact of a transition to parenting program on co-parenting, depression, parent-child relationship, and infant regulation. *Journal of Family Psychology*, **22**, 253–263.

Feinberg, M.E., Jones, D.E., Kan, M.L., and Goslin, M. (2010). Effects of family foundations on parents and children: 3.5 years after baseline. *Journal of Family Psychology*, **24**,532–542.

Feinberg, M.E., Kan, M.L., and Goslin, M. (2009). Enhancing co-parenting, parenting, and child self-regulation: effects of family foundations 1 year after birth. *Prevention Science*, **10**, 276–285.

Fenwick, J., Bayes, S., and Johansson, M. (2012). A qualitative investigation into the pregnancy expectations of Australian fathers-to-be. *Sexual & Reproductive Healthcare*, **3**, 3–9.

Flach, C., Leese, M., Heron, J., et al. (2011). Antenatal domestic violence, maternal mental health and subsequent child behavior: a cohort study. *British Journal of Gynaecology: An International Journal of Psycho-Analysis*, **118**, 1381–1391.

Fletcher, R., Mathey, S., and Marley, C. (2006). Addressing depression and anxiety among new fathers. *Medical Journal of Australia*, **18**, 461–463.

Lawrence, E., Rothman, A.D., Cobb, R.J., Rothman, M.T., and Bradbury, T.N. (2008). Marital satisfaction across the transition to parenthood. *Journal of Family Psychology*, **22**, 41–50.

Lewis, G. and Drife, J. (2005). *Why Mothers Die 2000–2002: Report on Confidential Enquiries into Maternal Deaths in the United Kingdom*. London: CEMACH.

Loring, J., Hughes, M., and Unterstaller, U. (2001). Post-traumatic stress disorder (PTSD) in victims of domestic violence: a review of the research. *Trauma, Violence, Abuse*, **2**, 99–119.

Marmot, M., Allen, J., Goldblatt, P., et al. (2010). *Fair Society, Healthy Lives: The Strategic Review of Health Inequalities in England post-2010*. London: The Marmot Review. Available at: http://www.instituteofhealthequity.org/resources-reports/fair-society-healthy-lives-the-marmot-review/fair-society-healthy-lives-full-report-pdf.pdf.

Office for National Statistics (2012). Divorces in England and Wales, 2012. [online] Available at: http://www.ons.gov.uk/ons/dcp171778_351693.pdf [Accessed 20 Jan. 2016].

Petch, J. and Halford, W.K. (2008). Psycho-education to enhance couples' transition to parenthood. *Clinical Psychology Review*, **28**, 1125–1137.

Pinquart, M. and Teubert, D. (2010). A meta-analytic study of couple interventions during the transition to parenthood. *Family Relations*, **59**, 221–231.

Ramchandani, P., Stein, A., Evans, J., and O'Connor, T.G. (2005). Paternal depression in the postnatal period and child development: a prospective population study. *The Lancet*, **365**, 2201–2205.

Ramchandani, P.G., Stein, A., O'Connor, T.G., et al. (2008). Depression in men in the postnatal period and later child psychopathology: a population cohort study. *Journal of the American Academy of Child and Adolescent Psychiatry*, **47**, 390–398.

Raphael-Leff, J. (1992). *Psychological Processes of Childbearing*. London: Chapman and Hall.

Røsand, G.M., Slinning, K., Eberhard-Gran, M., Røysamb E., and Tambs, K. (2011). Partner relationship satisfaction and maternal emotional distress in early pregnancy. *BMC Public Health*, **11**, 161.

Schrader McMillan, A., Barlow, J., and Redshaw, M. (2009). *Birth and Beyond: A Review of Evidence about Antenatal Education*. London: Department of Health.

Stein, A., Pearson, R.M., Goodman, S.H., et al (2014). Effects of perinatal mental disorders on the fetus and child. *The Lancet*, **384**, 1800–1819.

Taft, A. (2002). *Violence against Women in Pregnancy and after Childbirth: Current Knowledge and Issues in Healthcare Responses*. Paper 6. Sydney: Australian Domestic and Family Violence Clearing House, University of New South Wales.

Trillingsgaard, T., Baucom, K. J.W., Heyman, R.E., and Elklit, A. (2012). Relationship interventions during the transition to parenthood: issues of timing and efficacy. *Family Relations*, **61**, 770–783.

Section 3

Primary prevention and health promotion in childhood

Chapter 8

Primary prevention and health promotion in childhood

Cheryll Adams and Sarah Cowley

Summary

This chapter:

◆ builds on earlier explanations about why prevention needs to start in early childhood

◆ considers some of the practicalities of providing primary prevention services

◆ explains key principles and practice approaches that have been found helpful to the preventive effort

◆ discusses some effective approaches to health promotion for families and promoting effective parenting.

Introduction

Early child development, a period defined as conception up to the age of 7 years (Irwin et al., 2007), is recognized as the basis for determining individuals' future health and educational status. Early child development has massive potential to affect health inequalities across the whole of society (Shonkoff et al., 2012; Black et al., 2017) with a return on investment that has been shown to far outweigh the benefits of later interventions (Heckman, 2007), as shown in Figure 8.1. Providing primary prevention and health promotion in these early years is likely to yield greater improvements in health inequalities than activities at any other stage of life (Marmot et al., 2010).

The 'foundations of health', summarized in Table 8.1, refer to domains that establish a context for nourishing the early roots of physical and mental well-being (Center on the Developing Child at Harvard University, 2010; Britto et al., 2017).

Primary prevention includes not only averting the occurrence of a disease or disability, but also reducing risk factors and promoting resources that enhance health, strength, and resilience in the face of challenges to mental and social well-being. Health is the ability to adapt and self-manage (Huber et al., 2011), and is linked with the idea of health promotion. This is 'the process of enabling people to increase control over, and to improve, their health' (World Health Organization, 1998, p. 1). Health improvement, health equity, and sustainable development are linked concepts that have, at

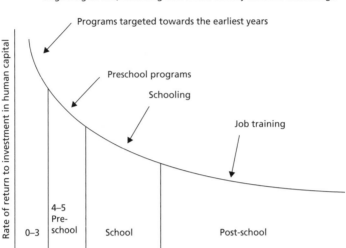

Fig. 8.1 Investing in early childhood development.

Table 8.1 Foundations of health

Center on the Developing Child at Harvard University (2010)*	Lancet Early Child Development Series 3, Britto et al. (2017)†
◆ Stable and responsive environment of relationships providing consistent nurturing, allowing the development of well-regulated stress response systems ◆ Safe and supportive emotional and physical environments, including opportunities for safe exploration and support for families ◆ Sound and appropriate nutrition including food and eating habits, and future mothers' preconception nutritional status	Nurturing care: defined as an overarching concept incorporating a stable environment that is sensitive to a child's: ◆ health ◆ nutrition ◆ security and safety ◆ responsive caregiving ◆ early learning It is supported by a large array of social contexts including home, childcare, schooling, community, work, and policy

their heart, a conviction that health is a fundamental right, with each infant and child having the right to grow and develop their full potential, so as to live a flourishing life.

Health inequalities in the UK are such that avoidable ill health and lost opportunities continue to blight children's lives (Wolfe et al., 2014). Drawing on global reviews of evidence about health inequalities, Marmot et al. (2010) recommend 'proportionate universalism', that is, having a system that provides a primary preventive service to everyone, using this base to identify and target anyone needing additional provision. Action needs to be taken 'at scale', through a national system for the universal delivery of primary prevention (Britto et al., 2017), ideally through a system offering targeted provision from within a universal service (Daro and Dodge, 2010). British health visiting services use specific professional skills in providing such proportionate universal services (Cowley et al., 2015).

Assessing the need for primary prevention

This section offers examples of three different approaches to needs assessment, described as an epidemiological approach, a structured approach (including screening), and professional or clinical judgement (Cowley and Houston, 2004). In practice, they tend to overlap, being integral to a form of working that aims to increase and maximize uptake of preventive services and health-promoting activities. They form part of a comprehensive process of assessment and may lead to any one of a range of outcomes, shown in Figure 8.2, which also emphasizes the importance of taking service users' views into account.

An epidemiological assessment of need is required to decide a necessary focus for services. One example concerns the initiation and continuation of breastfeeding (Rollins et al., 2016). Specifically, in the UK, supporting mothers who are exclusively breastfeeding 1 week after the birth to continue breastfeeding until 4 months could save at least £11 million annually (Pokhrel et al., 2015). Breastfeeding for 26 weeks or longer is associated with a 51% reduction in the risk of obesity at 9 years of age (Cathal and Layte, 2012).

Organized support, which is predictable, scheduled, and includes ongoing visits with trained health professionals or trained volunteers, helps women breastfeed their babies for longer (McFadden et al., 2017). Such 'support' is complex and multifaceted, incorporating building women's esteem, giving information and practical support, and being available to respond in a timely way if problems are encountered (McFadden et al., 2017). Thus, it provides a basis from which to deliver targeted as well as primary prevention, enabling identification of those who need additional support. Relationships established while focusing on one topic can have a 'spillover' effect on others, encouraging openness to other health-promoting messages.

Universal services also allow routine screening and the opportunity to identify needs by using validated assessment instruments for specific concerns, such as maternal postnatal depression (PND). PND has a significant impact on the mother's ability to develop a stable, responsive relationship with her baby. Morrell et al.'s (2009) cluster randomized trial demonstrated that health visitors were effective in early identification and treatment (through listening visits) of PND. In addition, mothers receiving

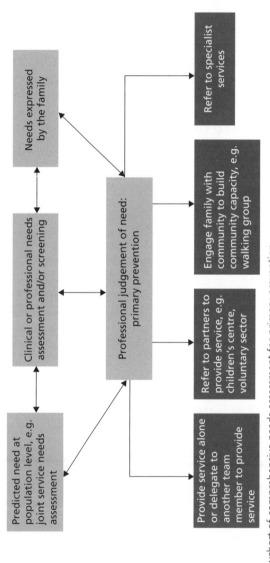

Fig. 8.2 A flowchart of comprehensive needs assessment for primary prevention.

Adapted from 'Needs Assessment Model' courtesy of Professor Viv Bennett.

a cost-effective universal service from health visitors who had developed higher-level skills for the trial, had significantly lower levels of PND (Brugha et al., 2010; Henderson et al., 2018). Thus, targeted interventions may lead to primary prevention, by opening discussion of a sensitive topic and raising awareness in suitably trained staff.

Validated, structured instruments can be very valuable for identifying specific concerns such as PND, but are less helpful for assessing the need for preventive intervention across an undifferentiated population, such as those in receipt of universal services. Some needs are hidden or stigmatized, such as domestic violence and abuse, solvent misuse, family poverty and debt, status of migrants, and many other challenges that may affect the parents' ability to provide a safe and secure environment, supportive of child development. In these circumstances, in place of structured instruments, sensitivity, relationship formation, partnership working, and a sophisticated level of professional knowledge are all essential for informing clear assessments and future interventions with parents.

This more open approach to assessment requires considerable professional knowledge and skill, along with the confidence to be able to respond sensitively to any topic raised by the parents. Primary care is a serial activity, in which professional judgements include both a process and an outcome. Appleton and Cowley (2003, p. 219) suggest health visitors encompass and integrate needs assessments with decision-making, reaching a judgement following 'an accumulation and careful deliberation of evidence: it is informed by a broad spectrum of professional and life experiences, knowledge, instinct and common sense'. The process of assessment may encompass intervention, where discussion opens opportunities for anticipatory guidance, advice, or information that may not have been expected prior to the contact, perhaps engaging them about their aspirations as new parents, and how this matches their experience, and any barriers or support mechanisms they can call upon.

Principles of health promotion

Health-promoting services need to be delivered in partnership with colleagues, working across sectors (such as health and social care, education, and housing). They build capacity by developing knowledge, skills, commitment, structures, systems, and leadership (Smith et al., 2006). Health promotion needs to take account of the whole culture and situation in which families live, including family, community, and schools, using a finely honed set of skills and attributes and a positive 'health-creating' (salutogenic) approach (Cowley and Billings, 1999). This includes notions of social inclusion (Beresford and Branfield, 2006), community health assets (Hufford et al., 2009), and strengths-based practice (Darbyshire and Jackson, 2004).

Skills and qualities

However effective a programme or intervention may be, it will only work for families that receive it (Whittaker and Cowley, 2012). Particular abilities are required to enable all families to benefit from services, regardless of their situation. Primary prevention and health promotion services are offered to parents, rather than being provided in response to a request for help, which is unusual in healthcare and creates two challenges to practitioners. First, they need to somehow convey their vision of how much parents and/or their child could benefit from accepting approved health advice, without appearing to preach or intrude in ways that are off-putting and therefore counterproductive. Second, they need to achieve this in a way that enables families to express, and have met, their own views of their needs and understanding of health and parenting. Meeting these challenges requires humility and respect for families, as well as expert communication, relationship-building skills, and knowledge of different cultural beliefs and parenting approaches (Davis and Day, 2010).

Universality helps to promote take-up, as it avoids stigma and any sense of being 'picked on' or 'singled out' for attention, since everyone is equally valued. Families who are the most in need by any normative criteria may find official provision intimidating or hard to access. Parent–professional relationships are important in enabling parents to use services, especially if they feel valued and respected, rather than judged, and are given time and opportunities to open up about their own needs (Donetto and Maben, 2014). It helps if professionals focus not only on individuals' needs, but explicitly expand their interest to the whole family and local community, who provide that vital early environment for the new infant or young child in their care.

One-to-one approaches to health promotion

One-to-one approaches for health promotion can take place in a range of settings including the home, the clinic, group settings, children's centres, and the community at large. The appropriateness and effectiveness of each site will depend on the issue that needs to be addressed. The home setting provides many advantages, especially for individuals who may feel less comfortable in clinic or group settings. Wiggins et al.'s (2005) trial showed that 94% of new mothers accepted the offer of monthly health visitor home visits for a year, compared to only 19% who took up the offer of community group support. Those receiving home visits were more relaxed and made better use of services. Dodge et al.'s (2013) trial, similarly, showed that universal home visiting to new parents significantly reduces the use of emergency medical care.

Home visits allow for more complex situations to be explored with the family by a professional who is trained to do so, such as a health visitor (see Box 8.1). The

---

Box 8.1 At-risk parents

Home visiting interventions for at-risk families show positive benefits, including for parent–child interaction, parenting behaviour, and children's cognitive and socio-emotional development. The National Institute for Health and Care Excellence (2012) guideline PH40 on social and emotional well-being in the early years recommends that appropriately trained health visitors, nurses, or midwives should offer a series of intensive home visits to parents assessed to be in need of additional support. Activities should be based on a set curriculum and cover issues such as maternal sensitivity, home learning, and parenting skills (Axford, 2015).

professional can both respond to perceived needs reported by the parents, and allude to needs noticed through observation of the family's living environment, or matters of immediate concern that may have been identified and reported by another professional.

Interventions

Working with children and families requires evidence-based approaches to promoting primary prevention, risk avoidance, and behavioural change, using approaches that practitioners are trained in. A number of approaches popular with many health visitors and early years professionals in the UK have good evidence of effectiveness (see Chapter 10). Others have a more limited evidence base, for example, the Solihull Approach, a popular approach based on a powerful theoretical framework addressing primary prevention through containment, reciprocity, and behavioural management (Douglas et al., 2004). Qualitative data from one study (Adams, 2006) suggested that counselling skills were considered one of the most helpful parts of a health visitor's toolkit. Another example of emerging evidence is the 'HENRY' approach to promoting 'Health, Exercise, and Nutrition for the Really Young'. Evaluation using routine pre- and post- programme data demonstrated the effectiveness of this combination of parenting support and accessible information on food choices and activities (Willis et al., 2016).

Emerging technologies, such as smartphone technology and apps, show much promise, particularly in engaging young early adopters of social media (Kratze et al., 2012). There is little strong evidence available about the benefits or potential harm of these approaches as yet, particularly in the UK, but it makes sense to warn parents about the potential bias within commercially sponsored support pages (e.g. associated with particular brands of baby goods). The best networking support pages are moderated, to ensure particularly vulnerable parents can be identified and supported offline if needed. Some high-quality apps are available, such as the 'Baby Buddy' app from Best Beginnings (2018). This is one of a suite of apps developed with strong professional and research evidence to ensure accuracy and appropriate advice, with rigorous evaluations underway.

Promotional interviewing

Promotional interviewing can form part of the professional needs assessment conducted usually in the home. It draws on the Family Partnership Model, a relational approach, based on partnership working. It was tested in a Europe-wide evaluation study (Davis et al., 2005) with primary care professionals (health visitors in the UK). The professionals were trained to use an antenatal and postnatal promotional guide to work in partnership with parents to explore their feelings, attitudes, and expectations for becoming a parent (antenatally) and to explore and support parental behaviours and feelings that can impact their relationship with their infant or child (postnatally). Barlow and Coe (2013) showed the importance of using a planned approach to its introduction, ensuring the availability of referral pathways and making available appropriate training.

Motivational interviewing

Motivational interviewing (MI) is centred on the parent, aiming to build on their intrinsic motivation for change by helping them to overcome what is preventing them from making the suggested change. In one systematic review of MI for parent–child health interventions, it was associated with significant improvements in health behaviours (e.g. oral health, diet, physical activity, reduced screen time, smoking cessation, and reduced second-hand smoke) and a reduction in body mass index (Borrelli et al., 2015).

Engaging fathers

Research shows clearly that, when engaged, fathers have a substantial impact on child development, well-being, and family functioning. Panter-Brick et al.'s (2014) review concluded that it was essential that parenting programmes find ways of engaging fathers/co-parenting couples as well as mothers. Seven key barriers to engaging fathers in parenting programmes are cultural, institutional, professional, operational, content, resource, and policy considerations in their design and delivery. Fathers are susceptible to perinatal mental illness making it all the more important to include them in primary preventative activities, as with the mother. One systematic review reported depression of 10.4% in fathers both ante- and postnatally (Paulson and Bazemore, 2010).

Families who find services hard to reach

There are many groups of families who, for a range of reasons, are less likely than others to access preventive children's services. Boag-Munroe and Evangelou (2012) reviewed the expansive literature on families that appear 'hard to reach' by service providers, noting the lack of a single definition for people 'who were not coming in to receive the service provided or those who had to be contacted by means other than routine information notices' (p. 211).

In the course of recruiting for a randomized controlled trial, Barlow et al. (2004) identified some key reasons that woman declined an early intervention service. These included perceptions about vulnerability, particularly that they were either not in need of support or were sufficiently well provided for with their existing network of family and friends. Some were simply not interested enough to engage with the provision. Others felt already so burdened (by pregnancy, depression, or other worries) that they could not conceive of how accepting a service could possibly help. Misperceptions or lack of knowledge about the service and mistrust of officialdom accounted for refusals by many others. On the other hand, universal services that are clearly explained and understood, that allow the development of a non-judgemental parent–professional relationship, offering both visits to the home and provision at a friendly children's centre or other convenient venue, can overcome initial misgivings (Donetto and Maben, 2014).

It is essential to design and offer services to match the needs and preferences of service-users. Axford et al. (2015) found evidence suggesting that brief, intensive engagement interventions, at the point of entry to treatment, can be effective in improving engagement in early sessions, if they target both practical (e.g. schedules, transport) and psychological (e.g. family members' resistance, beliefs about the treatment process) barriers.

Group-based approaches for health promotion

Perinatal group-based approaches for health promotion have been covered extensively in Chapter 7, which examines the evidence for preparation for parenting programmes. These programmes can lead to improved parenting quality, quality of parental relationships, levels of maternal depression and anxiety, and also co-parenting when both parents attend. Programmes should be provided by two people, including at least one professional skilled in working with parents and with groups, and should be at least five sessions in length. A successful programme developed with a different population, or in a different country, will not necessarily transfer as successfully to the UK or to a different local context. The actual programme may be less important than applying the success factors for running groups to its delivery—for example, the skill of the person leading it, the time of day when it takes place, where it takes place, the number of sessions, whether one or both parents are present, the strength of evidence base for what is included, and how (Davis et al., 2005).

Many useful interventions are delivered by the voluntary sector and others (e.g. story time in libraries or children's centres to promote reading to children), though these may not have been evaluated (see Box 8.2). A promising approach is the Institute of Health Visiting-led programme, Ready Steady Mums, a national network of walking groups (http://www.rsm.org). Each group is initiated by a health visitor but led by a local mother. The groups motivate mothers to undertake low- to medium-intensity physical activity, such as walking in the outdoors, and support the evidence (Chapter 12) that this will offer a boost to their physical, emotional, and social health.

Box 8.2 Health promotion in day care settings

There is moderate evidence that programmes in educational and day care settings for young children can have a positive impact on various outcomes, including cognitive development, school readiness, behaviour, and attainment. The National Institute for Health and Care Excellence (2012) recommends that children's services (including health visitors) should ensure that all vulnerable children can benefit from high-quality childcare outside the home on a part- or full-time basis and can take up their entitlement to early childhood education, where appropriate. Services should aim to enhance children's social and emotional well-being and build their capacity to learn (Axford et al., 2015).

Promoting effective parenting

Whittaker et al. (2014), using qualitative research, has described surface and depth approaches to supporting parenting. The surface approach deals with pressing issues, but without the in-depth approach may not have any long-term and sustainable impact on the causes of the issues. Working at depth requires a trusting relationship, with the practitioner taking a strengths-based approach, understanding the family's needs and working in the context of the family's real-life circumstances. Effectiveness depends on the resources available and staff approach, also the training and supervision of staff (Axford et al., 2015)—see Chapter 10.

Community and group-based approaches for parenting

There are numerous parenting programmes available, although few of the promising and popular UK ones have been subjected to rigorous evaluation. Children's centres and health visitors often run informal groups which can provide a stepping stone to more formal groups (secondary prevention) (Whittaker and Cowley, 2012). These provide a good opportunity for providing anticipatory guidance and peer support for parents, particularly those least likely to seek out classes for themselves. Research in Scotland reported that mothers experiencing disadvantage are *less likely* to attend antenatal classes, parenting classes, and parent and baby/toddler groups; while younger parents, lone parents, and parents with lower levels of income and education are less comfortable engaging with formal support services and more likely to believe that there is a stigma attached to them (Scottish Government, 2015, p. 20).

Axford et al. (2015) provide an overview of the evidence for different types of programmes for different circumstances but make the point that these programmes must be implemented with fidelity to be effective. Barlow and Schrader McMillan (2010, p. 131) have reviewed the principles of effective programmes for the prevention of maltreatment (see Box 8.3), which can equally be applied to parenting

---

Box 8.3 The principles of effective programmes

Programme design and content is theory driven, of sufficient dosage and intensity, comprehensive, and actively engaging.

The *programme is relevant*: it is developmentally appropriate, appropriately timed, and socio-culturally relevant.

The *programme is delivered* by well qualified, trained, and supportive staff, and focused on fostering good relationships.

Programme assessment and quality assurance is in place and well documented. There is a commitment to evaluation and refinement.

Source: data from Small S. et al. 'Evidence-informed program improvement: using principles of effectiveness to enhance the quality and impact of family-based prevention programs,' *Family Relations*, Volume 58, Issue 1, pp.1–13, Copyright © 2009 by the National Council on Family Relations.

programmes. However evidence-based interventions alone are not sufficient, they must be built into local systems so they can reach all who might benefit from them (Cuthbert, 2011).

To summarize, this chapter has highlighted the need for, and benefits from, anticipating needs so that timely guidance can be offered to support parenting and early child development. Some of the practicalities of providing primary prevention and health promotion have been explored along with key, evidence-based examples illustrating how the principles can be applied in practice.

Learning links

- Center on the Developing Child, Harvard University: https://developingchild. harvard.edu/resources/
- Institute of Health Visiting—'Resource Library A–Z': http://ihv.org.uk/for-health-visitors/resources/resource-library-a-z/ (paywall)
- Institute of Health Visiting—'Top Tips for Parents': http://ihv.org.uk/families/top-tips/ (open access)
- Institute of Health Visiting—'Good Practice Points': http://ihv.org.uk/for-health-visitors/resources/good-practice-points/ (some paywall)
- Institute of Health Visiting—e-Learning: http://ihv.org.uk/for-health-visitors/resources/e-learning/ (open access)
- Institute of Health Visiting—'iHV Training Programme': https://ihv.org.uk/training-and-events/training-programme/.

Recommendations

- Provide health professionals in universal services with sufficient time to develop relationships, identify needs and respond to them, and to provide opportunities for health promotion and anticipatory guidance. (*Evidence: moderate.*)
- Support the whole family to reduce the onset and development of physical, social, and emotional health issues in the child and improve the long-term impact on the health economy and government fiscal spend. (*Evidence: moderate.*)
- Consider working with individuals and the community to provide primary prevention and health promotion approaches to deliver the required outcomes. (*Evidence: moderate.*)
- Home visiting should be an intervention of choice when working with young families as it allows for a more accurate assessment of family need and remains the best evidenced approach to reach the families that will benefit the most from services. (*Evidence: moderate.*)

References

Adams, C. (2006). *Mental Health Promotion in Families with Pre-School Children: The Role and Training Needs of Health Visitors.* Unpublished doctoral thesis, University of Portsmouth.

Appleton, J.V. and Cowley, S. (2003). Valuing professional judgement in health visiting practice. *Community Practitioner,* **26**, 215–220.

Axford, N., Barlow, J., Coad, J., et al. (2015). *Rapid Review to Update Evidence for the Healthy Child Programme 0–5.* London: Public Health England.

Barlow, J. and Coe, C. (2013). New ways of working. Promotional interviewing in health visiting practice *Journal of Health Visiting,* **1**, 44–50.

Barlow, J. and Schrader McMillan, A. (2010). *Safeguarding Children from Emotional Maltreatment: What Works.* London: Jessica Kingsley Publishers.

Barlow, J., Kirkpatrick, S., Stewart-Brown, S., and Davis, H. (2004). Hard-to-reach or out-of-reach? Reasons why women refuse to take part in early interventions. *Children and Society,* **19**, 199–210.

Beresford, P. and Branfield, F. (2006). Developing inclusive partnerships: user-defined outcomes, networking and knowledge – a case study. *Health & Social Care in the Community,* **14**, 436–444.

Best Beginnings (2018). About Baby Buddy. [online] Available at: https://www.bestbeginnings. org.uk/about-baby-buddy.

Black, M.P., Walker, S.P., Fernhold, L.C.H., et al. (2017). Early childhood development coming of age: science through the life course. *The Lancet,* **389**, 77–90.

Boag-Munroe, G. and Evangelou, M. (2012). From hard to reach to how to reach: a systematic review of the literature on hard-to-reach families. *Research Papers in Education,* **27**, 209–239.

Borrelli, B., Tooley, E.M., and Scott-Sheldon, L.A.J. (2015). Motivational interviewing for parent-child health interventions: a systematic review and meta-analysis. *Pediatric Dentistry,* **37**, 254–265.

Britto, P.R., Lye, S.J., Proulx, K., et al. (2017). Nurturing care: promoting early childhood development. *The Lancet,* **389**, 91–102.

Brugha, T.S., Morrell, C.J., Slade, P., and Walters, S.J. (2010). Universal prevention of depression in women postnatally: cluster randomized trial evidence in primary care. *Psychological Medicine,* **41**, 739–748.

Cathal, M.C. and Layte, D.R. (2012). Breastfeeding and risk of overweight and obesity at nine years of age. *Social Science and Medicine,* **75**, 323–330.

Center on the Developing Child at Harvard University (2010). The Foundations of Lifelong Health Are Built in Early Childhood. [online] http://developingchild.harvard.edu/wp-content/uploads/2010/05/Foundations-of-Lifelong-Health.pdf [Accessed 21 Sep. 2017].

Cowley, S. and Billings, J.R. (1999). Resources revisited: salutogenesis from a lay perspective. *Journal of Advanced Nursing,* **29**, 994–1004.

Cowley, S. and Houston, A. (2004). Contradictory agendas in health visitor needs assessment. A discussion paper of its use for prioritizing, targeting and promoting health. *Primary Health Care Research and Development,* **5**, 240–254.

Cowley, S., Whittaker K., Malone M., et al. (2015). Why health visiting? Examining the potential public health benefits from health visiting practice within a universal service: a narrative review of the literature. *International Journal of Nursing Studies,* **52**, 465–480.

Cuthbert, C., Raynes, G., and Stanley, K. (2011). *All Babies Count: Prevention and Protection for Vulnerable Babies*. London: NSPCC.

Darbyshire, P. and Jackson, D. (2004). Using a strengths approach to understanding resilience and build health capacity in families. *Contemporary Nurse*, **18**, 211–212.

Daro, D. and Dodge, K.A. (2010). Strengthening home visitation intervention policy: expanding reach, building knowledge. In: Haskins, R. and Barnett, W.S. (Eds.), *Investing in Young Children: New Directions in Federal Preschool and Early Childhood Policy*, pp. 79–88. Washington, DC: Centre on Children and Families at Brookings and the National Institute for Early Education Research. Available at: https://www.brookings.edu/wp-content/uploads/2016/07/1013_investing_in_young_children_haskins_ch7.pdf.

Davis, H. and Day, C. (2010). *Working in Partnership: The Family Partnership Model*. London: Pearson Education Ltd.

Davis, H., Dusoir, T., Papadopoulou, K., et al. (2005). Child and family outcomes of the European early promotion project. *International Journal of Mental Health Promotion*, **7**, 63–81.

Dodge, K.A., Goodman, W.B., Murphy, R.A., et al. (2013). Randomized controlled trial of universal postnatal nurse home visiting: impact on emergency care. *Pediatrics*, **132**, S140.

Donetto, S. and Maben, J. (2014). 'These places are like a godsend': a qualitative analysis of parents' experiences of health visiting outside the home and of children's centres services. *Health Expectations*, **18**, 2559–2569.

Douglas, H. and Brennan, A. (2004). Containment, reciprocity and behaviour management: Preliminary evaluation of a brief early intervention (the Solihull approach) for families with infants and young children. *Infant Observation: International Journal of Infant Observation and Its Applications*, **7**, 89–107.

Heckman, J.J. (2007). The economics, technology and neuroscience of human capability formation. *Proceedings of the National Academy of Sciences of the United States of America*, **104**, 13250–13255.

Henderson, C., Dixon, S., Bauer, A., et al. (2018). Cost-effectiveness of PoNDER health visitor training for mothers at lower risk of depression: findings on prevention of postnatal depression from a cluster-randomised controlled trial. *Psychological Medicine*, 1–11. doi: 10.1017/S0033291718001940

Huber, M., André Knottnerus, J., Green, L., et al. (2011). How should we define health? *BMJ*, **343**, d4163.

Hufford, L., West, D.C., Paterniti, D.A., and Pan, R.J. (2009). Community-based advocacy training: applying asset-based community development in resident education. *Academic Medicine*, **84**, 765–770.

Irwin, L.G., Siddiqi A., and Hertzman, C. (2007). *Early Child Development: A Powerful Equalizer. A Report for the WHO Commission on Social Determinants of Health*. Geneva: World Health Organization.

Kratzke, C. and Cox, C. (2012). Smartphone technology and apps: rapidly changing health promotion. *International Electronic Journal of Health Education*, **15**, 72–82.

Marmot, M., Allen, J., Goldblatt, P., et al. (2010). *Fair Society, Healthy Lives: Strategic Review of Heath Inequalities in England post-2010*. London: Institute of Health Equity.

McFadden, A., Gavine, A., Renfrew, M.J., et al. (2017). Support for healthy breastfeeding mothers with healthy term babies. *Cochrane Database of Systematic Reviews*, **2**, CD001141.

Morrell, C.J., Warner, R., Slade, P., et al. (2009). Psychological interventions for postnatal depression: cluster randomised trial and economic evaluation. The PONDER trial. *Health Technology Assessment*, **13**, 1–176.

National Institute for Health and Care Excellence (2012). *Social and Emotional Wellbeing: Early Years*. PH40. London: National Institute for Health and Care Excellence.

Panter-Brick, C., Burgess, A., Eggerman, M., et al. (2014). Practitioner Review: Engaging fathers – recommendations for a game change in parenting interventions based on a systematic review of the global evidence. *Journal of Child Psychology and Psychiatry*, **55**, 1187–1212.

Paulson, J. and Baxemore, S. (2010). Prenatal and postpartum depression in fathers and its association with maternal depression: a meta-analysis. *JAMA*, **303**, 1961–1969.

Pokhrel, S., Quigley, M.A., Fox-Rushby, J., et al. (2015). Potential economic impacts from improving breastfeeding rates in the UK. *Archives of Disease in Childhood*, **100**, 334–340.

Rollins, N.C., Bandari, N., Hajeebhoy, N., et al. (2016). Lancet Breastfeeding Series: Why invest, and what it will take to improve breastfeeding practices in less than a generation? *The Lancet*, **387**, 491–504.

Scottish Government (2015). *Tackling Inequalities in the Early Years: Key Messages from 10 Years of the Growing Up in Scotland Study*. Edinburgh: Scottish Government. Available at: http://www.gov.scot/Resource/0048/00486755.pdf [Accessed 9 Aug. 2016].

Shonkoff, J.P., Akil, H., Chang, H.I., et al. (2012). From Neurons to Neighborhoods: An Update. Washington, DC: National Academies Press.

Smith, B.J., Tang, K.C., and Nutbeam, D. (2006). WHO Health Promotion Glossary: new terms. *Health Promotion International*, **21**, 340–345.

Whittaker, K.A., Cox, P., Thomas, N., and Cocker, K. (2014). A qualitative study of parents' experiences using family support services: applying the concept of surface and depth. *Health & Social Care in the Community*, **22**, 479–487.

Whittaker, K. and Cowley, S. (2012). An effective programme is not enough: a review of factors associated with poor attendance at and engagement with parenting support programmes. *Children and Society*, **26**, 138–149.

Wiggins, M., Oakley, A., Roberts, I. et al. (2005). Postnatal support for mothers living in disadvantaged inner city areas: a randomised controlled trial. *Journal of Epidemiology and Community Health*, **59**, 288–295.

Willis, T.A., Roberts, K.P.J., Berry, T.M., et al. (2016). The impact of HENRY on parenting and family lifestyle: a national service evaluation of a preschool obesity prevention programme. *Public Health*, **136**, 101–108.

Wolfe, I., Macfarlane, A., Donkin, A., et al. (2014). *Why Children Die: Death in Infants, Children, and Young People in the UK*. London: Royal College of Paediatrics and Child Health, National Children's Bureau, British Association for Child and Adolescent Public Health.

World Health Organization (1998). *Health Promotion Glossary*. Geneva: World Health Organization.

Chapter 9

Promoting child development

James Law and Alan Emond

Summary

This chapter:

- reviews the evidence on the interconnectedness of child development and emphasizes the value of taking a 'developmental approach' in a child health programme
- stresses that promoting child development requires a partnership approach with the family
- describes how professionals have a key role in providing appropriate information about child development to families, and also in mediating what is available on the internet
- emphasizes that the outcome of promoting early child development should be seen in terms of improving school readiness, and enhancing children's well-being.

Introduction

Children's development is strongly determined by genetic inheritance and follows predictable patterns, but there is also plenty of evidence that many of the competencies that go to make up child development can be very sensitive to social factors (Maggi et al., 2010), and that wide social disparities have opened up by the time children have reached compulsory schooling (Mani et al., 2013). Child development is associated with child well-being more generally, and delayed or abnormal development can have substantive policy implications for health, social, and educational services and on long-term health (Engle et al., 2007). Promoting child development involves anticipatory guidance to make parents aware of their child's next developmental stage, enhancing the skills themselves and reducing the impact of factors negatively affecting child development, and then measuring the impact on the child and the family.

Recent research in child development

Models for promoting child development are evolving with our understanding of the basic biological and neurobiological processes underpinning child development.

Box 9.1 Key facts about early brain development

- ◆ A fully grown adult brain has an estimated 86 billion neurons, the majority of which are already formed in the womb.

- ◆ From birth to age two, the brain goes through a period of rapid development and growth. During the first two years of life the brain displays a remarkable capacity to absorb information and adapt to its surroundings.

- ◆ By age one, the size of a child's brain is already 72% of adult volume on average and by age two it has grown to 83% of an adult's volume on average.

- ◆ At age two, the connections that are being formed in a child's brain are happening about twice as fast as in an adult's brain.

- ◆ At age three, a child's brain is estimated to be about twice as active as an adult's brain. At age five, a child's brain uses almost twice as much energy as an adult's brain to support brain development.

Reproduced from Finnegan, J. (2016), *Lighting up young brains: How parents, carers and nurseries support children's brain development in the first five years*. London: Save the Children, with permission from Save the Children.

Early neuropsychological and biological development has been one of the greatest 'growth' areas in recent years. In their recent report 'Lighting up young brains' (Finnegan, 2016), Save the Children identified a number of key take-home messages about these findings (see Box 9.1).

The interconnectedness of different aspects of child development

Child development covers a wide variety of competencies which manifest across childhood. These are commonly grouped into physical (fine and gross motor), socio-emotional and behavioural (well-being, emotional regulation, attention, etc.), and communication (speech and language development and interaction skills). These skills emerge gradually over time, driven by a combination of biological and social processes. These skills are commonly described in terms of specific milestones (Sharma and Cockerill, 2007) and there are numerous websites (e.g. www.nhs.uk/tools/pages/birthtofive.aspx) available for parents and professionals to check whether behaviour x is appropriate at age y. However, the reality is that while an individual child may experience delays in one aspect of development or another, these skills are closely intertwined and are likely to have a cumulative effect on key outcomes such as school readiness. Importantly, these milestones may not be the same for children from different populations, and care may be needed in their interpretation in different ethnic and cultural groups (Kelly et al., 2006).

It is also important for all families, of whatever cultural background, to understand the importance of 'sensitive periods' in their child's development, when it is easy for the child to acquire key new skills, building on existing developmental attainments. One example of a sensitive period is the introduction of solid food in weaning between 6 and 9 months, as the late introduction of lumpy food has been shown to be associated with later feeding difficulties (Coulthard et al., 2009). Another is the initiation of toilet training between 18 and 24 months: delaying starting until after 24 months is associated with an increased risk of daytime wetting in school-aged children (Joinson et al., 2009). Many of the sensitive periods last only a few months, and practitioners should be aware of the vulnerability of children who are unwell, or experience family disruption or other traumatic life events during these crucial months—their parents will need support and guidance in persisting with helping their child to practise the new developmental skill to avoid problems later.

When is the best time to promote child development?

The obvious answer is 'as early as possible' and the recent policy has emphasized the importance of pregnancy and the first 3 years. In the UK, good examples are the 'First 1,000 Days' (Nct.org.uk, 2017) campaign by the NCT and the cross-party parliamentary children's manifesto 'The 1001 Critical Days' (1001criticaldays.co.uk, 2016). However, the messages given are often rather deterministic, and the focus on the very early years has been criticized because children continue to adjust to their environment long past their third birthday (Bruer, 1999). Early experiences clearly matter, especially when in the context of sustained social disadvantage (Lloyd et al., 2010), but they are not the only factor driving child development. Concentrating on the first 1000 days, however, does facilitate the early identification of families under stress and children who are not going to be ready for school, allowing the targeting of resources.

Promoting child development in the UK

All four countries in the UK have specific policy guidance about the health contacts offered to families with babies and young children. Although these contacts often focus on specific screening measures, most tests of child development do not fulfil the criteria for a screening test, and there has been considerable debate about which measures to use for assessing development and the quality of the evidence underpinning such assessments (Wallace et al., 2015; Warren et al., 2016). All well child programmes share the objective of making sure children are prepared for school, and the recommended health and developmental need to cover a comprehensive range of topics to assess risk and protective factors, and establishing where further support is required. Promoting child development requires a partnership approach with the family. Interaction between professionals and parents is key to promoting child development and a critical first step in engaging parents with developmental difficulties (Kaiser and Hancock, 2003). Bellman and colleagues (2013) highlighted some simple messages from routine consultations with families to help identify developmental issues (see Box 9.2).

> ## Box 9.2 Key features of the developmental consultation
>
> - Every consultation is an opportunity to ask flexible questions about a child's development as part of comprehensive medical care.
> - Parents who voice concerns about their child's development are usually right.
> - Loss of previously acquired skills (regression) is a red flag and should prompt rapid referral for detailed assessment and investigation.
> - Parents and carers are usually more aware of norms for gross motor milestones, such as walking independently, than for milestones and patterns of normal speech, language acquisition and play skills; consider targeted questioning.
> - Consider use of developmental screening questionnaires and measurement tools to supplement clinical judgement.

The role of the family

Although children are meant to be regularly monitored, the reality for many parents is that this does not happen (Rice et al., 2014) and decisions about a child's development depend on the parents' engagement with the information that is readily available and their own interest and resources. Historically, much of this was delivered via the television, and with visual materials such as DVDs provided to new parents which have been shown to be more effective methods of health promotion than written materials (Lee et al., 2013). Most parents now use the internet as the prime source of information, but concerns have been raised about the quality of information about child development that is available online to parents (Williams et al., 2008). Practitioners working as part of the child health programme have a responsibility to signpost families to reliable sources of information such as the 'Birth to five development timeline' on NHS choices (nhs.uk, 2016), and the resources available on Talking Point (talkingpoint. org.uk, 2017) and on the website of the Center on the Developing Child (https:// developingchild.harvard.edu/). Materials about child development should be sensitive to the culture and religious beliefs of the parents. For example the 'Approachable Parenting' organization in Birmingham specifically produces materials targeting Muslim families (http://approachableparenting.org.uk/). The 'Baby Buddy' (Best Beginnings, 2017) is a free smartphone app targeted at vulnerable mums which has been endorsed by the Department of Health to provide information in video format to guide mothers through pregnancy and the first 6 months of the baby's life. The results of a multicentre evaluation are awaited.

Attempts to engage parents using telehealth approaches via the internet have proved to be quite successful when they have focused on specific conditions (Wade et al., 2011). However, as Shonkoff (2010) states: 'the provision of information on child development and advice on parenting is not sufficient for mothers and fathers with low income and limited education if the parents themselves are having considerable difficulty coping with the stresses of poverty, depression, substance abuse, food inse-curity, homelessness and/or neighbourhood violence'.

In most families, fathers and the extended family have important roles in pro-moting children's development. Although published evidence often focuses on what the mother is doing to stimulate the child, development is everyone's business and there is now ample evidence that fathers have a pivotal role in promoting the develop-ment of their children (Lamb, 2004). Fathers' positive involvement with their child's play and development leads to improved outcomes, and studies of paternal depression have indicated ways in which fathers influence their children's development (Barker et al., 2017). Specific resources for fathers are available from the Fatherhood Institute (Fatherhoodinstitute.org, 2017).

Health visitors remain the most common source of guidance on matters to do with child development, closely followed by friends and family. Community groups, tod-dler groups, and preschool nurseries also play a critical role in the upbringing of chil-dren, and provide opportunities to promote social development and to respond to parental concerns and self-help endeavours (Donetto and Maben, 2015).

An example of an approach explicitly focusing on child development, with the out-come of improving school readiness is Stoke Speaks Out (2017). This programme of work was first initiated in 2004 to address the reported high rates of early language difficulties in young children in Stoke-on-Trent. The key feature of this approach was public health messaging, training, and resources for parents and for over 5500 early years practitioners such as health visitors and staff in nurseries. The programme has an explicit theory of change (see Figure 9.1).

Although this programme has not been evaluated with a trial, it has been subject to a return on investment study. Focusing on improved school readiness as the outcome, the authors reported that relative to statistical neighbours the return on investment

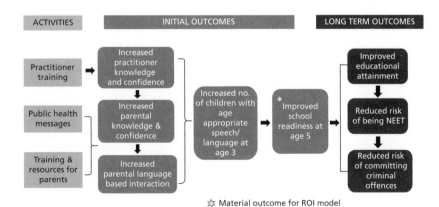

☆ Material outcome for ROI model

Fig. 9.1 High-level theory of change for Stoke Speaks Out.

Reproduced with permission from the NEF Consulting (part of the New Economics Foundation) report for the Royal College of Speech and Language Therapists: *Stoke Speaks Out: Pilot Return on Investment (ROI),* Copyright ©2016 RCSLT, available from https://www.rcslt.org/news/news/2016_news_archive/stoke_speaks_out_roi2016.

ratio was 1:1.9, so for each £1 of investment delivered an extra £1.19 worth of value was created. This analysis was then scaled up to predict the programme's potential return in reducing the likelihood of not being in employment, education, or training (NEET) at 16, and the return then goes up to £4.26 for every £1 invested.

A more ambitious programme to enhance early development in children living in deprived areas is the A Better Start programme, which is described in more detail in Chapter 32.

Social marketing: tailoring messages to different populations

One area which has attracted considerable attention in recent years is *social marketing*, defined as 'the systematic application of marketing concepts and techniques to achieve specific behavioural goals relevant to improving health and reducing health inequalities' (French and Blair-Stevens, 2006). A systematic review (Gordon et al., 2006) highlighted that social marketing interventions can be effective in health, and there is reasonably strong evidence of their effectiveness for nutrition, alcohol, tobacco, and illicit drug use (with mixed results for physical activity). Social marketing has also been applied in relation to parents and children, with positive results, for example, in promoting breastfeeding (Lowry et al., 2011). An approach that specifically applied social marketing techniques to the identification of developmental delays in early childhood is Learn the Signs, Act Early (LSAE) from Atlanta, US, which campaigned to help every child reach his or her full potential. It aimed to increase the early identification and treatment of autism and other developmental disorders through an application of a social marketing approach to both parents of children under 4 years and practitioners. Fear-based autism warning messages quickly turned parents away, while messages around general milestones positively engaged parents (Daniel et al., 2009).

Expected outcomes of promoting child development

One of the key issues in promoting child development is the identification of the most appropriate outcomes. On the one hand, one might argue that the aim should be to enhance some specific competencies—such as speech and language development—or reducing challenging behaviours, on the grounds that these are the antecedents of later difficulties. On the other hand, there is a broader agenda for building familial resilience, encouraging readiness for the next stage in the child's development—that is, the transition to primary school—promoting a broader sense of familial well-being, and preventing downstream problems. The former is often more immediately attainable and the latter rarely recorded.

In practice, the longer-term outcomes are rarely recorded in routine data even if the children are explicitly followed up for a further 6 months to check whether gains are maintained. From a societal perspective, it is likely to be more important to establish whether the intervention in the early years has a substantive impact on 'school readiness' (see Chapter 31) as this determines future life chances. In the US, the evaluation of the Head Start programmes have used longer-term societal goals such as staying on at school, avoiding teenage pregnancy, and not getting in trouble with the criminal justice system. Another target, rarely considered in the health literature but more commonly a concern in education, is the reduction in the performance gap between the children from more and less socially disadvantaged backgrounds. There is ample evidence to suggest that such gaps are well established by the time children enter compulsory schooling. But they represent something of a challenge for those developing truly universal services, because those concerned have to demonstrate effects at the more disadvantaged end without showing comparable enhancement at the top end, hence the focus on selected targeted interventions. The challenge, as has been demonstrated elsewhere, is that genuinely universal interventions can have the effect of widening rather than closing such a gap (White et al., 2009).

Parents often want more holistic goals for their children: when parents of children with speech and language difficulties were asked what they wanted for their children, they focused less on the specific skills targeted by the professionals (expressive and receptive language, speech, etc.) and instead emphasized the needs of their children to be happy and to gain their independence (Roulstone et al., 2012).

The evaluation of programmes to promote child development

Whether programmes promoting child development can be said to work depends on the programme, the level of investment, the context in which the intervention is delivered, and the way it has been evaluated. Children who have marked learning or neurodevelopmental difficulties are unlikely to benefit from universal or selected targeted interventions. Their difficulties are likely to need more intensive targeted and individualized interventions than are commonly offered in broad community programmes. Nevertheless, all parents are likely to benefit from general information about child development and what to expect of their children in different stages of their development. The first stage in engaging parents in more intensive interventions is often engaging them in these earlier stages.

There have been a variety of recent reviews of evidence related to interventions aimed at socio-emotional and cognitive development, some delivered by parents (Axford et al., 2015), and others by a range of different agents (Asmussen et al., 2016). The quality of the evidence ranges considerably, many programmes are at a relatively early stage in their development, but others are much better developed with good underpinning empirical evidence. Overall, the short-term effects of early childhood programmes on cognitive and achievement scores have small (approximately 0.2 standard deviations) effect sizes (Shonkoff, 2016). Whether such gains are sufficient depends a little on how they can be generalized. Such effect sizes are relatively common in an educational context where the results have the potential to reach whole populations. But successful replication of programmes that have shown positive outcomes for small numbers of children demands adaptations for different populations, and more research is needed on the implementation and upscaling of such initiatives.

Learning links

- Module 6 ('Development and Behaviour') of the Healthy Child Programme provides guidance when dealing with challenges around feeding, sleeping, and toileting as well as common emotional and behavioural problems: https://www.e-lfh.org.uk/programmes/healthy-child-programme/
- Harvard Developing Child resources: https://developingchild.harvard.edu/resources.

Recommendations

- All practitioners working with young children need to have a sound understanding of normal child development, and the skills to work sensitively with parents from different social and cultural backgrounds. (*Evidence: strong.*)
- Practitioners should take a 'developmental' perspective on the child health programme, and be aware of sensitive periods in child development and the importance of developmental transitions. (*Evidence: moderate.*)
- Every contact with a parent as part of a well child programme is an opportunity to discuss child development. When parents do express concerns they ought to be taken seriously. (*Evidence: strong.*)
- All practitioners should work in partnership with parents to enable them to help their children acquire the skills and self-regulation needed to benefit from formal education, and to identify children who need further assessment and support. (*Good practice.*)

Acknowledgements

Text extracts from Shonkoff J.P., Building a new biodevelopmental framework to guide the future of early childhood policy, *Child Development*, Volume 81, Issue 1, pp. 357–367, Copyright © the Author(s). Journal Compilation © 2010, Society for Research in Child Development, Inc. Reproduced with permission from John Wiley and Sons.

Text extracts from French and Blair-Stevens (2006) *Big pocket guide: social marketing* reproduced with permission from the National Social Marketing Centre.

References

1001criticaldays.co.uk (2016). Manifesto: 1001 critical days. [online] Available at: http://www.1001criticaldays.co.uk/manifesto [Accessed 25 Sep. 2017].

Asmussen, K., Feinstein, L., Martin, J., and **Chowdry, H.** (2016). Foundations for life: what works to support parent child interaction in the early years. Early Intervention Foundation.

[online] Available at: http://www.eif.org.uk/publication/foundations-for-life-what-works-to-support-parent-childinteraction-in-the-early-years/ [Accessed 12 Nov.18].

Axford, N., Barlow, J., Coad, J., et al. (2015). *Rapid Review to Update Evidence for the Healthy Child Programme 0–5*. London: Public Health England.

Barker, B., Iles, J., and Ramchandani, P. (2017). Fathers, fathering and child psychopathology. *Current Opinion in Psychology*, **15**, 82–87.

Bellman, M., Byrne, O., and Sege, R. (2013). Clinical review: developmental assessment of children. *BMJ*, **346**, e8687.

Best Beginnings (2017). Baby Buddy online. [online] Available at: https://www.bestbeginnings.org.uk/baby-buddy-online [Accessed 25 Sep. 2017].

Bruer, J.T. (1999). *The Myth of the First Three Years: A New Understanding of Early Brain Development and Lifelong Learning*. New York: The Free Press.

Coulthard, H., Harris, G., and Emmett, P. (2009). Delayed introduction of lumpy foods to children during the complementary feeding period affects children's food acceptance and feeding at 7 years of age. *Maternal and Child Nutrition*, **5**, 75–85.

Daniel, K.L., Prue, C., Taylor, M.K., Thomas, J., and Scales, M. (2009). "Learn the signs. Act early': a campaign to help every child reach his or her full potential. *Public Health*, **123**(Suppl. 1), e11–e16.

Donetto, S. and Maben, J. (2015). 'These places are like a godsend': a qualitative analysis of parents' experiences of health visiting outside the home and of children's centre services. *Health Expectations*, **18**, 2559–2569.

Engle, P.L., Behrman, J.R., Cabral de Mello, M., et al. (2007). Strategies to avoid the loss of developmental potential in more than 200 million children in the developing world. *The Lancet*, **369**, 229–242.

Fatherhoodinstitute.org (2017). The Fatherhood Institute: The UK's fatherhood think tank. [online] Available at: http://www.fatherhoodinstitute.org/ [Accessed 25 Sep. 2017].

Finnegan, J. (2016). *Lighting up Young Brains: How Parents, Carers and Nurseries Support Children's Brain Development in the First Five Years*. London: Save the Children.

French, J. and Blair-Stevens, C. (2006). *Big Pocket Guide: Social Marketing*. London: National Social Marketing Centre.

Gordon, R., McDermott, L., Stead, M., and Angus, K. (2006). The effectiveness of social marketing interventions for health improvement: What's the evidence? *Public Health*, **120**, 1133–1139.

Joinson, C., Heron, J., Von Gontard, A., et al. (2009). A prospective study of the age at initiation of toilet training and subsequent daytime bladder control in school age children. *Journal of Developmental and Behavioural Pediatrics*, **30**, 385–393.

Kaiser A.P. and Hancock T.B. (2003). Teaching parents new skills to support their young children's development. *Infants & Young Children*, **16**, 9–21.

Kelly, Y., Sacker, A., Schoon, S., and Nazroo, J. (2006). Ethnic differences in achievement of developmental milestones by 9 months of age: the Millennium Cohort Study. *Developmental Medicine & Child Neurology*, **48**, 825–830.

Lamb, M. (2004). *The Role of the Father in Child Development* (4th edn.). London: Wiley.

Lee, P., Foley, S., and Mee, C. (2013). Getting it right from the evaluation of a DVD and booklet for new parents. *Community Practitioner*, **86**, 32–36.

Lloyd, J.E.V., Li, L., and Hertzman, C. (2010). Early experiences matter: lasting effect of concentrated disadvantage on children's language and cognitive outcomes. *Health & Place*, **16**, 371–380.

Lowry, R., Austin, J., and Patterson, M. (2011). Using social marketing to improve breast-feeding rates in a low socioeconomic area. *Social Marketing Quarterly*, **2**, 64–75.

Maggi, S., Irwin, L.J., Siddiqi, A., and Hertzman, C. (2010). The social determinants of early child development: an overview. *Journal of Paediatrics and Child Health*, **46**, 627–635.

Mani, A., Mullainathan, S., Shafir, E., and Zhao, J. (2013). Poverty impedes cognitive function. *Science*, **341**, 976–980.

Nct.org.uk (2017). *First 1,000 Days*. [online] Available at: https://www.nct.org.uk/about-nct/first-1000-days [Accessed 25 Sep. 2017].

Nhs.uk (2016). Birth to five development timeline. [online] Available at: http://www.nhs.uk/Tools/Pages/birthtofive.aspx [Accessed 25 Sep. 2017].

Rice, C., Van Naarden Braun, K., Kogan, M.D., et al. (2014). Screening for developmental delays among young children – National Survey of Children's Health, United States, 2007. *Morbidity and Mortality Weekly Report*, **63**(Suppl 2), 27–35.

Roulstone, S., Coad, J., Ayre, A., Hambley, H., and Lindsay, G. (2012). *The Preferred Outcomes of Children with Speech, Language and Communication Needs and their Parents*. London: Department for Education.

Sharma, A. and Cockerill, H. (2007). *From Birth to Five Years: Children's Developmental Progress* (3rd edn.). London: Routledge and Kegan Paul.

Shonkoff, J.P. (2016). Capitalizing on advances in science to reduce the health consequences of early childhood adversity. *JAMA Pediatrics*, **170**, 1003–1007.

Shonkoff, J.P. (2010). Building a new biodevelopmental framework to guide the future of early childhood policy. *Child Development*, **81**, 357–367.

Stoke Speaks Out (2017). Homepage. [online] Available at: https://www.stokespeaks.org/ [Accessed 25 Sep. 2017].

Talkingpoint.org.uk (2017). Free Activities. [online] Available at: http://www.talkingpoint.org.uk/directory/free-resources-parents/free-activities [Accessed 25 Sep. 2017].

Wade, S.L., Oberjohn, K., Conaway, K., Osinska, P., and Bangert, L. (2011). Live coaching of parenting skills using the internet: implications for clinical practice. *Professional Psychology: Research and Practice*, **42**, 487–493.

Wallace, I.F., Berkman, N.D., Watson, L.R., et al. (2015). Screening for speech and language delay in children 5 years old and younger: a systematic review. *Pediatrics*, **136**, e448–e462.

Warren, R., Kenny, M., Bennett, T., et al. (2016). Screening for developmental delay among children aged 1–4 years: a systematic review. *CMAJ Open*, **J4**, E20–E27.

White, M., Adams, J., and Heywood, P. (2009). How and why do interventions that increase health overall widen inequalities within populations? In: Babones, S. (Ed.), *Social Inequality and Public Health*, pp. 64–81. Bristol: Policy Press.

Williams, N., Mughal, S., and Blair, M. (2008). 'Is my child developing normally?': a critical review of web-based resources for parents. *Developmental Medicine and Child Neurology*, **50**, 893–897.

Chapter 10

Promoting infant and child mental health through support for parenting

Jane Barlow

Summary

This chapter:

- provides an overview of the nature and prevalence of early regulatory problems affecting children

- describes some of the main universal and targeted intervention approaches that have been developed to address such problems

- summarizes the evidence about their effectiveness in improving outcomes for both parents and children.

Introduction

Mental health in the early years is underpinned by the capacity of young children for emotion regulation, and the child's early relational context (i.e. the parenting that they receive) has been identified as being key to the development of such abilities. However, many children show signs of regulatory difficulties including sleeping and crying disturbances, and emotional and behavioural problems in the early years, and a high proportion of such problems are stable over time, and are associated with later problems. The early years of a child's life are, as such, an important window of opportunity for both primary and secondary preventive approaches aimed at optimizing parenting, and preventing early parent–child relationship problems.

This chapter will start by examining the nature and prevalence of early regulatory problems, and will describe two key models that have been developed to explain their development. It will go on to examine some of the main universal and targeted intervention approaches that have been developed to address such problems, and the evidence about their effectiveness in improving outcomes for both parents and children. The chapter will conclude by examining key workforce skills and training issues. Although this chapter hasn't included a review of methods of identification, all child health programmes involve a range of statutory visits that begin in pregnancy and are most frequent during the early years. These are the first and most crucial step in the provision of both universal and targeted services, primarily because they provide a key opportunity to offer universal support to parents without stigma, but also to identify and intervene with families who may be in need of additional input. It is, as such, highly important that all families receive these visits.

Nature and prevalence of mental health problems in early childhood

Mental health in infancy and childhood refers to the capacity of the child to achieve optimal social, emotional, and behavioural functioning, and is underpinned by the child's developing capacity during the early years of life to regulate their emotional states, and to develop trusting relationships with the individuals around them.

In terms of development in very early childhood, infant regulatory disturbances, such as excessive crying, feeding or sleeping difficulties, and bonding/attachment problems are common, and are one of the major reasons for seeking professional support (Smart and Hiscock, 2007; St James-Roberts and Peachey, 2011) as well as being the main reasons for referral to infant mental health clinics (Keren et al., 2001), and a significant source of parental distress (Smark and Hiscock, 2007). The Copenhagen Child Cohort Study (including 6090 infants) found a population prevalence of such regulatory problems (including emotional and behavioural, eating, and sleeping disorders) in children aged 1.5 years in the region of 18% (Skovgaard et al., 2008; Skovgaard, 2010). Although many of these problems are developmental and, as such, resolve over time, a high proportion are stable over time, with one study suggesting that as many as 49.9% of infants and toddlers (aged 12–40 months) show a continuity of emotional and behavioural problems 1 year after initial presentation (Briggs-Gowan et al., 2006). Problems of this nature can also be significant predictors of longer-term difficulties including delays in motor, language, and cognitive development, and continuing parent–child relational problems (DeGangi et al., 2000). Difficult temperament, non-compliance, and aggression in infancy and toddlerhood (aged 1–3 years) are associated with internalizing and externalizing psychiatric disorders at 5 years of age (Keenan et al., 1998). Insecure attachment in infancy is also associated with less optimal outcomes in childhood across a range of domains such as emotional, social and behavioural adjustment, school achievement, and social status with peers (Sroufe, 2005), while disorganized attachment is associated with later psychopathology, including externalizing (Fearon et al., 2010), and personality disorders (Steele et al., 2010).

Studies of the prevalence of behaviour problems in preschool children, using cut-off scores on standardized measures to define the disorder, show that approximately 10–15% of children have mild to moderate problems (Campbell, 1995). Aggressiveness, conduct problems, and antisocial behaviours are also the most frequent cause of child and adolescent clinical referral encompassing between one-third to one-half of all child and adolescent clinic referrals (Kazdin et al., 1992). In addition to having a high prevalence, behaviour problems are stable over time (e.g. Rutter, 1996).

Epidemiology of early child mental health problems

The Copenhagen Child Cohort Study found that early childhood emotional and behavioural problems can best be understood in a relational context, and that disturbances to the parent–child relationship and parental psychosocial adversity are significant risk factors for early emotional, behavioural, eating, and sleeping disorders (Skovgaard et al., 2008; Skovgaard, 2010).

Two models have been developed to explain this. The first is underpinned by social learning theory, which posits a relationship between coercive parenting practices (originally developed by Patterson et al., 1989) and child emotional and behavioural problems. For example, parenting practices characterized by parental monitoring, psychological control, and negative behaviours such as rejection and hostility, have been shown to be associated with an increased risk of a range of poor outcomes, including delinquency and substance abuse (Hoeve et al., 2009).

The second model, which is underpinned by attachment theory, suggests that many of the family correlates of aggressive child behaviour are present in infancy before the onset of the type of coercive cycles described above (Lyons-Ruth, 1996). For example, insecure and disorganized attachment status are common at 12 months of age and are strongly associated with significant behavioural problems (Fearon and Silver, 2010). A range of parental behaviours have been identified as being important in terms of infant attachment security, including parental sensitivity (De Wolff and van IJzendoorn, 1997); the specific nature or quality of the attunement or contingency between parent and infant (Beebe et al., 2010); the parent's capacity for what has been termed 'maternal mind-mindedness' (Meins et al., 2001) or 'reflective function' (Slade et al., 2001); and a range of atypical or anomalous parenting behaviours (Madigan et al., 2006).

A range of factors have been found to influence parenting capacity including poverty (Katz et al., 2007) and psychosocial factors (e.g. Skovgaard et al., 2008; Skovgaard, 2010) (e.g. parental mental health problems and domestic violence).

Interventions to promote parent–child interaction, and children's social and emotional development

[+]A range of approaches have been developed to promote the mental health of young children either by improving the well-being and functioning of their parents or the relationship between parents and their children. These can be delivered as part of universal (primary prevention) or targeted/indicated (secondary/tertiary prevention) approaches, by practitioners such as health visitors during home visits, or in child health clinics and children's centres. They have been categorized below according to the main method of administration (i.e. media, self-administered, dyadic, one-to-one, and group based). The following section does not cover preparation for parenthood programmes, which are described fully in Chapter 7, programmes targeting parental

---

[+] Section adapted with permission from Axford N. et al. *The Best Start at Home: A Report on what works to improve the quality of parent-child interactions from conception to age 5.* Early Intervention Foundation. Copyright © 2015. Available from http://www.eif.org.uk/publication/the-best-start-at-home/.

mental health problems, which are described in Chapter 5 and group-based parenting programmes, which are discussed only briefly here but more fully in Chapter 8.

Most of the available evidence regarding the effectiveness of the interventions described below has been evaluated in terms of outcomes for mothers, or using mother-reported data about the child. However, a review of studies that have examined the effectiveness of these programmes (including infant massage, observation and modelling of behaviour with infant, kangaroo care, participation with child in a preschool programme, discussion groups, and parent training programmes) with fathers (Magill-Evans et al., 2006), found that interventions that involve active participation with or observation of the father's own child can be effective. Other methods for engaging and retaining fathers in programmes have also been identified (http://www.academia.edu/3522325/Fathers_and_Parenting_Interventions_-_what_works).

Media-based programmes

[+]Over the past decade, a range of media-based methods have been developed to provide information to parents during the first few years of life. Media-based information for parents involves the delivery of written materials (e.g. a regular newsletter or resource pack), tailored to the child's age, and/or screen-based material (DVD/video) with related learning materials. A range of approaches have been developed including newsletters (e.g. Baby Express) and their embedding within an assertive outreach model that involves home visiting (Baby Express Outreach) (C4EO, 2017) and the use of books and DVDs (e.g. *The Social Baby*) (Cooper et al., 2009). Newly developed approaches include websites (e.g. Getting to Know Your Baby) and apps (e.g. Baby Buddy).

Universal (level 1) Triple P also involves the use of media and informational strategies (e.g. newspaper and local radio articles), informational flyers, and brochures, which can be distributed widely to community centres, advocacy organizations, and individual family households.

Evidence for the impact of *universal media-based strategies* on attachment and parental sensitivity and responsiveness is limited due to a lack of evaluation and equivocal results from the few evaluations that exist. One randomized controlled trial (RCT) of an intervention involving the dissemination of newsletters (Baby Express) found improvement for some aspects of early parenting (perceived hassles, appropriate expectations) that are associated with attachment security, but no impact on parental empathy towards the child's needs (Waterston et al., 2009). The Triple P universal programme has also been found to be effective in reducing population levels of abuse (Prinz et al., 2009).

Self-administered programmes

[+]A number of both universal (e.g. Triple P (Prinz et al., 2009)) and targeted (e.g. Incredible Years (Webster-Stratton et al., 1988)) programmes offer self-administered

---

[+] Section adapted with permission from Axford N. et al. *The Best Start at Home: A Report on what works to improve the quality of parent-child interactions from conception to age 5.* Early Intervention Foundation. Copyright © 2015. Available from <http://www.eif.org.uk/publication/the- best-start-at-home/>.

versions. For example, targeted programmes such as Incredible Years include the use of videotape modelling in which filmed actors model good and bad parenting practices. There is systematic review-level evidence to show that *self-administered parenting programmes* can have the level of benefit attributed to more intensive therapist-led interventions (O'Brien and Daley, 2011).

Dyadic

[+]Dyadic programmes (e.g. attachment and psychodynamic/mentalization-based interventions) are characterized by the fact that they work with both the parent and child together (i.e. rather than working with the parent or child on their own) and are of two main types (i.e. attachment and psychotherapeutic/mentalisation-based approaches).

Attachment-based dyadic programmes

[+]Dyadic programmes are typically used as part of a targeted/indicated approach with parents who are experiencing problems in terms of sensitivity and/or attachment, and some can be used both with infants and older children. They are characterized by the use of live demonstration with the parent and infant/child (e.g. infant massage) concerned in order to increase parental sensitivity, and ultimately infant attachment security. They aim to help parents become aware of their infant's or child's developmental and interactive capabilities with a view to enhancing parental responsiveness.

Other programmes in this category involve the use of video feedback techniques, and include VIPP/VIPP-SD (Video feedback Intervention to promote Positive Parenting/ and Sensitive Discipline) (Van Zeijl et al., 2006), Circle of Security (Cassidy et al., 2011), and Attachment and Biobehavioural Catchup (Lind et al., 2014). Video feedback generally involves a professional videotaping up to 10 minutes of interaction between the carer and baby/child, returning subsequently to examine the tape with the parent, and using the videotape to point out examples of positive parent–infant interaction. VIPP-SD includes sessions that focus on the delivery of sensitive discipline (e.g. Van Zeijl et al., 2006). There is systematic review-level evidence to support the use of video feedback particularly in terms of its impact on parenting behaviours including parental sensitivity (Fukkink, 2008), although the evidence about its impact on attachment is less strong. There is also evidence from a number of RCTs regarding the effectiveness of VIPP (e.g. Velderman et al., 2006) and VIPP-SD (e.g. Van Zeijl et al., 2006).

Attachment and Biobehavioural Catchup has also been found to be effective in a small number of RCTs in terms of attachment in the short term (Bernard et al., 2012) and improvements in negative affect expression in parents, lower overall levels of anger, lower levels of anger towards the parent, and lower levels of global anger/ sadness on the part of the child (Lind et al., 2014). There is currently limited rigorous evidence on the group-based version of Circle of Security, but a study of its use on an individual basis showed improved attachment organization but only for infants identified as being irritable at baseline (Cassidy et al., 2011).

[+] Section adapted with permission from Axford N. et al. *The Best Start at Home: A Report on what works to improve the quality of parent-child interactions from conception to age 5.* Early Intervention Foundation. Copyright © 2015. Available from <http://www.eif.org.uk/publication/the- best-start-at-home/>.

Parent–Child Interaction Therapy (Chaffin et al., 2004) also works with the parent and child together and is also used with parents experiencing significant social problems. It involves two components that focus on basic interactions and that utilize *in vivo* techniques to support the parent's interaction with the child. A number of evaluations have demonstrated the effectiveness of parent–child interaction therapy (e.g. Chaffin et al., 2004).

Psychotherapeutic/mentalization-based programmes

[+]Parent–infant psychotherapy can be used with parents who are reporting problems with bonding or the infant having problems with feeding or sleeping, or the treatment of mothers experiencing mental health problems. Early models of parent–infant/child psychotherapy were known as 'representational' and focused on the development of a supportive relationship with the therapist and discussions based on what the therapist observed in the interaction between the parent and baby, to increase the parents' understanding about the way in which past relationships have influenced their current relationship with the child.

More recent approaches have been modified to include behavioural 'infant-led' components that encourage the parent to 'Watch, Wait, Wonder' about their infant's play and interactions, and to follow the infant's lead (Cohen et al., 1999). The therapist works at representational and interactional levels through observation and comments to help the mother clarify and alter distorted perceptions, and to link current experience with the mother's childhood experience. Some parent–child psychotherapy programmes have also incorporated the use of video feedback (e.g. the Anna Freud Centre Parent Infant Project). Parent–child psychotherapy interventions can also be used with children who have experienced traumatic events such as abuse, violence, or bereavement, and who are consequently experiencing behaviour, attachment, or mental health problems including post-traumatic stress disorder (e.g. Child Parent Psychotherapy) (e.g. Lieberman et al., 2005).

Parent–infant/child psychotherapy is mostly clinic-based, although it can be home-based, or delivered in other settings (e.g. the Anna Freud Parent Infant Project has been delivered in children's centres, hospitals, and a homeless hostel). It is provided during 60–90-minute sessions that take place over the course of 5–12 sessions, although the programmes are adapted to meet the needs of individual parent–child pairs (dyads) and may, as such, continue for much longer (e.g. up to a year). Parent–child psychotherapy is led by a psychotherapist who receives regular (weekly) supervision.

There is good evidence regarding the effectiveness of dyadic methods of working. In terms of *parent–infant/toddler psychotherapy* a systematic review found that there is some evidence to suggest that it is effective in improving infant attachment security in high-risk families although there was no evidence of effectiveness in improving other outcomes (e.g. parental depression) (Barlow et al., 2015).

[+] Section adapted with permission from Axford N. et al. *The Best Start at Home: A Report on what works to improve the quality of parent-child interactions from conception to age 5.* Early Intervention Foundation. Copyright © 2015. Available from <http://www.eif.org.uk/publication/the- best-start-at-home/>.

A second type of programme in this category is mentalization-based programmes that are aimed primarily at improving the mother's capacity for reflective functioning (i.e. her ability to think about and understand her child's behaviour in terms of their internal feeling states). Minding the Baby, for example, is a manualized, mentalization-based, interdisciplinary home visiting programme delivered by two specially trained practitioners (a nurse and a social worker) in the home setting over an extended period; mothers are visited for an hour a week beginning in the third trimester of pregnancy through to the child's first birthday, at which point visits take place bi-weekly through to the child's second birthday. Session length can vary based on each family's need (Sadler et al., 2013). Clinicians support reflective parenting, promote the mother–infant attachment relationship, and model and foster a range of parenting skills.

There is also evidence from a limited number of RCTs to support the use of mentalization-based programmes such as Minding the Baby. A study of the newly developed Minding the Baby programme found improved attachment status in the intervention group (i.e. more secure and less disorganized) although no improvements in reflective functioning (Sadler et al., 2013).

Home visiting programmes

[+]Over 250 evaluations of named home visiting programmes for pregnant women and families with children aged 0–5 years have been published in English since 1989 (Paulsell et al., 2010). They range widely in their approach in terms of their content/curriculum, duration, and underpinning theory (Boller, 2012). Core features of such early childhood home visiting programmes, are an intensive series of home visits beginning prenatally (e.g. Family Nurse Partnership or soon after the child's birth (e.g. Family Action) and continuing during the child's first 2 years of life. They are typically delivered by specially trained personnel—usually professionals but sometimes volunteers, who provide information, support, and training regarding child health, development, and care. Programmes vary in terms of the issues they address, being largely driven by their theoretical underpinnings. Common themes include early infant care, infant health and development, and parenting skills, but they may also include maternal health and well-being, diet, smoking, drug/alcohol use, exercise, transition to parenthood, and the parent's relationship with their partner. Overall, the programmes place a strong emphasis on building a good relationship within the family, tailoring the intervention to the needs of the family, and developing the parents' social support network.

Numerous systematic reviews have summarized the available evidence on the effectiveness of home visiting programmes, most of which conclude overall that the impact of home visiting is variable, with some programmes showing no evidence of effectiveness, and other programmes being effective for some outcomes (see http://pediatrics.aappublications.org/content/101/3/486). The Nurse Family Partnership programme is possibly one of the best-evidenced programmes to date.

[+] Section adapted with permission from Axford N. et al. *The Best Start at Home: A Report on what works to improve the quality of parent-child interactions from conception to age 5.* Early Intervention Foundation. Copyright © 2015. Available from <http://www.eif.org.uk/publication/the- best-start-at-home/>.

One-to-one parenting programmes (including crying and sleeping interventions)

[+]The evidence suggests that most infants wake during the night, but that younger infants (e.g. under 6 months) tend to require parental intervention, while older infants are more capable of self-soothing (Goodlin-Jones et al., 2001). Good practice is now recognized to include supporting parents to develop a bedtime routine as early as 6–8 weeks of age that involves a regular set of activities (e.g. bath, book, lullaby, gentle massage, and kissing goodnight; https://www.babycentre.co.uk/a553895/bedtime-routines-for-babies). In addition, a number of behaviourally based sleeping interventions have been developed with the aim of supporting parents experiencing difficulty in this area. A behavioural sleep intervention involves teaching the parent to implement one or more of the following practices: delayed response to infant signals or cues (i.e. 'graduated extinction', controlled crying, and gradual retreat, which all involve variations of the requirement for parents to leave their children alone for strictly timed intervals, ignoring any protests and cries), regulation of feed times, algorithms for sleep durations and bedtimes, or other strategies, all of which aim to condition the infant to fall asleep in the absence of feeding or bodily contact with the carer (Douglas and Hill, 2013). Concern about the use of these approaches has focused on the potential impact on both the infant's attachment development, which requires responsiveness to infant distress, and their stress response system, which also requires adult input to help reduce cortisol levels (see below for further discussion). Findings from the most recent systematic review suggest that controlled crying and gradual retreat are successful in treating infant sleep disturbances, with gradual retreat causing the least distress in the child; and that there is some evidence that learning about these techniques can also be successfully delivered in a group setting (Mancz and Wigley, 2017) and using the internet (Mindell, 2011). There is also evidence that these brief interventions can have a significant positive impact on maternal mood, and as such should be targeted at high-risk groups, and that where improvements in child sleep duration were achieved, a positive impact on child body mass index, nutrition, and physical activity was also observed (Yoong et al., 2016).

The above research also found, however, that unmodified extinction techniques should not be used because of the distress caused and the high parental dropout, and that when examining physiological cues in infants undergoing even modified extinction techniques, cortisol levels continued to be elevated after behavioural cues had reduced, and the authors suggest that further research is on this important topic is undertaken (Yoong et al., 2016). A further overview of systematic reviews (Field, 2017) identified two reviews that focus explicitly on infants under 6 months (Douglas and Hill, 2013; Chrichton and Symon, 2016), and one focusing on both prevention and treatment in infants less than 12 months. While Chrichton and Symon (2016) conclude based on 11 studies that 8 showed evidence of improved sleep outcomes, Douglas and

---

[+] Section adapted with permission from Axford N. et al. *The Best Start at Home: A Report on what works to improve the quality of parent-child interactions from conception to age 5.* Early Intervention Foundation. Copyright © 2015. Available from <http://www.eif.org.uk/publication/the- best-start-at-home/>.

Hill (2013) are critical of this body of literature concluding that studies showing evidence of effectiveness in infants under 6 months have failed to identify and control for issues such as feeding difficulties, and that they also don't distinguish between the neurodevelopmentally different first and second halves of the first year of life.

The third review that included nine RCTs evaluating the effectiveness of preventive ($n = 7$) and treatment interventions ($n = 2$ including behavioural techniques such as controlled crying) with infants less than 12 months, found overall improvement in sleep time, but not in night wakings (Kempler et al., 2016).

This evidence is as such confusing, particularly with regard to infants less than 12 months of age, and there is some evidence of adverse consequences in terms of cortisol, and a lack of evidence about the impact of such behavioural techniques on attachment security. For example, with regard to the latter, research suggests that more infants who are insecure resistant (anxious) experience more night wakings compared with insecure avoidant children, and are more likely to develop sleep problems (McNamara et al., 2003). The use of behavioural interventions could arguably contribute to the maintenance of such problems.

Most experts recommend that parents are helped to find techniques that meet their own needs in terms of stress and sleep, and tolerance for leaving an infant crying. In terms of the latter, for example, the 'no cry techniques' involve rocking and feeding the infant to sleep, with the parent providing comforting responses to crying including night wakings (https://sleeplady.com/baby-sleep/sleep-training-methods-demystified/). Good practice should involve the use of this type of routine with all young children (i.e. less than 12–15 months of age), with the introduction of other behavioural techniques, if and when this doesn't work.

In terms of young children, there is moderate-level evidence to support the use of behavioural interventions for paediatric insomnia, but low level evidence for older children, adolescents, and those with special needs (Meltzer and Mindell, 2014). The most recent review of interventions for children aged 1–12 years concluded that there was evidence to support the use of age-appropriate bedtimes, schedules, and routines; limiting access to electronics during and after bedtime; and support of children needing to learn to settle to sleep in their own beds without parents (Allen et al., 2016).

The reasons for excessive crying in early childhood are numerous and include circadian rhythm alterations, central nervous system immaturity, and alterations in the intestinal microbiota (Halpern and Coelho, 2016). A number of treatments have been described, including behavioural measures, manipulation techniques, use of medication, and acupuncture. However, the evidence for most of these is inconclusive (Halpern and Coelho, 2016). The Period of PURPLE Crying˚ is, however, an evidence-based prevention programme offered by the National Center on Shaken Baby Syndrome (NCSBS). The programme approaches the prevention of abusive head trauma, also known as shaken baby syndrome, by helping parents to understand normal infant crying and reduce incidence of shaken baby syndrome. The acronym *PURPLE* is used to describe specific characteristics of an infant's crying during this phase and let parents and caregivers know that what they are experiencing is indeed normal and, although frustrating, is simply a phase in their child's development that will pass. The word 'Period' is important because it tells parents that it is only temporary and will come to an end (http://purplecrying.info/what-is-the-period-of-purple-crying.php). The information can be shared at numerous time-points (e.g. prior to discharge from hospital, first and later postnatal visits by health visitors and/or general practitioners). An RCT of this programme found that it is effective in improving both parental knowledge and some behaviours that are thought to be important for the prevention of shaking in parents of newborn babies (Barr et al., 2009a, 2009b).

A number of other one-to-one parenting programmes are being delivered as part of targeted approaches. For example, Parents Under Pressure targets substance-dependent parents and utilizes the teaching of mindfulness strategies alongside a range of other parenting techniques, with the aim of improving parental functioning and parenting practices (Dawe and Harnett, 2007). The programme is underpinned by an ecological model that involves addressing wider problems (e.g. housing and finance). It has now been extended to include parents of children under 2 years of age (Barlow et al., 2012), and the 12 modules can be delivered flexibly over 12–20 weeks. One RCT found that the Parent Under Pressure programme produced improvements in parents' stress and methadone consumption, and in children's behavioural adjustment (Dawe and Harnett, 2007). A more recent RCT found that the Parents Under Pressure Programme produced improvements in the functioning of substance dependent parents of children under 36 months of age (Barlow et al., 2018).

Group-based parenting programmes

[+]Although possibly the best-known group-based parenting programmes are Incredible Years and Triple P, there are now a range of programmes that have been developed to meet the needs of different children in terms of age (e.g. under 3 years, 3–14 years, and adolescents) and problems (e.g. behavioural problems, attention deficit hyperactivity disorder (ADHD), autism, and disabilities). While many of the early parenting programmes were largely behavioural in orientation, many are now eclectic, drawing on a range of theories (e.g. attachment, cognitive behavioural therapy, and family therapy) in addition to social learning theory. They are still largely provided over 4–12 weeks in a variety of community-based settings, and by a variety of practitioners (e.g. health visitors, social workers, psychologists, etc.).

Evidence from a range of systematic reviews has confirmed that *group-based parenting training programmes* are effective in improving the emotional and behavioural adjustment of children aged 0–3 years (Barlow et al., 2015) and 3–14 years (Furlong et al., 2012). There is also evidence of their effectiveness in preschoolers at risk of ADHD (Charach et al., 2013) and older children with ADHD (Daley et al., 2014), and in improving a range of aspects of parental psychosocial functioning (Barlow et al., 2015).

[+] Section adapted with permission from Axford N. et al. *The Best Start at Home: A Report on what works to improve the quality of parent-child interactions from conception to age 5.* Early Intervention Foundation. Copyright © 2015. Available from <http://www.eif.org.uk/publication/the- best-start-at-home/>.

Workforce skills and training

+All of the interventions described in this chapter that involve direct work with families and children (e.g. not including media-based or self-directed programmes) require additional training and supervision on the part of the practitioner, the latter being an ongoing requirement while working with families. Most of the training programmes required for the delivery of these interventions are fairly brief, affordable, and accessible for existing practitioners (e.g. midwives, health visitors, nursery nurses, family centre workers, social workers, and psychologists) such as video-interaction guidance (https://www.videointeractionguidance.net/training), Parents Under Pressure (http://www.pupprogram.net.au/training--supervision.aspx), Circle of Security (https://www.circleofsecurityinternational.com/trainings) etc., although a few require to be delivered by specialist practitioners (e.g. parent–infant/child psychotherapy).

Learning links

- The Institute of Health Visiting have three e-learning modules on 'Infant Mental Health': https://ihv.org.uk/for-health-visitors/resources-for-members/resource/e-learning/infant-mental-health-e-learning-module-1/
- The Royal College of General Practitioners has an e-learning course on 'Child and Adolescent Mental Health': http://elearning.rcgp.org.uk/course/view.php?id=111
- Early Intervention Foundation Guidebook of early intervention: http://guidebook.eif.org.uk/.

Recommendations

- Prioritize early recognition and intervention by the universal services to support the development of healthy emotional regulation. (*Evidence: strong.*)
- Consider commissioning of primary and secondary preventive approaches to parents to address early problems (media-based and self-administered programmes, infant massage, video feedback, and parent–infant psychotherapy). (*Evidence: moderate.*)
- Consider targeting when based on early signals of risk in child development (targeted/indicated). (*Evidence: moderate.*)

+ Section adapted with permission from Axford N. et al. *The Best Start at Home: A Report on what works to improve the quality of parent-child interactions from conception to age 5.* Early Intervention Foundation. Copyright © 2015. Available from http://www.eif.org.uk/publication/the-best-start-at-home/.

References

Allen, S., Howlett, M., Coulombe, J., and **Corkum, P.** (2016). ABCs of sleeping: a review of the evidence behind pediatric sleep practice recommendations. *Sleep Medicine Review*, **29**, 1–14.

Axford, N., Sonthalia, S., Wrigley, Z., et al. (2015). The best start at home: what works to improve the quality of parent-child interactions from conception to age 5 years. [online] Early Intervention Foundation. http://www.eif.org.uk/wp-content/uploads/2015/03/The-Best-Start-at-Home-report.pdf.

Barr, R.G., Barr, M., Fujiwara, T., Conway, J., Catherine, N., and Brant, R. (2009a). Do educational materials change knowledge and behaviour about crying and shaken baby syndrome? A randomized controlled trial. *Canadian Medical Association Journal*, **180**, 727–733.

Barr, R.G., Rivara, F.P., Barr, M., et al. (2009b). Effectiveness of educational materials designed to change knowledge and behaviors regarding crying and shaken-baby syndrome in mothers of newborns: a randomized, controlled trial. *Pediatrics*, **123**, 972–980.

Barlow, J., Bennett, C., Midgley, N., Larkin, S., and Yinghui, W. (2015). Parent-infant psychotherapy for improving parental and infant mental health. *Cochrane Database of Systematic Reviews*, **1**, CD010534.

Barlow, J., Sembi, S., Parsons, H., Kim, S., Petrou, S., Harnett, P., Dawe, S.A. (2018). A randomized controlled trial and economic evaluation of the Parents under Pressure Program for parents in substance abuse treatment. *Drug and Alcohol Dependence,* **194**, 184–194.

Barlow, J., Smailagic, N., Ferriter, M., Bennett, C., and Jones, H. (2010). Group-based parent-training programmes for improving emotional and behavioural adjustment in children from birth to three years old. *Cochrane Database of Systematic Reviews*, **3**, CD003680.

Barlow, J., Smailagic, N., Huband, N., Roloff, V., and Bennett, C. (2012). Group-based parent training programmes for improving parental psychosocial health. *Cochrane Database of Systematic Reviews*, **6**, CD002020.

Beebe, B., Jaffe, J., Markese, S., et al. (2010). The origins of 12-month attachment: a microanalysis of 4-month mother-infant interaction. *Attachment & Human Development*, **12**, 3–141.

Bernard, K., Dozier, M., Bick, J., Lewis-Morrarty, E., Lindhiem, O., and Carlson, E. (2012). Enhancing attachment organization among maltreated children: results of a randomized clinical trial. *Child Development*, **83**, 623–636.

Boller, K. (2012). Evidence for the role of home visiting in child maltreatment prevention. [online] Encyclopedia on Early Childhood Development. Available at: http://www.child-encyclopedia.com/sites/default/files/textes-experts/en/912/evidence-for-the-role-of-home-visiting-in-child-maltreatment-prevention.pdf.

Briggs-Gowan, M.J., Carter, A.S., Bosson-Heenan, J., Guyer, A.E., and Horwitz, S.M. (2006). Are infant-toddler social-emotional and behavioral problems transient? *Journal of the American Academy of Child and Adolescent Psychiatry*, **45**, 849–858.

C4EO (2017). Centre for Excellence and Outcomes in Children and Young People's Services. [online] http://archive.c4eo.org.uk/themes/earlyyears/vlpdetails.aspx?lpeid=471 [Accessed 27 March 2017].

Campbell, S.B. (1995). Behaviour problems in preschool children: a review of recent research. *Journal of Child Psychology and Psychiatry*, **36**, 113–149.

Cassidy, J., Woodhouse, S.S., Sherman, L.J., Stupica, B., and Lejuez, C.W. (2011). Enhancing infant attachment security: an examination of treatment efficacy and differential susceptibility. *Development and Psychopathology*, **23**, 131–148.

Chaffin, M., Kelleher, K., and Hollenberg, J. (1996). Onset of physical abuse and neglect: psychiatric, substance abuse, and social risk factors from prospective community data. *Child Abuse & Neglect*, **20**, 191–203.

Chaffin, M., Silovsky, J.F., Funderburk, B., et al. (2004). Parent-child interaction therapy with physically abusive parents: efficacy for reducing future abuse reports. *Journal of Consulting and Clinical Psychology*, **72**, 500–510.

Charach, A., Carson, P., Fox, S., Ali, M.U., Beckett, J., and Lim, G. (2013). Interventions for preschool children at high risk for ADHD: a comparative effectiveness review. *Pediatrics*, **131**, 1584–1604.

Cohen, N.J., Muir, E., Lojksek, M., et al. (1999). Watch, wait, and wonder: testing the effectiveness of a new approach to mother-infant psychotherapy. *Infant Mental Health Journal*, **20**, 429–451.

Cooper, P.J., Tomlinson, M., Swartz, L., et al. (2009). Improving quality of mother-infant relationship and infant attachment in socioeconomically deprived community in South Africa: randomised controlled trial. *BMJ*, **338**, b974.

Crichton, G.E. and Symon, B. (2016). Behavioral management of sleep problems in infants under 6 months—what works? *Journal of Developmental and Behavioral Pediatrics*, **37**, 164–171.

Daley, D., van der Oord, S., Ferrin, M., et al. (2014). Behavioral interventions in attention-deficit/hyperactivity disorder: a meta-analysis of randomized controlled trials across multiple outcome domains. *Journal of the American Academy of Child and Adolescent Psychiatry*, **53**, 835–847.

Dawe, S. and Harnett, P. (2007). Reducing potential for child abuse among methadone-maintained parents: results from a randomized controlled trial. *Journal of Substance Abuse Treatment*, **32**, 381–390.

DeGangi, G.A., Breinbauer, C., Roosevelt, J.D., Porges, S., and Greenspan, S. (2000). Prediction of childhood problems at three years in children experiencing disorders of regulation during infancy. *Infant Mental Health Journal*, **21**, 156–175.

De Wolff, M.S. and van IJzendoorn, M.H. (1997). Sensitivity and attachment: a meta-analysis on parental antecedents of infant attachment. *Child Development*, **68**, 571–591.

Douglas, P. and Hill, P. (2013). Behavioral sleep interventions in the first six months of life do not improve outcomes for mothers or infants: a systematic review. *Journal of Developmental and Behavioral Pediatrics*, **34**, 497–507.

Fearon, R.P., Bakermans-Kranenburg, M.J., Van IJzendoorn, M.H., Lapsley, A.M., and Roisman, G.I. (2010). The significance of insecure attachment and disorganization in the development of children's externalizing behavior: a meta-analytic study. *Child Development*, **81**, 435–456.

Field, T. (2017). Infant sleep problems and interventions: a review. *Infant Behavior & Development*, **47**, 40–53.

Fukkink, R.G. (2008). Video feedback in widescreen: a meta-analysis of family programs. *Clinical Psychology Review*, **28**, 904–916.

Furlong, M., McGilloway, S., Bywater, T., Hutchings, J., Smith, S.M., and Donnelly, M. (2012). Behavioural and cognitive-behavioural group-based parenting programmes for early-onset conduct problems in children aged 3 to 12 years. *Cochrane Database of Systematic Reviews*, **2**, CD008225.

Goodlin-Jones, B.L., Burnham, M., Gaylor, E., and Anders, T.M. (2001). Night waking, sleep-wake organisation, and self-soothing in the first year of life. *Journal of Developmental and Behavioral Pediatrics*, **22**, 226–232.

Halpern, R. and Coelho, R. (2016). Excessive crying in infants. *Jornal de Pediatria*, **92**(3 Suppl. 1), S40–S45. Available at: http://www.scielo.br/pdf/jped/v92n3s1/0021-7557-jped-92-03-s1-0S40.pdf.

Hoeve, M., Dubas, J.S., Eichelsheim, V.I., van der Laan, P.H., Smeenk, W., and Gerris, J.R.M. (2009). The relationship between parenting and delinquency: a meta-analysis. *Journal of Abnormal Child Psychology*, **37**, 749–775.

Katz, I., Corlyon, J., Vincent La Placa, V., and Hunter, S. (2007). *The Relationship Between Poverty and Parenting*. York: Joseph Rowntree Foundation.

Kazdin, A.E., Siegel, T.C., and Bass, D. (1992). Cognitive problem-solving skills training and parent management training in the treatment of antisocial behavior in children. *Journal of Consulting and Clinical Psychology*, **60**, 733–747.

Keenan, K., Shaw, D., Delliquadri, E., Giovannelli, J., and Walsh, B. (1998). Evidence for the continuity of early problem behaviors: application of a developmental model. *Journal of Abnormal Child Psychology*, **26**, 441–454.

Kempler, L., Sharpe, L., Miller, C.B., and Bartlett, D.J. (2016). Do psychosocial sleep interventions improve infant sleep or maternal mood in the postnatal period? A systematic review and meta-analysis of randomized controlled trials. *Sleep Medicine Reviews*, **29**, 15–22.

Keren, M., Feldman, R., and Tyano, S. (2001). Diagnoses and interactive patterns of infants referred to a community-based infant mental health clinic. *Journal of the American Academy of Child and Adolescent Psychiatry*, **40**, 27–35.

Lieberman, A.F., Van Horn, P., and Ghosh Ippen, C. (2005). Toward evidence-based treatment: child-parent psychotherapy with pre-schoolers exposed to marital violence. *Journal of the American Academy of Child and Adolescent Psychiatry*, **44**, 1241–1248.

Lind, T., Bernard, K., Ross, E., and Dozier, M. (2014). Intervention effects on negative affect of CPS-referred children: results of a randomized clinical trial. *Child Abuse and Neglect*, **38**, 1459–1467.

Lyons-Ruth, K. (1996). Attachment relationships among children with aggressive behavior problems: the role of disorganized early attachment patterns. *Journal of Consulting and Clinical Psychology*, **64**, 64–73.

Madigan, S., Bakermans-Kranenburg, M., Van IJzendoorn, M., Moran, G., Pederson, D., and Benoit, D. (2006). Unresolved states of mind, anomalous parental behavior and disorganized attachment: a review and meta-analysis. *Attachment and Human Development*, **8**, 89–111.

Magill-Evans, J., Harrison, M.J., Rempel, G., and Slater, L. (2006). Interventions with fathers of young children: systematic literature review. *Journal of Advanced Nursing*, **55**, 248–264.

Mancz, G. and Wigley, W. (2017). Long-term outcomes of techniques used to manage sleep disturbance in the under-5s. *Journal of Health Visiting*, **5**, 16–24.

McNamara, P., Belsky, J., and Fearon, P. (2003). Infant sleep disorders and attachment: sleep problems in infants with insecure-resistant versus insecure-avoidant attachments to mother. *Sleep & Hypnosis*, **5**, 7–16.

Meins, E., Fernyhough, C., Fradley, E., and Tuckey, M. (2001). Rethinking maternal sensitivity: mothers' comments on infants' mental processes predict security of attachment at 12 months. *Journal of Child Psychology and Psychiatry*, **42**, 637–648.

Meltzer, L.J. and Mindell, J.A. (2014). Systematic review and meta-analysis of behavioral interventions for pediatric insomnia. *Journal of Paediatric Psychology*, **39**, 932–948.

Mindell, J.A., DuMond, C.E., Sadeh, A., Telofski, L.S., Kulkarni, N., and Gunn, E. (2011). Efficacy of an internet-based intervention for infant and toddler sleep disturbances. *Sleep*, **34**, 451–458.

O'Brien, M. and Daley, D. (2011). Self-help parenting interventions for childhood behaviour disorders: a review of the evidence. *Child Care, Health and Development*, **37**, 623–637.

Panter-Brick, C., Burgess, A., Eggerman, M., McAllister, F., Pruett, K., and Leckman, J.F. (2014). Practitioner review: engaging fathers – recommendations for a game change in parenting intervention based on a systematic review of the global evidence. *Journal of Child Psychology and Psychiatry*, **55**, 1187–1212.

Patterson, G.R., DeBa Ryshe, D., and Ramsey, E. (1989). A developmental perspective on antisocial behavior. *American Psychiatry*, **44**, 329–335.

Paulsell, D., Avellar, S., Sama Miller, E., and Del Grosso, P. (2010). *Home Visiting Evidence of Effectiveness: Executive Summary*. Princeton, NJ: Mathematica Policy Research.

Prinz, R.J., Sanders, M.R., Shapiro, C.J., Whitaker, D.J., and Lutzker, J.R. (2009). Population-based prevention of child maltreatment: the U.S. Triple P System population trial. *Prevention Science*, **10**, 1–12.

Rutter, M. (1996). Transitions and turning points in developmental psychopathology: as applied to the age span between childhood and mid-adulthood. *International Journal of Behavioral Development*, **19**, 603–626.

Sadler, L.S., Slade, A., Close, N., et al. (2013). Minding the Baby: enhancing reflectiveness to improve early health and relationship outcomes in an interdisciplinary home-visiting program. *Infant Mental Health Journal*, **34**, 391–405.

Sanders, M.R., Kirby, J.N., Tellegen, C.L., and Day, J.J. (2014). The Triple P-Positive Parenting Program: a systematic review and meta-analysis of a multi-level system of parenting support. *Clinical Psychology Review*, **34**, 337–357.

Skovgaard, A.M. (2010). Mental health problems and psychopathology in infancy and early childhood. An epidemiological study. *Danish Medical Bulletin*, **57**, B4193.

Skovgaard, A.M., Olsen, E.M., Christiansen, E., et al. (2008). Predictors (0–10 months) of psychopathology at age 11/2 years – a general population study in The Copenhagen Child Cohort CCC 2000. *Journal of Child and Adolescent Psychiatry*, **49**, 553–562.

Slade, A., Grienenberger, J., Bernbach, E., Levy, D., and Locker, A. (2001). Maternal reflective functioning and attachment: considering the transmission gap. In: *Proceedings of the Biennial Meeting of the Society for Research in Child Development, April 19–22*, Minneapolis, MN. Minneapolis, MN: Society for Research on Child Development.

Smart, J. and Hiscock, H. (2007). Early infant crying and sleeping problems: a pilot study of impact on parental well-being and parent-endorsed strategies for management. *Journal of Paediatrics and Child Health*, **43**, 284–290.

Sroufe, A.L. (2005). Attachment and development: a prospective longitudinal study from birth to adulthood. *Attachment and Human Development*, **7**, 349–367.

St James-Roberts, I. and Peachey, E. (2011). Distinguishing infant prolonged crying from sleep-waking problems. *Archives of Disease in Childhood*, **96**, 340–344.

Steele, H. and Siever, L. (2010). An attachment perspective on borderline personality disorder: advances in gene-environment considerations. *Current Psychiatry Reports*, **12**, 61–67.

Van Zeijl, J., Mesman, J., Van IJzendoorn, M.H., Bakermans-Kranenburg, M.J., Juffer, F., and Stolk, M.N. (2006). Attachment-based intervention for enhancing sensitive discipline in mothers of 1-to 3-year-old children at risk for externalizing behavior problems: a randomized controlled trial. *Journal of Consulting and Clinical Psychology*, **74**, 994–1005.

Velderman, M.K., Bakermans-Kranenburg, M.J., Juffer, F., Van IJzendoor, M.H., Mangelsdorf, S.C., and Zevalkink, J. (2006). Preventing preschool externalizing behavior problems through video-feedback intervention in infancy. *Infant Mental Health Journal*, **27**, 466–493.

Waterston, T., Welsh, B., Keane, B., et al. (2009). Improving early relationships: a randomized, controlled trial of an age-paced parenting newsletter. *Pediatrics*, **123**, 241–247.

Webster-Stratton, C., Hollinsworth, T., and Kolpacoff, M. (1988). Self-administered videotape therapy for families with conduct problem children: comparison with two cost-effective treatments and control group. *Journal of Consulting and Clinical Psychology*, **56**, 558–566.

Yoong, S.L., Chai, L.K., Williams, C.M., Wiggers, J., Finch, M., and Wolfenden, L. (2016). Systematic review and meta-analysis of interventions targeting sleep and their impact on child body mass index, diet, and physical activity. *Obesity (Silver Spring)*, **24**, 1140–1147.

Chapter 11

Promoting healthy nutrition

Charlotte M. Wright

Summary

This chapter:

- addresses the key nutritional issues affecting preschool children, of which breastfeeding has the greatest public health and practical significance, while complementary feeding is a common topic of concern

- addresses the two important potential micronutrient deficiencies in this age group: iron and vitamin D

- provides an overview of what constitutes a healthy diet and eating pattern in preschool children.

Sources of evidence

The evidence cited for this review, where possible, is to be found within existing national or international guidelines or evidence reviews. However, randomized trials in this discipline are scarce and thus most of the evidence underpinning even these documents still relies largely on observational studies and in some aspects on expert opinion.

Breastfeeding

Breast milk is the sole food required for the first 6 months of an infant's life and provides energy, via sugar (lactose), protein, and fat, as well as vitamins and minerals, though the exact composition varies with the infant's age, the stage of each feed, and maternal diet. However, it is also a complex biologically active substance which is vital for infant and maternal health.

The role of breast milk in supporting immunity and development

Breast milk could be said to act as the young infant's immune system, at a time when the infant's own immune system is immature. It confers passive immunity via immunoglobulin A, macrophages, T cells, stem cells, and lymphocytes. In addition, breast milk contains hundreds of other biologically active substances. For example, alpha-lactalbumin has both antibacterial and immunostimulatory properties, lacto-ferrin binds iron in competition with bacterial pathogens, and oligosaccharides se-lectively encourage the growth of beneficial (probiotic) organisms (Ballard and Morrow, 2013).

Because breast milk plays such an important immune protective role, even in high-income countries, infants fed with formula show increased rates of infection and mor-tality, and these effects are not explained by social class (Victora et al., 2016). There is also robust observational evidence of the role breast milk plays in gut maturation and healing, particularly in preterm infants, in the development of the brain, and the prevention of dental caries (Scientific Advisory Committee on Nutrition (SACN), 2018). In addition, breastfeeding protects the mother's health, by spacing pregnancies, aiding weight loss after birth, and reducing the risk of cancer of the breast and ovaries (Victora et al., 2016). This is why the World Health Organization (WHO) and all UK health departments recommend exclusive breastfeeding for around the first 6 months of life, as well as continued breastfeeding for at least 1 year, preferably for up to 2 years, as breast milk continues to provide immune protection for as long as breastfeeding continues.

Breastfeeding in the UK

After a low point in the 1970s, rates of breastfeeding in the UK rose and now around 80% of UK mothers give at least some breast milk initially. However, when last recorded in 2010, only around 40% of babies were still breastfed at the age 4 months and less than 1% were exclusively breastfed at 6 months (McAndrew et al., 2012). Thus, much more could be done to promote and protect ongoing breastfeeding (SACN, 2018).

Many mothers use formula milk as well as breastfeeding (mixed feeding) and this is strongly associated with premature cessation of breastfeeding (McAndrew et al., 2012). Because formula milk allows feeding in the absence of the mother, families tend to discount or disbelieve the risks associated with formula feeding and in particular the risk mixed feeding poses to the supply of breast milk. Thus, most children receive only a fraction of the potential protective benefits of breast milk that they need. This is a crucial equity issue, as less educated mothers or those living in poverty, are both less likely to start and to continue breastfeeding (Rollins et al., 2016). Mothers from Asian, black, and Chinese or other ethnic groups are more likely to breastfeed, though South Asian mothers tend to revert to formula feeding by 6 months (McAndrew et al., 2012).

Supporting successful lactation

Knowledge of how the production and supply of breast milk is controlled and how to recognize problems with feeding are essential in order to offer practical advice (Entwistle, 2013). Lactation depends upon milk production in the lactocytes, stimu-lated by prolactin, and its release due to secretion of oxytocin, both in response to stimulation of the nipple. As the breast fills, a feedback inhibitor secreted with the milk then inhibits milk production until the breast is emptied. Thus milk is only made and released in response to suckling. Skin-to-skin contact immediately after birth is vital for the initiation of lactation, as is keeping mother and baby together to allow unrestricted, frequent feeds (Demott et al., 2006).

The infant draws the milk out of the breast by drawing the nipple deep into the mouth and then emptying the breast by compressing rather than sucking on it (see Figure 11.1). Good positioning is essential to ensure effective milk removal and prevent painful suckling and nipple trauma. Prompt recognition of problems with attachment and issues such as tongue tie (see Chapter 21) can forestall problems (Demott et al., 2006). True lactation failure is very rare and most breastfeeding problems reflect difficulties with milk transfer or lack of stimulus for milk production. If unresolved these may lead to secondary lactation failure, particularly if mothers then 'supplement' with formula milk, which will further compromise their milk supply.

A sensitive, reciprocal, 'responsive' relationship between a mother and her baby is important, so that the mother can recognize her baby's feeding cues (Entwistle, 2013). Breastfeeding initially requires the mother to be near the baby 24 hours per day and is demanding (Wright et al., 2006), making support for new mothers essential in the weeks after birth. Health staff need to explain the value and importance of frequent, though often irregular, feeding, particularly overnight, and that breastfed babies cannot be overfed or 'spoiled' (Entwistle, 2013). The use of dummies is discouraged due to concern about creating 'nipple confusion', though limited trial evidence does not suggest that they are actually harmful to breastfeeding (Jaafar et al., 2016).

It is important to recognize that breastfeeding is a maternal and infant behaviour that has to be learned by the mother–infant dyad and this may be challenging in a culture where breastfeeding skills have been lost. Staff and parents need to accept that sometimes weight gain is slow at first, but be prepared to discount this against the long-term benefits of successfully establishing lactation, for this child, for the mother, and for future pregnancies (National Institute for Health and Care Excellence (NICE), 2017). Supplementary bottle feeding may allay short-term anxiety, but at a much greater long-term risk.

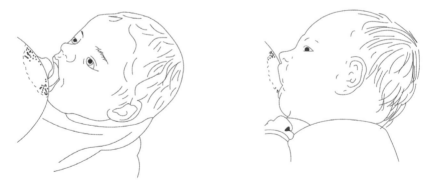

Fig. 11.1 Correct attachment pattern for successful breastfeeding.

Expressing breast milk

Expressing of breast milk (pumping) is an important aid to breastfeeding where for any reason direct milk transfer to the infant is not possible, as it empties the breast and promotes milk production. It can be done manually or using a hand or electric pump (Demott et al., 2006). In younger infants, expressing can be helpful where suckling is proving hard to establish and it is vital to express in parallel where the infant has to be artificially fed for any reason. Expressing is an increasingly important aid for when a mother goes back to work, as milk can be frozen for up to 6 months (Johns et al., 2013).

Formula feeding

When mothers choose not to breastfeed or to stop breastfeeding, they should use only infant formula meeting the compositional requirements of European Union legislation until the age of 1 year. Guidance regarding the safe preparation, storage, and handling of infant formula should always be followed. There is no evidence to support the use of follow-on milks (NHS Choices, 2016).

Complementary feeding

As infants grow, their nutrient requirements increase, and more nutrient-dense foods are required alongside breast milk. The transition from milk feeding to supplementary solid foods begins at around 6 months, but is not complete until after the age of 1 year and should complement, but not displace, breastfeeding. The term *weaning* is unhelpful, though still widely used in the UK, as it suggests stopping breastfeeding, rather than starting solid food.

The optimal timing of first solids

Until the age of 6 months, infants lack the developmental and motor skills required to sit up, swallow, and put food to the mouth and the supply of breast milk is sufficient to supply all nutritional requirements. In the early weeks, the gut and kidneys may not be sufficiently mature to handle the extra solute load. Beyond the age of 6 months, breast milk will not be able to keep pace with increasing energy requirements and stores of micronutrients such as iron are largely depleted, so that there is an increasing risk of micronutrient deficiency, reduced fat stores, and slow growth. If solids are given before 6 months, they displace rather than complement breast milk (Kramer and Kakuma, 2012).

In 2003, the WHO concluded that until 6 months the consequent loss of immune protection outweighed the potential nutritional benefits of solid feeding. While this was much disputed at the time, an updated review by the same authors found an even stronger evidence base and drew the same conclusions (Kramer and Kakuma, 2012). In the meantime, the consistent change in advice since 2003 has resulted in a substantial increase in the average age of first solids, with only a minority now starting before 4 months (McAndrew et al., 2012).

Once established, complementary foods should be offered two or three times per day initially, rising to three meals and two nutritious snacks per day by the age of 12–24 months. These will usually supply only around one-quarter of energy requirements at 6–8 months, rising to around two-thirds by 12–24 months (Dewey, 2003).

What foods to give

In the UK, most mothers start with a cereal such as baby rice or pureed fruit or vegetables. In fact, there is little evidence in favour of any particular foods and the WHO simply recommend 'a variety of foods to ensure that nutrient needs are met' and to give meat, fish, or eggs daily if possible (Dewey, 2003). UK recommendations are that these should have no added salt or sugar. Parents were previously advised to defer offering potentially allergenic foods, for fear of inducing allergy. However, recent trial evidence suggests that infants at risk of allergy are protected by exposure in the first year and that allergenic foods should be introduced one by one with weaning solids after the age of 6 months (SACN, 2018).

The early solid feeding period is an important opportunity to introduce children to a range of tastes and types of foods. It had been hypothesized that there was a critical period for the development of tastes and feeding skills around 4 months, but a recent review found no evidence for this (SACN, 2018).

Infants have an innate capacity to suck, swallow, and open and close their jaw in order to empty the breast, but in order to take solid foods they need to acquire more complex oromotor skills to allow them to move food around the mouth and chew. Traditionally, feeding starts with thin purees, with the consistency gradually increased to stimulate oromotor development. However, by around the age of 6 months most infants also have head and some trunk control and are beginning to hold objects and mouth them. Thus starting solids at the optimum age should allow more rapid progression onto family foods. At around 6 months most children can reach out for and attempt to feed themselves finger food (SACN, 2018). To avoid choking, these can be provided either in bite-sized pieces or in a form that can be held and bitten. Proponents of 'baby-led weaning' argue that by the age of 6 months infants can learn to feed solely by self-feeding and it has been suggested that that spoon feeding overrides the child's natural appetite, leading to obesity (SACN, 2018), but a recent trial found no protective effect against obesity, though it did lead to less food fussiness and greater participation in family foods and meals (Taylor et al., 2017).

Micronutrients

Vitamins and minerals are nutrients with essential functions in metabolism, tissue synthesis, and cell function. Most micronutrients have a dynamic relationship with the tissues using them, so that even where the level of the micronutrient can be measured in serum, an individual's true status can be hard to fully assess meaningfully. In practice, even apparently low-quality foods are rich in two of the micronutrients most essential for young children (vitamin A, zinc), so that in the UK, there are only two deficiency states that are found with any frequency: iron and vitamin D (SACN, 2018).

Iron deficiency

Iron is important for the synthesis of haemoglobin, but also for neurodevelopment. The iron content of breast milk is low (though highly bioavailable) but most infants have substantial iron stores at birth, so there is no need for dietary iron in the early weeks (Domellöff et al., 2014). By the age of 6 months, these stores are depleted and iron-containing complementary foods become important. Iron bound into haem from red meat and oil-rich fish is the most easily absorbed source of iron. Unbound iron is poorly absorbed, though absorption may be enhanced by vitamin C, for example, in fruit (SACN, 2010). In practice, the most common sources of iron for children are breakfast cereals and formula milks, which are fortified with non-haem iron (Lennox et al., 2013). Unmodified cow's milk is a very poor source of iron and children who drink a lot of milk to the exclusion of solid foods are at high risk of iron deficiency.

Thus in order to prevent iron deficiency, mothers should be advised to include meat, eggs, beans, pulses, and dried fruit into the complementary diet from 6 months of age. Vegetarians (NHS Choices, 2018a) should be able to obtain sufficient iron from non-meat sources. For most children there is no need to continue formula milk after the age of 1 year, but intake of unmodified (doorstep) milk should be restricted to no more than 500 mL per day.

Vitamin D

Vitamin D is particularly important for the growth and maturation of the skeleton, but unlike other vitamins, in natural circumstances it is predominantly synthesized in the skin by the action of sunlight containing ultraviolet B (UVB) radiation. However, where there is little sunlight exposure, or where the sunlight contain little UVB, as in Northern British winters, dietary sources become important (SACN, 2016). There are few natural food sources of vitamin D, but many foods eaten by infants and toddler are fortified with vitamin D, notably formula milk and margarine and some commercial baby foods (Lennox et al., 2013). Serum levels below the recommended lower limit (25(OH)D <25 nmol/L) have been found in up to 8% of children under 3 years and 24% of children aged 4–10 years (Lennox et al., 2013). However, symptomatic deficiency (rickets) is much less common and predominantly seen in children with low exposure to sunlight, in children with dark skins, and in children with limited diets (SACN, 2016). Supplementation with vitamin D has long been recommended for toddlers, but uptake has been consistently low (Lennox et al., 2013). A recent report now recommends vitamin D supplementation for all children from birth (SACN, 2016). Vitamin drops are provided free for children under 4 years of age in families eligible for Healthy Start. These also contain vitamin A, so should not be given to infants taking more than 500 mL of formula milk per day as there is a risk of vitamin A toxicity. It is particularly important to encourage vitamin D supplementation as well as outdoor activities in high-risk groups.

Calcium

A sufficient intake of calcium is required in order for vitamin D to be utilized. Most toddlers achieve ample intake of calcium from milk and dairy products. Children on a milk-free diet are at risk of calcium deficiency as well as potentially having difficulty meeting their energy requirements, therefore a milk-free diet should not be adopted without clear clinical indications. If this is truly required, the family should be referred for dietary advice (NICE, 2011).

Promoting a healthy diet

Preschool children have relatively high energy requirements (Dewey, 2003), so adult recommendations regarding a low-fat diet should not generally be adopted before the age of 2 years and semi-skimmed milk should not be introduced until 2 years of age. From the age of 2 years, children should gradually move to eating the same foods as the rest of the family, in the proportions shown in the Eatwell Guide (Gov. uk, 2016).

Young toddlers have small stomachs and still usually need three meals and two nutritious snacks per day (Dewey, 2003). However, grazing on sweet snacks or drinks between meals places children at risk of dental caries (NICE, 2008), becoming overweight (NICE, 2014), and may spoil the appetite and cause food refusal at meal times. Parents commonly report feeding behaviour problems in toddlers, but these are rarely associated with any limitations of weight gain or nutritional deficiency (Wright et al., 2007). Children commonly develop neophobia (avoidance of new foods) in the toddler years, but offers of small quantities of novel foods, repeated on several days, increase the likelihood of eventual acceptance (Hausner et al., 2012). The exact number of offers required will depend upon the palatability of the food and the tastes of the child.

A diverse intake of fruit and vegetables is associated with better adult health and exposing and familiarizing young children to fruit and vegetables at an early stage may help establish healthy eating habits. There is some evidence that early exposure leads to preferences that track over time, but also that some individuals are inherently more likely to like sour or bitter foods. Toddlers actually consume more vegetables than older children, suggesting that early exposure does not guarantee later intake (Lennox et al., 2013).

As with other behaviour issues, recognizing good eating behaviour and not overreacting to bad is the most effective approach. For more challenging problems, families can be advised to place a realistic limit on meal duration (20–30 minutes), reduce serving size, and leave the child to self-feed. Eating together with other children (e.g. at nursery) also helps model appropriate eating behaviour.

Parents of overweight children (for definitions please see Chapter 18) should be offered specific advice aimed at preventing further weight gain, via limiting portion sizes and reducing intake of high-energy foods as well as promoting physical activity (NICE, 2015). Parents who find it difficult to place limits on intake or who use food as a reward may benefit from a parenting programme or a family-based group child healthy weight programme, if these are available (NICE, 2013).

Table 11.1 Evidence-based advice for practitioners

Strong evidence	Moderate evidence	Good practice
Breastfeeding		
Recommend exclusive breastfeeding to age 6 month, continued for at least 1 year (Kramer and Kakuma, 2012)	Continued breastfeeding to age 2 years (SACN, 2018)	
Mixed breast and bottle feeding should be discouraged before 6 months (SACN, 2018)	If alternative feeds are necessary, mothers should express breast milk in parallel, to maintain milk supply (Entwistle, 2013)	
Complementary feeding		
Should be started at around 6 months (Kramer and Kakuma, 2012)	New foods should be reoffered on up to ten occasions (SACN, 2018)	Savoury vegetable foods recommended at first, with a range of textures and tastes (NHS Choices, 2018b)
Should include foods containing iron, such as meat, eggs, beans, pulses, and dried fruit (SACN, 2011)		Finger foods should be offered from 6 months, once a child is reaching out for food and can put food to the mouth (NHS Choices, 2018b)
Preventing iron and vitamin D deficiency		
Advise against the use of unmodified cow's milk as a drink before the age of 12 months (SACN, 2018)	Encourage the use of Healthy Start vitamins, particularly in children with low exposure to sunlight, dark skins, and limited diets (SACN, 2016)	
Toddler diet		
	Children aged 1–4 should be offered three meals and two nutritious snacks each day (Dewey, 2003)	Between ages of 2–5, children should progress to eating the same foods as the family, in the proportions shown in the Eatwell Guide (Public Health England, 2016)
Discourage sweet snacks and drinks between meals (SACN, 2015)	Where there are concerns about feeding behaviour, measure weight and height and calculate body mass index centile (see Chapter 18)	Families with children with body mass index >99.6th centile should be offered specific advice aimed at preventing further weight gain (see Chapter 18)

Learning links

- Healthy Child Programme, Module 8—'Growth and Nutrition': https://www.e-lfh. org.uk/programmes/healthy-child-programme/
- Institute of Health Visiting—'Healthy Weight Healthy Nutrition' e-learning modules: http://ihv.org.uk/for-health-visitors/resources/e-learning/
- Institute of Health Visiting—'Top Tips for Parents', factsheets with expert advice for parents: http://ihv.org.uk/families/top-tips/.

Recommendations

Commissioners

- Improve breastfeeding initiation by obtaining and maintaining breast-feeding initiatives, such as UNICEF Baby Friendly accreditation. (*Evidence: moderate.*)
- Ensure that services reflect national guidance, including regular and suitable training of staff. (*Evidence: moderate.*)

Practitioners

- Practitioners should follow the guidance in Table 11.1 as it reflects the current evidence of effectiveness. (*Evidence: moderate to strong.*)

References

Ballard, O. and Morrow, A.L. (2013). Human milk composition: nutrients and bioactive factors. *Pediatric Clinics of North America*, **60**, 49–74.

Demott, K., Bick, D., Norman, R., et al. (2006). *Clinical Guidelines and Evidence Review for Post Natal Care: Routine Post Natal Care of Recently Delivered Women and their Babies*. NICE Guideline. London: National Collaborating Centre for Primary Care and Royal College of General Practitioners.

Dewey, K. (2003). *Guiding Principles for Complementary Feeding of the Breastfed Child*. Washington, DC: Pan American Health Organization.

Domellöff, M., Bregger, C., Campoy, C., et al. (2014). Iron requirements of infants and toddlers. *Journal of Pediatric Gastroenterology and Nutrition*, **58**, 119–129.

Entwistle, F. (2013). The evidence and rationale for the UNICEF UK Baby Friendly Initiative standards. [online] UNICEF UK. Available at: https://www.unicef.org.uk/babyfriendly/wp-content/uploads/sites/2/2013/09/baby_friendly_evidence_rationale.pdf [Accessed 13 April 2018].

Gov.uk (2016). The Eatwell Guide. [online] Available at: https://www.gov.uk/government/publications/the-eatwell-guide [Accessed 26 Sep. 2017].

Hausner, H., Hartvig, D.L., Reinbach, H.C., Wendin, K., and **Bredie, W.L.P.** (2012). Effects of repeated exposure on acceptance of initially disliked and liked Nordic snack bars in 9-11 year-old children. *Clinical Nutrition*, **31**, 137–143.

Jaafar, S.H., Ho, J.J., Jahanfar, S., and **Angolkar, M.** (2016). Effect of restricted pacifier use in breastfeeding term infants for increasing duration of breastfeeding. *Cochrane Database of Systematic Reviews*, **8**, CD007202.

Johns, H.M., Forster, D.A., Amir, L.H., and **McLachlan, H.L.** (2013). Prevalence and outcomes of breast milk expressing in women with healthy term infants: a systematic review. *BMC Pregnancy and Childbirth*, **13**, 212.

Kramer, M.S. and **Kakuma, R.** (2012). Optimal duration of exclusive breastfeeding. *Cochrane Database of Systematic Reviews*, **8**, CD003517.

Lennox, A., Sommerville, J., Ong, K., Henderson, H., and **Allen, R.** (2013). *Diet and Nutrition Survey of Infants and Young Children, 2011*. London: Department of Health and Social Care.

McAndrew, F., Thompson, J., Fellows, L., Large, A., Speed, M., and **Renfrew, M.** (2012). *Infant Feeding Survey 2010*. London: The Health and Social Care Information Centre.

NHS Choices (2016). Types of infant formula. [online] Available at: http://www.nhs.uk/Conditions/pregnancy-and-baby/Pages/types-of-infant-formula.aspx#followon [Accessed 13 April 2018].

NHS Choices (2018a). Vegetarian and vegan babies and children. [online] Available at: https://www.nhs.uk/conditions/pregnancy-and-baby/vegetarian-vegan-children/ [Accessed 13 April 2018].

NHS Choices (2018b). Your baby's first solid foods. [online] Available at: https://www.nhs.uk/conditions/pregnancy-and-baby/solid-foods-weaning/ [Accessed 13 April 2018].

National Institute for Health and Care Excellence (NICE) (2008). Maternal and child nutrition. Public health guideline [PH11] (Last updated Nov. 2014). [online] Available at: https://www.nice.org.uk/guidance/ph11.

National Institute for Health and Care Excellence (NICE) (2011). Food allergy in under 19s: assessment and diagnosis. Clinical guideline [CG116]. [online] Available at: https://www.nice.org.uk/guidance/cg116.

National Institute for Health and Care Excellence (NICE) (2013). Weight management: lifestyle services for overweight or obese children and young people. Public health guideline [PH47]. [online] Available at: https://www.nice.org.uk/guidance/ph47.

National Institute for Health and Care Excellence (NICE) (2014). Obesity: identification, assessment and management. Clinical guideline [CG189]. [online] Available at: https://www.nice.org.uk/guidance/cg189.

National Institute for Health and Care Excellence (NICE) (2015). Preventing excess weight gain. NICE guideline [NG7]. [online] Available at: https://www.nice.org.uk/guidance/ng7.

National Institute for Health and Care Excellence (NICE) (2017). Faltering growth: recognition and management of faltering growth in children. NICE guideline [NG75]. [online] Available at: https://www.nice.org.uk/guidance/ng75.

Public Health England (2016). The Eatwell Guide [Online]. NHS Choices. Available at: https://www.nhs.uk/Livewell/Goodfood/Pages/the-eatwell-guide.aspx [Accessed 13 April 2018].

Rollins, N.C., Bhandari, N., Hajeebhoy, N., et al. (2016). Why invest, and what it will take to improve breastfeeding practices? *The Lancet*, **387**, 491–504.

Scientific Advisory Committee on Nutrition Scientific Advisory Committee on Nutrition (SACN) (2010). *Iron and Health*. London: Public Health England.

Scientific Advisory Committee on Nutrition (SACN) (2015). *The Scientific Advisory Committee on Nutrition Recommendations on Carbohydrates, Including Sugars and Fibre.* London: Public Health England.

Scientific Advisory Committee on Nutrition (SACN) (2016). *Vitamin D and Health.* London: Public Health England.

Scientific Advisory Committee on Nutrition (SACN) (2018). *Feeding in the First Year.* London: Public Health England.

Taylor, R.W., Williams, S.M., Fangupo, L.J., et al. (2017). Effect of a baby-led approach to complementary feeding on infant growth and overweight: a randomized clinical trial. *JAMA Pediatrics,* **171**, 838–846.

Victora, C.G., Bahl, R., Barros, A.J., et al. (2016). Breastfeeding in the 21st century: epidemiology, mechanisms, and lifelong effect. *Lancet,* **387**, 475–490.

Wright, C.M., Parkinson, K., and Scott, J. (2006). Breast-feeding in a UK urban context: who breast-feeds, for how long and does it matter? *Public Health Nutrition,* **9**, 686–691.

Wright, C.M., Parkinson, K.N., Shipton, D., and Drewett, R.F. (2007). How do toddler eating problems relate to their eating behavior, food preferences, and growth? *Pediatrics,* **120**, e1069–e1075.

Chapter 12

Promoting physical activity

Anna Chalkley and Lauren Sherar

Summary

This chapter:

- presents some of the current research on why physical activity is so important for our children's health
- describes the minimum amount of physical activity children need to maintain good health
- explores some of the factors influencing children's physical activity and how active children actually are.

Introduction

Physical activity is defined as any bodily movement produced by skeletal muscles that requires energy expenditure (Caspersen et al., 1985). It includes all forms of bodily movement such as everyday walking or cycling to get from one place to another, active recreation, household chores, as well as organized and structured activities such as competitive sport. Physical inactivity (not meeting physical activity guidelines) is a modifiable risk factor for a range of diseases including cardiovascular disease, type 2 diabetes, cancer (colon and breast), obesity, hypertension, osteoporosis and osteoarthritis, and depression (Warburton et al., 2006). As such, physical activity has been described as 'the best buy for public health' (Morris, 1994).

Of particular significance is the strong evidence of a dose–response relationship between physical activity disease and all-cause mortality (Warburton et al., 2006). That is, the greater the volume of physical activity undertaken, the greater the health benefits that are obtained (see Figure 12.1). From a population perspective, the greatest gains in public health will be achieved by helping those who are most inactive to become moderately active.

In addition to being physically active, there is also a growing awareness of and interest in the role of sedentary behaviour for health. Sedentary behaviour is not simply a lack of physical activity but is a cluster of sitting/reclining behaviours during waking hours which require low energy expenditure (Tremblay et al., 2017), for example, sitting while reading, watching television, using a computer, or travelling in

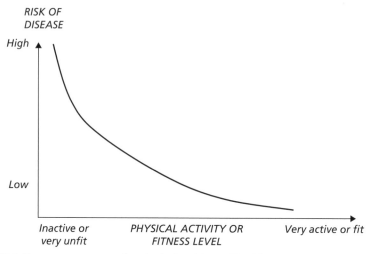

Fig. 12.1 Dose–response curve for physical activity and health.

Adapted from Department of Health, *At least 5 a week: Evidence on the impact of physical activity and its relationship to health. A report from the Chief Medical Officer*, © Crown Copyright 2004 under the Open Government Licence v3.0.

a car. Physical inactivity is not the same as being sedentary, indeed it is now well recognized that physical activity and sedentary behaviour can coexist, that is, an individual who is active and meets the recommendations for physical activity, can also accumulate a lot of time sitting for the remaining part of the day (Pearson et al., 2014). There is now good evidence to suggest that high amounts of sedentary behaviour during adulthood pose a distinct risk for a range of negative health outcomes including type 2 diabetes, cardiovascular disease, and all-cause mortality, regardless of participation in moderate-to-vigorous-intensity physical activity (MVPA) (Biswas et al., 2015).

Physical activity and health in children and young people

Given the opportunities and free choice, most young children will take part in active play which may involve hopping, chasing, jumping, dancing, skipping, climbing, and running. As children progress through childhood into adolescence, they are more likely to participate in formal (in clubs and teams) or informal ('pick-up' sports in the back garden, school playground, or in parks) organized sports. Strong evidence exists which shows that physical activity can play a major role in improving the future health and well-being of our children (Department of Health, 2004). The relationship between physical activity and physical health is now established beyond doubt with high-quality evidence from many international and large-scale reviews demonstrating the direct benefits of physical activity for children, such as improvements to cardiometabolic health and muscular strength (Physical Activity Guidelines

Advisory Committee, 2008), bone health (Macdonald et al., 2007), cardiorespiratory fitness (Physical Activity Guidelines Advisory Committee, 2008), and more favourable body composition (Janssen and Leblanc, 2010). Physical activity is an important feature of healthy development from birth, and inactivity is now recognized as a major public health concern, having been identified as the fourth leading risk factor for non-communicable diseases (Lee et al., 2012), many of which develop during childhood or adolescence.

While focus is placed on the physical health benefits of activity in children, a growing body of evidence exists relating to a wide variety of well-being outcomes. A rapid review from Public Health England (Chalkley et al., 2015) found strong evidence for a number of psychosocial outcomes in children and young people including self-esteem (Sallis et al. 2000; Cataldo et al., 2013); anxiety/stress (Biddle and Asare, 2011; Dimech and Seiler, 2011); academic achievement (Tremblay et al., 2000; Haapala, 2012; Booth et al., 2013); cognitive functioning (Sibley and Etnier, 2003; Biddle and Asare, 2011); attention/concentration (Trudeau and Shephard, 2008; Erwin et al., 2012); confidence (Wiersma and Fifer, 2008; Zarrett et al., 2009; Holt et al., 2011); and peer acceptance (Fitzgerald et al., 2012). Physical activity is thought to accelerate the development of many of these dimensions in a unique and comprehensive way.

Although not a focus of this chapter, it is worth noting that increases in children's sedentary behaviour is becoming an increasingly worrying public health issue. Interest in sedentary behaviour as a research area has grown since early studies of television viewing in children in the 1980s. Sedentary behaviour is particularly relevant in contemporary society with an increased lure of sedentary pursuits around technology (Ofcom, 2016) and perhaps heightened academic pressures. The importance of sedentary behaviour and its effect on health have been recognized and is reflected in the current national recommendations for physical activity (Department of Health, 2011).

A pervasive finding in the literature is that physical activity declines with age from childhood through adolescence and into adulthood, with boys being more active than girls at all ages (Klasson-Heggebø and Anderssen, 2003). Furthermore, there is evidence to support that active children will also be active in adulthood (Telama, 2009). Given the wide physical, psychological, and social benefits that physical activity affords, childhood is considered a uniquely important time and window of opportunity in the development or predispositions to be physically active, which will influence health status in later life.

Although schools and community settings have an important role in promoting physical activity in children and young people, family members, in particular parents, are important players (Taylor et al., 1994). Encouraging parents and carers to play and interact with their child from birth can help nurture a sense of well-being that is important throughout childhood and contributes to children's enjoyment of physical activity and promotes the value of parents as role models for activity (Vaughn et al., 2013). Furthermore, there is now strong evidence to suggest a bidirectional relationship between activity-related parenting practices and child physical activity with parents and children mutually influencing each other's behaviour (Sleddens et al., 2017).

Current recommendations for physical activity in childhood

While there are not enough data to produce definitive guidelines on the minimum amounts of physical activity that children need to gain particular health benefits, it is clear that all children should participate in certain types of physical activity from birth to improve their health. In 2011, the four Chief Medical Officers of the UK's *Start Active, Stay Active* report provided a set of age-specific guidelines pertaining to the minimum amount of physical activity needed by different population groups for health benefits (Department of Health, 2011). For the first time ever, these included guidelines specifically for children from birth to 5 years old as well as specific mention of reducing sedentary behaviour for all age groups (see Table 12.1).

These guidelines have been translated into a set of infographics for professionals to use when communicating directly with children and their families (see Figures 12.2 and 12.3).

Table 12.1 UK physical activity guidelines for children from birth to 18 years old

Children from birth to 5 years old	Children and young people 5–18 years old
For infants who cannot walk, physical activity should be encouraged from birth, particularly through floor-based play and water-based activities in safe environments	All children and young people should engage in moderate-to-vigorous-intensity physical activity for **at least 60 minutes and up to several hours every day**
For example, tummy time, crawling, rolling, reaching/grasping for objects, and pushing or pulling up against furniture	For example, brisk walking, cycling, dance, swimming, most sports
Children of preschool age who are capable of walking unaided should be physically active for **at least 180 minutes (3 hours) spread throughout the day**	Vigorous-intensity activities, including those that strengthen muscle and bone, should be incorporated at least 3 days a week
For example, walking, cycling, or scooting, active purposeful play, everyday tasks such as tidying up toys and helping to prepare for mealtimes	For example, gymnastics, skipping, jumping, climbing, aerobics, and most sports
All under-fives should minimize the amount of time spent being sedentary (being restrained or sitting) for extended periods	All children and young people should minimize the amount of time spent being sedentary (sitting) for extended periods
For example, minimizing the amount of time sat restrained in high chairs, push chairs, or baby walkers	For example, minimizing the amount of time spent lounging or sitting while watching TV, playing computer games, and on the computer

Adapted from Department of Health. *Start Active, Stay Active: A report on physical activity in the four home countries' Chief Medical Officers*, © Crown Copyright 2011 under the Open Government Licence v3.0.

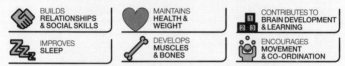

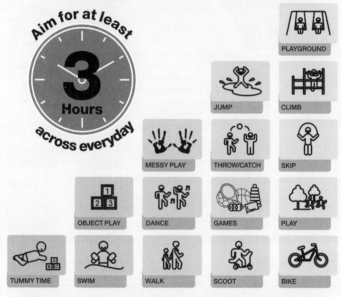

Fig. 12.2 UK Chief Medical Officers' physical activity infographic for the early years from birth to 5 years.

Reproduced from UK Government, *Start active, stay active: infographics on physical activity*, © Crown Copyright 2017, available from https://www.gov.uk/government/publications/start-active-stay-active-infographics-on-physical-activity, under the Open Government Licence v3.0.

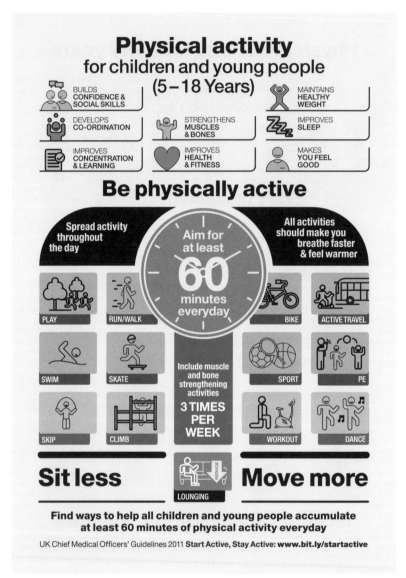

Fig. 12.3 UK Chief Medical Officers' physical activity infographic for children and young people (5–18 years).

Reproduced from UK Government, *Start active, stay active: infographics on physical activity*, © Crown Copyright 2017, available from https://www.gov.uk/government/publications/start-active-stay-active-infographics-on-physical-activity, under the Open Government Licence v3.0.

The Chief Medical Officers' physical activity guidelines and infographics should be used to:

- inform the professional development and training of those working with children and young people
- form the basis of any advice given to children, young people, and/or their parents/carers within different settings
- underpin the design and implementation of physical activity programmes
- provide a focus for campaigns designed to target children, young people, and their parents/carers
- inform educational materials (booklets, leaflets, mobile phone apps) and other forms of written and web-based advice and guidance for children, young people, and their parents/carers
- inform the marketing and promotion of local opportunities and programmes for children and their families.

When speaking to parents and carers, it is important to convey that at all ages (a) the benefits of being physically active outweigh the potential harm (risk); (b) some physical activity is better than none, but generally the more the better; and (c) by becoming more active throughout the whole day, in relatively simple ways, all children should be able to achieve the recommended physical activity levels.

Activity levels of children in the UK

Self-report is the most commonly used method to measure physical activity; its advantages are that it is easy to collect data from a large number of people at low cost. Indeed, all four home countries currently have a measure of physical activity included in their large-scale health surveys. Data from the most recent surveys are presented below, however it is worth noting that the measures used to assess and monitor children's physical activity across the UK are not aligned and therefore our ability to assess trends in activity over time and draw comparisons between the home countries is challenging and limited.

The most recent self-report data from the Health Survey for England (2015) found that, excluding school-based activities, 22% of children aged between 5 and 15 years met the physical activity guidelines. A higher proportion of boys than girls (23% and 20% respectively) were achieving at least 1 hour of MVPA per day. Of children aged 2–4 years of age, 9% (9% girls and 10% of boys) were achieving at least 3 hours of physical activity per day.

In Scotland, physical activity measurement is included in the Scottish Health Survey (Gov.scot, 2017) and includes a self-report measure of the proportion of children aged 2–15 years meeting the physical activity guidelines. The most recent data from the 2015 survey showed that 73% of children are meeting the physical activity recommendations when school-based activity is included. If excluded, this figure drops to 66%. The Scottish Health Survey, however, does not currently include a specific measure of physical activity for under-fives against the current physical activity recommendation.

In Wales, the 2015 Welsh Health Survey (Gov.wales, 2017) reported that 36% of children aged 4–15 years met the physical activity guidelines based on self-reported data. No data, however, is available for physical activity levels of under-fives.

In Northern Ireland, the latest available information comes from the 2017 Young Person's Behaviour and Attitudes survey (Foster et al., 2017) which provides self-reported information on sport and physical activity for children aged 11–16 years. It found that the number of young people who report attaining the physical activity recommendation has remained relatively stable since 2007, with boys twice as likely to attain this as girls (17% and 8% respectively). Unfortunately, there is no current measure of physical activity for children under five.

Collectively, these data indicate that there are still large numbers of children not participating in the recommended levels of physical activity across the UK and therefore losing out on the numerous benefits associated with activity. There is therefore still much work to be done to increase awareness of the physical activity guidelines and to identify and implement effective evidence-based interventions to increase levels of physical activity. Better surveillance measures providing a more accurate assessment of physical activity at a population level are needed to guide and inform the development of policies and programmes to increase activity levels.

Influences on physical activity in childhood

Children's physical activity is a complex, multidimensional behaviour influenced by a wide range of factors working at individual, social, family, and environmental levels. Other well-recognized influences include personal characteristics such as age, with younger children more likely to be active than older children or adolescents (Sallis et al., 2000). Indeed, there is now high-quality evidence from a recent longitudinal study which suggests children's total volume of physical activity is already declining by the age of 7 years in the UK (Reilly et al., 2017). Similarly, in almost all countries where objective measurement is available, sex has been identified as a correlate, with boys being consistently more active than girls (Sherar et al., 2011).

Children's physical activity has been shown to be associated with a number of demographic factors although the relationship between these demographic factors is not so clear. This may be in part due to the confounding effects of complexities in studying these variables and the lack of evidence relating to a UK context. For example, there is evidence that ethnicity is related to physical activity; the relationship is less consistent in children, with some weak evidence to suggest that white Caucasians are more active than other ethnic groups (Gustafson and Rhodes, 2006). Similarly, it is not clear whether there is a link between children's activity levels and socioeconomic status, while data has shown adolescents from higher socioeconomic groups tend to be more physically active than those from lower socioeconomic groups, with a 10% difference between low- and high-affluence households (Currie et al., 2012). However a number of social and economic factors mediate physical activity, resulting in marginalized groups being particularly disadvantaged in terms of access to opportunities to be physically active (Lee et al., 2009; Biddle et al., 2011). Furthermore, young children have relatively little control over their behaviours, therefore social and environmental characteristics are likely to be particularly important for this age group. Indeed, access to programmes and facilities such as parks, playgrounds, and green spaces as well as time spent outdoors have been shown to positively affect participation in physical activity (Ferreira et al., 2007; Sterdt et al., 2013).

Physical activity participation is affected (both positively and negatively) by the social support and role modelling provided by significant others; these include family and care givers, peers, friends, teachers, as well as health and exercise professionals. The family environment, in particular, is a key target for physical activity promotion as parents play an important role in the development of children's physical activity behaviours and attitudes (Trost and Loprinzi, 2011). Parents can influence children's physical activity through their own activity habits and their physical activity parenting behaviours such as modelling physical activity, facilitating opportunities for activity, and encouraging children to be active (Beets et al. 2010; Edwardson and Gorely, 2010).

Interventions to increase children's physical activity

Identifying and understanding the factors associated with physical activity also helps to focus the modifiable risk factors which could be targeted by interventions. Influencing these factors through well-designed programmes provides an opportunity to change behaviour and evidence suggests that behaviour change is more likely to be successful when multiple levels of influence are targeted at the same time and a multifaceted approach is adopted (Smith and Biddle, 2008). Addressing the widespread physical inactivity levels will require commitment to a combination of strategies and there is a clear need to educate, advise, motivate, and support children to be active in ways that are safe, accessible, and enjoyable (National Institute for Health and Care Excellence, 2009). Multicomponent interventions and 'whole-of-community' approaches have been identified as one of the seven best investments that work for physical activity (Global Advocacy for Physical Activity (GAPA) the Advocacy Council of the International Society for Physical Activity and Health (ISPAH) 2012).

Physical activity promotion efforts for children have predominantly focused on school-based programmes given their potential to address a broad range of public health issues and help children develop the knowledge, skills, and habits for healthy active living. There is some evidence to suggest that physical activity interventions are effective in increasing the number of children engaged in MVPA as well as how long they spend engaged in these activities (Kriemler et al., 2010). Similarly, a Cochrane review of 44 interventions (Dobbins et al., 2013) found some evidence to suggest effectiveness of school-based interventions in increasing duration of physical activity; however, the magnitude of the effect was relatively small. Despite this encouraging evidence, increases in physical activity, as a result of school-based approaches, do not always manifest in overall increases in daily levels of physical activity and they have largely been unsuccessful in increasing activity levels outside of the school setting. Therefore, there is increasing recognition of the importance of family- and community-level interventions involving multiple settings and sectors, focusing on where children and families live and spend their leisure time, in order to influence large numbers of people to be active.

Active travel, that is, walking, cycling, scootering, and any incidental activity associated with public transport, has been identified as the most practical and sustainable way to increase physical activity on a daily basis (Mackett and Brown, 2011) and can make a significant contribution to achieving the physical activity recommendation if embedded within a whole-of-community approach. Promoting and educating children and families about active travel and highlighting safe walking and cycling routes to and from early years settings, schools, and other popular destinations is an important way to establish active travel habits among children which will increase physical activity and benefit their health.

Conclusion

The past two decades have seen a noticeable increase in the quantity and quality of evidence linking physical inactivity and health outcomes in children. It is desirable that preventive measures, through encouraging and supporting physically active lifestyles, should begin early in life; however, economic and technological advancements have created an environment that discourages lifestyle physical activity and embraces sedentary behaviours, where the easy opportunities for children to be physically active are fast disappearing. Furthermore, marginalized groups are likely to be disadvantaged in terms of access to opportunities to be physical active. On a positive note, commitments are being made at many levels, reflecting an awareness of the importance of physical activity. However, as we move forward, only through multisectoral approaches and transformative and enlightened public policy regarding many facets of children's lives such as school curricula, transportation, safe play areas, and enhanced sports opportunities for all, will we see a halting/reversing of inactivity projections in the UK.

Learning links

- The Exercise and Health online module by the People's Open Access Education Initiative (Peoples-uni). Courses help healthcare professionals understand the size of the problem of physical inactivity, the role of physical inactivity in disease causation, and the benefits of exercise in treatment and prevention: http://ooc. peoples-uni.org/course/index.php?categoryid=3.

Recommendations

- Through increased advocacy work, raise awareness of the importance of physical activity from birth and the UK physical activity guidelines. (*Evidence: strong.*)
- Engage parents/carers and families in the planning and development of physical activity opportunities to ensure their needs are met and potential barriers can be addressed. (*Evidence: good practice.*)
- Consider providing training for healthcare professionals (e.g. health visitors and their support teams) and community partners (e.g. staff at children's centres)

on physical activity and how to promote and support physical activity in daily practice. (*Evidence: emerging.*)

♦ Provide safe, attractive, and accessible outdoor play facilities in local communities that facilitate physical activity for all children. (*Evidence: strong.*)

♦ Communicate the health and non-health benefits of physical activity for health and well-being and building self-esteem. (*Evidence: strong.*)

♦ Work with parents to identify opportunities during their daily routine to increase levels of physical activity and well as decrease their sitting time (e.g. by substituting passive activities with active ones such as walking rather than using the car or bus for short journeys). (*Evidence: good practice.*)

♦ Advise parents and carers about physical activity levels at the different stages of development (e.g. tummy time for non-walkers or energetic play for walkers). (*Evidence: good practice.*)

♦ Advise parents, carers, and their families on how to limit and reduce screen time. (*Evidence: good practice.*)

References

Beets, M.W., Cardinal, B.J., and **Alderman, B.L.** (2010). Parental social support and the physical activity-related behaviors of youth: a review. *Health Education & Behavior*, **37**, 621–644.

Biddle, S.J.H., Atkin, A.J., Cavill, N., and **Foster, C.** (2011). Correlates of physical activity in youth: a review of quantitative systematic reviews. *International Review of Sport and Exercise Psychology*, **4**, 25–49.

Biswas, A., Oh, P.I., Faulkner, G.E., et al. (2015). Sedentary time and its association with risk for disease incidence, mortality, and hospitalization in adults. *Annals of Internal Medicine*, **162**, 123–132.

Booth, J.N., Tomporowski, P.D., Boyle, J.M., et al. (2013). Associations between executive attention and objectively measured physical activity in adolescence: findings from ALSPAC, a UK cohort. *Mental Health and Physical Activity*, **6**, 212–219.

Caspersen, C.J., Powell, K.E., and **Christenson, G.M.** (1985). Physical activity, exercise, and physical fitness: definitions and distinctions for health-related research. *Public Health Reports (Washington, D.C.: 1974)*, **100**, 126–131.

Cataldo, R., John, J., Chandran, L., Pati, S., and **Shroyer, A.L.** (2013). Impact of physical activity intervention programs on self-efficacy in youths: a systematic review. *ISRN Obesity*, **2013**, 586497.

Chalkley, A., Milton, K., and **Foster, C.** (2015). *Change4Life Evidence Review: Rapid Evidence Review on the Effect of Physical Activity Participation Among Children Aged 5–11 Years.* London: Public Health England. Available at: https://www.gov.uk/government/uploads/system/uploads/attachment_data/file/440747/Change4Life_Evidence_review_26062015.pdf.

Currie, C., Zanotti, C., Morgan, A., et al. (2012). *Social Determinants of Health and Well-Being Among Young People. Health Behaviour in School-aged Children (HBSC) study: International Report from the 2009/2010 Survey.* World Health Organization Health Policy for Children and Adolescents, No 6. Geneva: World Health Organization. Available at: http://www.euro.who.int/en/health-topics/Life-stages/child-and-adolescent-health/publications/2012/social-determinants-of-health-and-well-being-among-young-people.-health-behaviour-in-school-aged-children-hbsc-study.

Department of Health (2004). *At Least Five a Week: Evidence on the Impact of Physical Activity and its Relationship to Health.* London: Department of Health. Available at: http://webarchive.nationalarchives.gov.uk/+/http://www.dh.gov.uk/en/Publicationsandstatistics/Publications/PublicationsPolicyAndGuidance/DH_4080994.

Department of Health (2011). *Start Active, Stay Active: Report on Physical Activity in the UK.* London: Department of Health and Social Care. Available at: https://www.gov.uk/government/publications/start-active-stay-active-a-report-on-physical-activity-from-the-four-home-countries-chief-medical-officers.

Dimech, A.S. and **Seiler, R.** (2011). Extra-curricular sport participation: a potential buffer against social anxiety symptoms in primary school children. *Psychology of Sport and Exercise*, **12**, 347–354.

Dobbins, M., Husson, H., DeCorby, K., and **LaRocca, R.L.** (2013). School-based physical activity programs for promoting physical activity and fitness in children and adolescents aged 6 to 18. *Cochrane Database of Systematic Reviews*, **2**, CD007651.

Edwardson, C.L. and **Gorely, T.** (2010). Activity-related parenting practices and children's objectively measured physical activity. *Pediatric Exercise Science*, **22**, 105–113.

Erwin, H., Fedewa, A., Beighle, A., and **Ahn, S.** (2012). A quantitative review of physical activity, health, and learning outcomes associated with classroom-based physical activity interventions. *Journal of Applied School Psychology*, **28**, 14–36.

Ferreira, I., van der Horst, K., Wendel-Vos, W., Kremers, S., van Lenthe, F.J., and **Brug, J.** (2007). Environmental correlates of physical activity in youth – a review and update. *Obesity Reviews*, **8**, 129–154.

Fitzgerald, A., Fitzgerald, N., and **Aherne, C.** (2012). Do peers matter? A review of peer and/or friends' influence on physical activity among American adolescents. *Journal of Adolescence*, **35**, 941–958.

Foster, A.C., Scarlett, M., and **Stewart, B.** (2017). *Young Persons' Behaviour and Attitude Survey 2016: Health Modules.* Belfast: Department of Health.

Global Advocacy for Physical Activity (GAPA) the Advocacy Council of the International Society for Physical Activity and Health (ISPAH) (2012). NCD prevention: investments that work for physical activity. *British Journal of Sports Medicine*, **46**, 709–712.

Gov.scot. (2017). The Scottish Health Survey 2015: Volume 1: Main Report. [online] Available at: http://www.gov.scot/Publications/2016/09/2764 [Accessed 25 Sep. 2017].

Gov.wales. (2017). Welsh Government/Welsh Health Survey. [online] Available at: http://gov.wales/statistics-and-research/welsh-health-survey/?lang=en [Accessed 25 Sep. 2017].

Gustafson, S.L. and **Rhodes, R.E.** (2006). Parental correlates of physical activity in children and early adolescents. *Sports Medicine (Auckland, N.Z.)*, **36**, 79–97.

Haapala, E. (2012). Physical activity, academic performance and cognition in children and adolescents. A systematic review. *Baltic Journal of Health and Physical Activity*, **4**, 53–61.

Holt, N.L., Kingsley, B.C., Tink, L.N., and **Scherer, J.** (2011). Benefits and challenges associated with sport participation by children and parents from low-income families. *Psychology of Sport and Exercise*, **12**, 490–499.

Janssen, I. and **LeBlanc, A.G.** (2010). Systematic review of the health benefits of physical activity and fitness in school-aged children and youth. *International Journal of Behavioral Nutrition and Physical Activity*, **7**, 40.

Klasson-Heggebø, L. and **Anderssen, S.A.** (2003). Gender and age differences in relation to the recommendations of physical activity among Norwegian children and youth. *Scandinavian Journal of Medicine & Science in Sports*, **13**, 293–298.

Kriemler, S., Zahner, L., Schindler, C., et al. (2010). Effect of school based physical activity programme (KISS) on fitness and adiposity in primary schoolchildren: cluster randomised controlled trial. *BMJ*, **340**, 785.

Lee, I.-M., Shiroma, E.J., Lobelo, F., et al. (2012). Effect of physical inactivity on major non-communicable diseases worldwide: an analysis of burden of disease and life expectancy. *Lancet*, **380**, 219–229.

Lee, R.E., Mama, S.K., Banda, J.A., Bryant, L.G., and **McAlexander, K.P.** (2009). Physical activity opportunities in low socioeconomic status neighbourhoods. *Journal of Epidemiology & Community Health*, **63**, 1021.

Macdonald, H.M., Kontulainen, S.A., Khan, K.M., and **McKay, H.A.** (2007). Is a school-based physical activity intervention effective for increasing tibial bone strength in boys and girls? *Journal of Bone and Mineral Research*, **22**, 434–446.

Mackett, R.L. and **Brown, B.** (2011). *Transport, Physical Activity and Health: Present Knowledge and the Way Ahead.* London: UK Transport Research Centre. Available at: https://www.ucl.ac.uk/news/pdf/transportactivityhealth.pdf.

Morris, J.N. (1994). Exercise in the prevention of coronary heart disease: today's best buy in public health. *Medicine and Science in Sports and Exercise*, **26**, 807–814.

National Institute for Health and Care Excellence (2009). *Physical Activity for Children and Young People.* London: National Institute for Health and Care Excellence. Available at: https://www.nice.org.uk/guidance/ph17.

Ofcom (2016). Children and parents: media use and attitudes report. [online] Available at: http://stakeholders.ofcom.org.uk/binaries/research/media-literacy/media-use-attitudes-14/Childrens_2014_Report.pdf [Accessed 25 Sep. 2017].

Pearson, N., Braithwaite, R.E., Biddle, S.J., van Sluijs, E.M., and **Atkin, A.J.** (2014). Associations between sedentary behaviour and physical activity in children and adolescents: a meta-analysis. *Obesity Reviews*, **15**, 666–675.

Physical Activity Guidelines Advisory Committee (2008). *Physical Activity Guidelines Advisory Committee Report 2008.* Washington, DC: US Department of Health and Human Services.

Sallis, J.F., Prochaska, J.J., and **Taylor, W.C.** (2000). A review of correlates of physical activity of children and adolescents. *Medicine and Science in Sports and Exercise*, **32**, 963–975.

Sherar, L.B., Griew, P., Esliger, D.W., et al. (2011). International children's accelerometry database (ICAD): design and methods. *BMC Public Health*, **11**, 485.

Sibley, B.A. and **Etnier, J.L.** (2003). The relationship between physical activity and cognition in children: a meta-analysis. *Pediatric Exercise Science*, **15**, 243–256.

Sleddens, E.F.C., Gubbels, J.S., Kremers, S.P.J., van der Plas, E., and **Thijs, C.** (2017). Bidirectional associations between activity-related parenting practices, and child physical activity, sedentary screen-based behavior and body mass index: a longitudinal analysis. *International Journal of Behavioral Nutrition and Physical Activity*, **14**, 89.

Smith, A.L. and **Biddle, S.** (2008). *Youth Physical Activity and Sedentary Behavior: Challenges and Solutions.* Champaign, IL: Human Kinetics.

Sterdt, E., Liersch, S., and Walter, U. (2013). Correlates of physical activity of children and adolescents: a systematic review of reviews. *Health Education Journal*, **73**, 1–18.

Taylor, W.C., Baranowski, T., and Sallis, J.F. (1994). Family determinants of childhood physical activity: a social cognitive model. In: Dishman, R.K. (Ed.), *Advances in Exercise Adherence*, pp. 319–342. Champaign, IL: Human Kinetics.

Telama, R. (2009. Tracking of physical activity from childhood to adulthood: a review. *Obesity Facts*, **2**, 187–195.

Tremblay, M.S., Aubert, S., Barnes, J.D., et al. (2017). Sedentary Behavior Research Network (SBRN) – Terminology Consensus Project process and outcome. *International Journal of Behavioral Nutrition and Physical Activity*, **14**, 75.

Tremblay, M.S., Inman, J.W., and Willms, D.J. (2000). The relationship between physical activity, self-esteem, and academic achievement in 12-year-old children. *Pediatric Exercise Science*, **12**, 312–323.

Trost, S.G. and Loprinzi, P.D. (2011). Parental influences on physical activity behavior in children and adolescents: a brief review. *American Journal of Lifestyle Medicine*, **5**, 171–181.

Trudeau, F. and Shephard, R.J. (2008). Physical education, school physical activity, school sports and academic performance. *International Journal of Behavioral Nutrition and Physical Activity*, **5**, 10.

Vaughn, A.E., Hales, D., and Ward, D.S. (2013). Measuring the physical activity practices used by parents of preschool children. *Medicine and Science in Sports and Exercise*, **45**, 2369–2377.

Warburton, D.E.R., Nicol, C.W., and Bredin, S.S.D. (2006). Health benefits of physical activity: the evidence. *CMAJ: Canadian Medical Association Journal*, **174**, 801–809.

Wiersma, L.D. and Fifer, A.M. (2008). "The schedule has been tough but we think it's worth it": the joys, challenges, and recommendations of youth sport parents. *Journal of Leisure Research*, **40**, 505–530.

Zarrett, N., Fay, K., Li, Y., Carrano, J., Phelps, E., and Lerner, R.M. (2009). More than child's play: variable- and pattern-centered approaches for examining effects of sports participation on youth development. *Developmental Psychology*, **45**, 368–382.

Chapter 13

Primary prevention and health promotion in oral health

Jenny Godson and Diane Seymour

Summary

This chapter reviews:

- why oral health is a priority
- the impact of poor oral health
- what the evidence tells us works to improve oral health
- how the healthy child programme can facilitate integrated action
- recommendations for action.

Why is oral health a priority?

Oral health is part of general health and well-being and contributes to the development of a healthy child and school readiness. The most common oral disease in young children is tooth decay and while the oral health of young children across the UK is improving, challenges remain. The National Dental Epidemiology Programme for England 2017 oral health survey of 5-year-old children (Public Health England, 2018) revealed that almost a quarter (23%) of 5-year-old children in England, will start school with tooth decay, even though it is preventable, and they will have on average three or four teeth affected. In the devolved nations, the prevalence of tooth decay is even higher with 31% of Primary 1 children having tooth decay in Scotland (NHS National Services Scotland, 2016), 35% in Wales (2014/15) (Morgan and Monaghan, 2016), and 40% in Northern Ireland (Pitts et al., 2015).

Although oral health is improving, significant inequalities remain, according to deprivation, geographic location, and ethnicity (Public Health England, 2015a). Tooth decay was the most common reason for hospital admission for children aged 5–9 years in 2013–2014 (Public Health England, 2017). During 2015–2016, there were 60,361 cases of children aged 0–19 years admitted for the removal of one or more teeth: among 0–4-year-olds, there were 9306 children admitted. This has a significant financial impact with hospital trusts spending an estimated £50.5 million on extraction of multiple teeth for children aged 0–19 years in 2015/16 and £7.8million for children under 5 years of age (Public Health England, 2017).

In 2014, Public Health England published their first report on the dental health of 3-year-olds (Public Health England, 2014a). It highlighted that for those at risk, it happens early in life, with 12% of 3-year-olds having visible tooth decay and those affected had on average three decayed teeth. Tooth decay in childhood is known as early childhood caries and is defined as one or more decayed, missing, or filled tooth surface in any primary tooth of children aged under 72 months (American Academy of Pediatric Dentistry, 2008). It is associated with pain and tooth loss, as well as impaired growth, decreased weight gain, and negative effects on speech, appearance, self-esteem, school performance, and quality of life (Chou et al., 2013). Early childhood caries is associated with long-term bottle use with sugar-sweetened drinks, especially when these are given on demand overnight or for long periods of the day.

Indicators of oral health are included in both the public health (Public Health England, 2016a, 2016b) and NHS outcomes frameworks (Department of Health, 2016).

Impact of poor oral health

Poor oral health impacts children's and families' well-being and is a marker of wider health and social care issues such as poor nutrition and obesity. It may also be related to the need for parenting support and, in some instances, safeguarding and neglect (see Figure 13.1, based on research by Goodwin et al. (2015)).

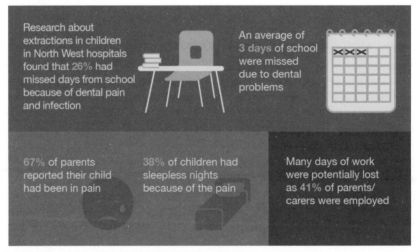

Fig. 13.1 Poor dental health harms school readiness.

Reproduced from Public Health England, *Guidance Health Matters: Child Dental Health*, 14 June 2017, available from https://www.gov.uk/government/publications/health-matters-child-dental-health/health-matters-child-dental-health, under the Open Government License v3.0. Source: data from Goodwin M *et al*. Issues arising following a referral and subsequent wait for extraction under general anaesthetic: impact on children. *BMC Oral Health*, Volume 15, Issue 3, Copyright © Goodwin *et al.*; licensee BioMed Central 2015.

Dental treatment is a significant cost (NHS England, 2014), with the NHS in England spending £3.4 billion per year on all ages for primary and secondary dental care (and an estimated additional £2.3 billion on private dental care).

Children who have high levels of dental disease in their deciduous dentition have an increased risk of disease in their permanent teeth. Teeth that are treated with fillings and other restorations will require maintenance throughout life (Public Health England, 2017).

Why do children have poor oral health?

Tooth decay occurs when a child consumes food or drink containing free sugars, from which cariogenic bacteria in the mouth over a period of time produce acid which demineralizes a susceptible tooth surface.

Risk factors for tooth decay include:

- poor nutrition and infant feeding including frequent exposure to free sugars and giving sugar–sweetened drinks in feeding bottles
- lack of access to fluoride including starting to brush teeth late, infrequently, and with low- or no-fluoride toothpaste
- evidence of previous tooth decay or extractions under general anaesthesia
- social inequalities
- those children identified as high risk by health and social care workers.

In addition, to those listed above, other groups may also be at risk of tooth decay. Individuals with a medical or physical disability may suffer harmful effects from the consequences of tooth decay (Scottish Intercollegiate Guidelines Network, 2014) and should receive additional support such as intensive preventive oral care.

What can be done?

We have good evidence of what works for oral health improvement, at both an individual and population level.

What works? Individual-level oral health improvement advice and treatment

The evidence-based messages from 'Delivering Better Oral Health', third edition (Public Health England, 2014b) outline preventive advice and treatments that work (shown in Table 13.1).

Access to fluoride

There is ample evidence that increasing fluoride availability to individuals and communities is effective at reducing levels of tooth decay. Fluoride is most effective if it is available at multiple times during the day, so sources of fluoride which are part of normal life are more likely to be effective. Fluoride can occur naturally in drinking water and some foods, and in toothpaste and professionally applied fluoride varnish.

Table 13.1 Prevention of tooth decay

	Evidence base*
Prevention of tooth decay in children aged up to 3 years	
Breastfeeding provides the best nutrition for babies	I
From 6 months of age infants should be introduced to drinking from a free-flow cup, and from the age of 1 year feeding from a bottle should be discouraged	III
Sugar should not be added to weaning foods or drinks	V
Parents or carers should brush or supervise tooth brushing	I
As soon as teeth erupt in the mouth, brush them twice daily with a fluoridated toothpaste	I
Brush last thing at night and on one other occasion	III
Use toothpaste containing no less than 1000 parts per million (ppm) fluoride	I
It is good practice to use only a smear of fluoride toothpaste	GP
The frequency and amount of sugary food and drinks should be reduced	III, I
Sugar-free medicines should be recommended	III
Prevention of tooth decay in children aged 3 to 6 years	
Brush at least twice daily, with a fluoridated toothpaste	I
Brush last thing at night and at least on one other occasion	III
Brushing should be supervised by a parent or carer	I
Use fluoridated toothpaste containing more than 1000 ppm fluoride.	I
It is good practice to use only a pea-sized amount of fluoride toothpaste	GP
Spit out after brushing and do not rinse, to maintain fluoride concentration levels	III
The frequency and amount of sugary food and drinks should be reduced	III, I
Sugar-free medicines should be recommended	III
Professional intervention	
All children aged 3–6 years should have fluoride varnish applied to their teeth two times a year (2.2% NaF)	I
Children aged 0–6 years giving concern (e.g. those likely to develop tooth decay, those with special needs)	
All advice as above plus: Use fluoridated toothpaste containing 1350–1500 ppm fluoride	I
It is good practice to use only a smear or pea-sized amount	GP
Where medication is given frequently or long term, request that it is sugar free, or used to minimize tooth decay	GP

(continued)

Table 13.1 Continued

	Evidence base*
Professional intervention	
Children aged 0–6 giving concern should have fluoride varnish applied to their teeth two or more times a year (2.2% NaF)	I
Investigate diet and assist adoption of good dietary practice in line with the Eatwell Guide	I

*Classification of strength of evidence (Gray, 1997): I, strong evidence from at least one systematic review of multiple well-designed randomized controlled trial/s. II, strong evidence from at least one properly designed randomized controlled trial of appropriate size. III, evidence from well-designed trials without randomization, single group pre–post, cohort, time series of matched case–control studies. IV, evidence from well-designed non-experimental studies from more than one centre or research group. V, opinions of respected authorities, based on clinical evidence, descriptive studies, or reports of expert committees. GP, good practice—specific evidence for statement if not available but it makes practical sense. References supporting each of the statements are provided in 'Delivering Better Oral Health' (Public Health England, 2014b).

Adapted from Public Health England, *Department of Health, Delivering better oral health: an evidence-based toolkit for prevention, third edition,* © Crown Copyright 2017, available from https://www.gov.uk/government/publications/delivering-better-oral-health-an-evidence-based-toolkit-for-prevention, under the Open Government Licence v3.0.

All water contains small amounts of naturally occurring fluoride; where it is naturally too low to provide dental benefits, a water fluoridation scheme raises it to the optimal concentration (one part per million or 1 mg fluoride per litre of water) to reduce decay levels and minimize severity. Currently, about 6 million people in England have a fluoridated water supply.

Nutritional advice

The Scientific Advisory Committee on Nutrition (SACN) reported in *Carbohydrates and Health* that high levels of sugar consumption are associated with a greater risk of tooth decay. For all age groups from 2 years upwards, the average intake of free sugars[1] should not exceed 5% of total dietary energy intake. The recommended maximum intake of free sugars is no more than 19 g per day = five sugar cubes for 4–6-year-olds, 24 g per day = six sugar cubes for 6–10-year-olds, and 30 g per day = seven sugar cubes for 11-year-olds and older. Younger children should have even less than this (Public Health England, 2015b, 2015c).

Healthier eating advice should routinely be given to promote good oral and general health. Key dietary messages to prevent tooth decay are to reduce the amount and frequency of consumption of foods and drinks that contain free sugars (Public Health England, 2014b). The 'Eatwell Guide' can be used to help children and families get a balance of healthier food (Public Health England, 2014b).

[1] Free sugars include all sugars added to foods and drinks by the manufacturer, cook or consumer, as well as sugars naturally present in honey, syrups and unsweetened fruit juices and smoothies. It does not include the sugar naturally found in milk (lactose) or the sugars found in whole fruit and vegetables.

An important factor contributing to tooth decay in children is the regular consumption of drinks high in free sugars. Sugar-sweetened drinks such as fizzy drinks, soft drinks, juice drinks, and squash have no place in a child's daily diet (Scientific Advisory Committee on Nutrition, 2015). Only *milk* or *water* should be drunk between meals and adding sugar to foods and drinks should be avoided. Sugary drinks should not be placed in baby bottles, feeder cups, or taken to bed as a night-time drink, as this means they will be in prolonged contact with the teeth. Only breast or formula milk or cooled, boiled water should be given in bottles. Breastfeeding up to 12 months of age is associated with a decreased risk of tooth decay (SACN, 2018). In order to support healthier eating, the National Institute for Health and Care Excellence (NICE, 2014) recommends that providers of public service environments such as leisure centres, nurseries and children's centres, schools, and other early years services should promote oral health by providing plain drinking water, a choice of sugar-free food, drinks (water or milk), and snacks (including fresh fruit), including from vending machines, and support breastfeeding. Sugars in *oral medicines* may cause decay if used frequently. Sugar-free formulations are available for most oral medicines and it is recommended that they are prescribed wherever possible and parents/carers advised to buy sugar free versions (if available).

What works? Population-level programmes

In 2014, both NICE (Public health guideline [PH55]), and Public Health England ('Commissioning Better Oral Health for Children and Young People') published key documents, which reviewed the evidence of effectiveness of population oral health improvement programmes.

Public Health England launched the Children's Oral Health Improvement Programme Board in 2016 to support this work, with a wide range of partners and stakeholders and a collective ambition that *every child grows up free from tooth decay* as part of every child having the best start in life. Currently in England, many local authorities already commission a variety of oral health improvement programmes. Scotland (Childsmile programme (NHS Health Scotland, 2018) and Wales (Designed to Smile (Welsh Government, 2014)) both have national oral health improvement programmes.

'Commissioning Better Oral Health for Children and Young People'

The final recommendations about oral health improvement programmes within 'Commissioning Better Oral Health for Children and Young People' (Public Health England, 2014c) were based on the totality of the evidence (including evidence of effectiveness, impact on reducing inequalities, cost/resource implications and implementation issues).

Recommended interventions

- Oral health training for the wider professional workforce.
- Integration of oral health into targeted home visits by health/social care workers.

- Targeted community-based fluoride varnish programmes. Fluoride varnish has been shown to be effective, easy to apply by suitably trained members of the dental team, acceptable to very young children, and has a high level of safety.
- Targeted provision of toothbrushes and toothpaste (i.e. postal or through health visitors).
- Supervised tooth brushing in targeted childhood settings.
- Healthy food and drink policies in childhood settings.
- Fluoridation of the public water supplies.
- Targeted peer (lay) support groups/peer oral health workers.
- Influencing local and national government policies.

Key oral health messages across the life course

The following are interventions that can be implemented within the child health programme, using identified contact points to promote key oral health messages and link to community-based programmes across the life course. These interventions detailed in Table 13.2 can also be found in the Public Health England resource 'Improving oral health for children and young people for health visitors, school nurses and practice nurses' (Public Health England, 2016c).

Table 13.2 Key oral health messages

Life course contact point	Individual advice	Community
Antenatal	**Midwives should inform parents:** • that mum is entitled to free NHS dental treatment during pregnancy and to free NHS dental treatment for 12 months after the baby is born • and encourage them to use the 'Red book', the parent-held Personal Child Health Record and 'e' health record which include oral health advice • to take their baby to the dentist as soon as the first tooth erupts at about 6 months of age for preventive advice • That breastfeeding provides the best nutrition for babies	
6 weeks	**The health visitor team should:** • identify families that may need additional support regarding their oral health (Scottish Intercollegiate Guidelines Network, 2014). • advise that breast milk is the only food or drink babies need for around the first 6 months of their life. First infant formula is the only suitable alternative • encourage dental attendance when the first tooth erupts at about 6 months of age	

(continued)

Table 13.2 Continued

Life course contact point	Individual advice	Community
6–12 months	**The health visitor team should advise:** ◆ parents/carers should brush their children's teeth as soon as they erupt ◆ use a smear of no less than 1000 parts per million (ppm) fluoride toothpaste ◆ for maximum protection from tooth decay or for children at risk, advice can be given to use fluoride toothpaste with 1350–1500 ppm fluoride using a smear of toothpaste. ◆ young children should always be supervised and supported when brushing ◆ to spit out after brushing and not to rinse with water ◆ to brush at least twice a day including last thing at night ◆ on reducing the frequency and consumption of free sugars in food and drink ◆ that from 6 months old, bottle-fed babies should drink from a non-valved free-flow cup ◆ that only breast milk, formula milk, or cooled boiled water should be given in feeding bottles ◆ not to bottle feed from 12 months of age ◆ that sugar-free medicines should be recommended ◆ mum that she is entitled to free dental care on any course of treatment started before the baby is 1 year old ◆ dental attendance when the first tooth erupts at about 6 months of age	◆ Health visitor team intervention with toothbrush and fluoride toothpaste and oral health advice at clinic visits ◆ This may be supplemented by targeted provision of toothbrushes and fluoride toothpaste through the post
2–2½	**As above plus:** ◆ parents/carers should brush or supervise tooth brushing until their child is at least 7 years old	Signpost to: ◆ any locally commissioned oral health programmes
3 years	**As above plus:** ◆ advise a pea-size amount of more than 1000 ppm fluoride toothpaste ◆ for maximum protection from tooth decay or for children at risk, advise toothpaste with 1350–1500 ppm fluoride using a pea-size amount. ◆ signpost all children to the dentist for the application of fluoride varnish to the teeth twice a year	Signpost to: ◆ early years setting supervised tooth brushing programme ◆ community fluoride varnish programme

(continued)

Table 13.2 Continued

Life course contact point	Individual advice	Community
4–5 years	**As above plus:** ♦ give information on eruption of permanent molars at age 6 years ♦ school nurses have a role in advising on children's oral health. Poor oral health can impact on school readiness	At school entry, school nurses signpost to: ♦ nursery/reception supervised tooth brushing programme ♦ community fluoride varnish programme
7–8 years	**As above plus:** ♦ Use fluoridated toothpaste (1350–1500 ppm fluoride) ♦ children should be able to brush their own teeth but should be helped or supervised by an adult	

Source: data from Public Health England, *Improving oral health for children and young people for health visitors, school nurses and practice nurses*, © Crown Copyright 2016. 2905764. Published October 2016. Gateway reference 2016367. Available from https://vivbennett.blog.gov.uk/wp-content/uploads/sites/90/2016/11/Improving-oral-health-for-children.pdf. Contains public sector information licensed under the Open Government Licence v3.0.

Public Health England (2016d, 2016e) has published a return on investment (ROI) tool that highlights the ROI of these community programmes at 5 and 10 years (Figure 13.2). This work highlights the important role of health visitors at the 6-month intervention, demonstrating a higher ROI when postal distribution of toothbrushes and toothpaste is in addition supported by health visitors

How will we know we are making progress?

Monitoring of the extent and severity of tooth decay is reported via the national oral health intelligence services' epidemiological surveys, as referenced in 'Why is oral health a priority?'

Workforce—skills and training

Promoting oral health improvement should be an integral part of the work of the children and young people's workforce as recommended by NICE (2014).

Learning links

♦ An oral health module is available on the e-Learning for Healthcare website in the Healthy School Child section of the Healthy Child Programme. The resource is aimed at the early years workforce including health visitors and school nurses: http://www.e-lfh.org.uk/programmes/healthy-school-child/.

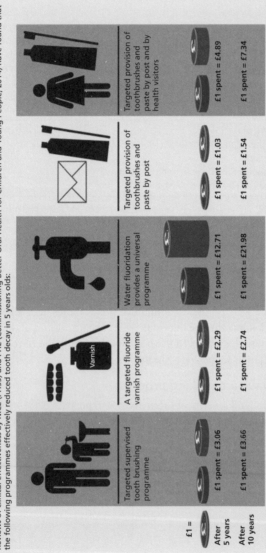

Fig. 13.2 Return on investment of oral health improvement programmes for 0–5-year-olds: infographic.

Recommendations

Commissioners and employers should ensure the following:

- ♦ That commissioned oral health improvement interventions follow evidence-based guidelines. (*Evidence: strong.*)
- ♦ That evidence-based oral health advice is incorporated within the commissioning of the mandated contacts in the Child Health Programme, and that providers have access to and receive relevant training. (*Evidence: strong.*)
- ♦ That the need for additional population-based oral health programmes has been considered, for example, supervised tooth brushing in early years settings, fluoride varnish, and water fluoridation. (*Evidence: strong.*)

Practitioners should:

- ♦ have knowledge of what the evidence tells us works to improve the oral health of young children and have access to regular training in supporting parents and carers (*Good practice*)
- ♦ facilitate dental attendance by signposting to local dental services as soon as the first tooth erupts and to any local population-based programmes (*Good practice*)
- ♦ encourage parents/carers to follow evidence based advice and to take their children to visit the dental team when the first tooth erupts, at about 6 months and then on a regular basis. (*Evidence: strong.*)

Acknowledgement

Chapter 13 'Primary prevention and health promotion in oral health' © is Crown Copyright and is reproduced with the permission of Public Health England under delegated authority from the Controller of HMSO.

References

American Academy of Pediatric Dentistry (2008). Definition of early childhood caries (ECC). [online] Available at: http://www.aapd.org/assets/1/7/D_ECC.pdf.

Chou, R., Cantor, A., Zakher, B., Mitchell, J.P., and **Pappas, M.** (2013). *Prevention of Dental Caries in Children Younger than Age 5 Years: Systematic Review to Update the US Preventive Services Task Force Recommendation*. Rockville, MD: Agency for Healthcare Research and Quality.

Department of Health (2016). NHS Outcomes Framework: at-a-glance 2016–2017. [online] Available at:https://www.gov.uk/government/uploads/system/uploads/attachment_data/file/513157/NHSOF_at_a_glance.pdf.

Goodwin, M., Sanders, C., Davies, G., Walsh, T., and **Pretty, I.** (2015). Issues arising following a referral and subsequent wait for extraction under general anaesthetic: impact on children. *BMC Oral Health*, **15**, 3.

Morgan, M. and **Monaghan, N.** (2016). Picture of Oral Health 2016: Dental Epidemiological Survey of 5 Year Olds 2014/15. [online] Available at: http://www.cardiff.ac.uk/__data/ assets/pdf_file/0006/218589/Picture-of-Oral-Health-2016.pdf.

National Institute for Health and Care Excellence (NICE) (2014). Oral health: approaches for local authorities and their partners to improve the oral health of their communities. Public health guideline [PH55]. [online] Available at: http://nice.org.uk/guidance/ph55.

National Institute for Health and Care Excellence (NICE) (2015). Oral health promotion in general dental practice. NICE guideline [NG30]. [online] Available at: https://www.nice. org.uk/guidance/ng30.

NHS England (2014). Improving dental care and oral health – a call to action. [online] Available at: https://www.england.nhs.uk/wp-content/uploads/2014/04/imprv-oral-health-info.pdf.

NHS Health Scotland (2018). Childsmile. [online] Available at: http://www.child-smile.org.uk/.

NHS National Services Scotland (2016). The National Dental Inspection Programme (NDIP) 2016. Report of the 2016 Detailed National Dental Inspection Programme of Primary 1 children and the Basic Inspection of Primary 1 and Primary 7 children. Publication date – 25 October 2016 Epidemiological Survey of 5 year olds 2014/2015. [online] Available at: https://www.isdscotland.org/Health-Topics/Dental-Care/Publications/2016-10-25/2016-10-25-NDIP-Report.pdf.

Pitts, N., **Chadwick, B.**, and **Anderson, T.** (2015). Children's Dental Health Survey 2013. Report 2: Dental Disease and Damage in Children: England, Wales and Northern Ireland. [online] Health and Social Care Information Centre. Available at: http://content.digital.nhs. uk/catalogue/PUB17137/CDHS2013-Report2-Dental-Disease.pdf.

Public Health England (2014a). Dental public health epidemiology programme. Oral health survey of three-year-old children 2013. A report on the prevalence and severity of dental decay. [online] Available at: http://www.nwph.net/dentalhealth/reports/DPHEP%20for%20 England%20OH%20Survey%203yr%202013%20Report.pdf.

Public Health England (2014b). Delivering better oral health: an evidence-based toolkit for prevention, 3rd edition. [online] Available at: https://www.gov.uk/government/uploads/ system/uploads/attachment_data/file/367563/DBOHv32014OCTMainDocument_3.pdf.

Public Health England (2014c). Commissioning Better Oral Health for Children and Young People. An evidence-informed toolkit for local authorities. [online] Available at: https://www.gov.uk/government/publications/ improving-oral-health-an-evidence-informed-toolkit-for-local-authorities.

Public Health England (2015a). Rapid review to update evidence for the Healthy Child Programme 0–5. [online] Available at: https://www.gov.uk/government/publications/ healthy-child-programme-rapid-review-to-update-evidence.

Public Health England (2015b). Sugar reduction: the evidence for action. [online] Available at: https://www.gov.uk/government/publications/ sugar-reduction-from-evidence-into-action.

Public Health England (2015c). Why 5%? An explanation of SACN's recommendations about sugars and health. [online] Available at: https://www.gov.uk/government/uploads/system/ uploads/attachment_data/file/489906/Why_5__-_The_Science_Behind_SACN.pdf.

Public Health England (2016a). Dental Public Health Intelligence Programme Hospital Episode Statistics: extractions data, 0–19 year olds, 2011/12 to 2015/16. [online] Available at:http://www.nwph.net/dentalhealth/Extractions.aspx.

Public Health England (2016b). Public Health Outcomes Framework: short statistical commentary, November 2016. [online] Available at: https://www.gov.uk/government/uploads/system/uploads/attachment_data/file/564111/PHOF_Official_Statistics_Summary_November_2016.pdf.

Public Health England (2016c). Improving oral health for children and young people for health visitors, school nurses and practice nurses. [online] Available at: https://vivbennett.blog.gov.uk/wp-content/uploads/sites/90/2016/11/Improving-oral-health-for-children.pdf.

Public Health England (2016d). Return on investment of oral health improvement programmes for 0 to 5 year olds: infographic. PHE Publication gateway number 2016321. [online] Available at: https://www.gov.uk/government/uploads/system/uploads/attachment_data/file/560973/ROI_oral_health_interventions.pdf.

Public Health England (2016e). Return on investment of oral health interventions tool. [online] Available at:https://www.gov.uk/government/publications/improving-the-oral-health-of-children-cost-effective-commissioning.

Public Health England (2017). Health Matters: Child dental health. [online]Available at: https://publichealthmatters.blog.gov.uk/2017/06/14/health-matters-child-dental-health/.

Public Health England (2018). National Dental Epidemiology Programme for England: oral health survey of five-year-old children 2017. A report on the inequalities found in prevalence and severity of dental decay. [online] Available at: http://www.nwph.net/dentalhealth/201617Survey5yearoldchildren/NDEP%20for%20England%20OH%20Survey%205yr%202017%20Report%20Gateway%20Approved%20v2.pdf

Scientific Advisory Committee on Nutrition (SACN) (2015). *Carbohydrates and Health*. London: The Stationery Office. Available at: https://www.gov.uk/government/publications/sacn-carbohydrates-and-health-report.

Scientific Advisory Committee on Nutrition (SACN) (2018). Feeding in the First Year of Life. Available at: https://assets.publishing.service.gov.uk/government/uploads/system/uploads/attachment_data/file/725530/SACN_report_on_Feeding_in_the_First_Year_of_Life.pdf.

Scottish Intercollegiate Guidelines Network (SIGN) (2014). Dental interventions to prevent caries in children. Edinburgh: SIGN. (SIGN publication no. 138). Available at: https://www.sign.ac.uk/sign-138-dental-interventions-to-prevent-caries-in-children.html.

Welsh Government (2014). Designed to Smile. A manual for delivering Designed to Smile. [online] Available at: http://www.designedtosmile.org/.

Chapter 14

Unintentional injuries and their prevention

Denise Kendrick

Summary

This chapter:

- quantifies the burden of childhood injuries and describes risk factors for child injury, levels and approaches to injury prevention, and recommendations for effective behaviour change

- summarizes evidence for preventing child injuries at home and on the roads

- discusses putting injury prevention into practice for practitioners and commissioners

- makes recommendations for the injury prevention content of the healthy child programme

- provides a resource list for practitioners, parents, and commissioners.

Unintentional injuries are a significant child health problem

In the UK, for each injury death among 0–15-year-olds, 151 children are admitted to hospital and 1947 attend emergency departments (EDs) (Walsh et al., 1996). Much less is known about the many injuries only receiving primary care or walk-in-centre treatment and those not medically attended. Fewer than half the injuries in school-age children are medically attended (Currie et al., 1996) (see Figure 14.1) and fewer than 10% of infant falls result in hospital attendance (Warrington et al., 2001).

In 2014/2015, there were 47,859 unintentional injury admissions among under-fives and 29,466 among 5–9-year-olds in England (NHS Digital, 2015), equivalent to 920 under-fives and 567 5–9-year-olds admitted each week. Data from 2002 (the most recent data available for UK ED injury attendances) shows over 617,000 unintentional injury attendances among under-fives (excluding road traffic injuries); equivalent to 11,875 per week (Royal Society for the Prevention of Accidents, 2002). As ED attendances almost doubled from 1987 to 2011 (Royal Society for the Prevention of Accidents, 2012), current figures are likely to exceed this.

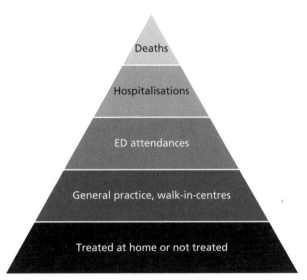

Fig. 14.1 The injury pyramid.

Childhood unintentional injury deaths are reducing over time: death rates in 0–18-year-olds declined by 50% to 70% across the four UK countries from 1980 to 2010 (Hardelid et al., 2013). Despite this, more than one child aged under five still dies each week from unintentional injuries in England and Wales (Office for National Statistics, 2015). In 1–4-year-olds, unintentional injuries account for 12.8% of all deaths, coming just behind neoplasms (15.4%), respiratory conditions (13.4%), and congenital malformations (13.4%).

However, this is only part of the story. All deaths are not preventable, but many unintentional injury deaths are. Recent English child death review data suggests 20% of deaths among 0–17-year-olds were preventable (defined as 'modifiable factors may have contributed to the death' (Fraser et al., 2014)), compared to 68% of trauma-related deaths (Fraser et al., 2014). The Royal Society for the Prevention of Accidents (RoSPA) (2015) estimates that unintentional injury accounts for most preventable deaths (Figure 14.2) and more than 85% of preventable hospital admissions from 0 to 9 years of age.

What types of unintentional injuries happen to children?

Most deaths and hospital admissions from unintentional injuries among the under-fives occur in or around the home. Deaths most commonly result from choking, suffocation, or strangulation (49%); drowning (22%); falls (8%); and smoke, fire, and flames (8%). Most admissions (52%) result from falls, being struck by objects (22%), poisoning (13%), and heat/hot substances (6%) (Public Health England (PHE), 2014a).

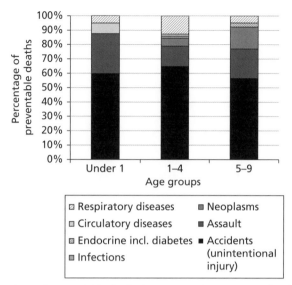

Fig. 14.2 Percentage of preventable deaths by cause and age group using Office for National Statistics data from 2012.

Reproduced with permission of Errol Taylor, The Royal Society for the Prevention of Accidents (RoSPA), Birmingham, UK

Above the age of 5 years, transport injuries are the most common fatal injury (51% in 5–14-year-olds) (Office for National Statistics, 2015), but falls (52%) are the most common cause of hospital admission (NHS Digital, 2015). Most transport deaths and serious injuries among 0–15-year-olds involve pedestrians (50% deaths, 68% serious injuries), motor vehicle occupants (38% deaths, 17% serious injuries), and cyclists (12% deaths, 15% serious injuries). These figures do not accurately reflect risks associated with these modes of travel—pedestrian and cyclist death rates per billion miles travelled are 20 and 17 times higher, respectively, than for motor vehicle occupants (Department for Transport, 2016).

Which children are most at risk of injury?

A large number of risk factors for child injury have been identified (see Table 14.1).

Preventing unintentional injuries: levels, approaches, and behavioural models

Actions to prevent injury can occur at three levels (see Figure 14.3). Within each level, different approaches can be used, commonly referred to as the 3 Es—education, engineering, and enforcement (see Figure 14.4).

More recently, a fourth 'E', empowerment, has been added. The World Health Organization (1998) defines this as 'a process through which people gain greater control over decisions and actions affecting their health'. Active or passive approaches can also be used to prevent injury. Active approaches need repeated actions (e.g. closing

Table 14.1 Risk factors for child injury

Risk factor	Evidence
Age	Injury incidence varies with age (Pearson et al., 2009), related to physical and cognitive development. Mortality rates are highest for under-ones, reduce until mid-teenage years, then increase (Sethi et al., 2008)
Gender	Boys have higher injury rates (Pearson et al., 2009), particularly road traffic injuries, drowning, and falls (Sethi et al., 2008)
Other child factors	Previous injury (Sellar et al., 1991), sensory impairment (Schwebel and Brezausek, 2010), physical or cognitive disability (Shi et al., 2015), and epilepsy (Pearson et al., 2009) increase injury risk
Socio-economic deprivation	Steeper socio-economic gradient for injury deaths than for any other cause of child death (Marmot et al., 2010). Gradient in hospital admissions steeper for 0–4-year-olds (Hippisley-Cox et al., 2002), pedestrian injury, poisoning, and burns (Hippisley-Cox et al., 2002; Orton et al., 2014). Gradients have reduced over time (Orton et al., 2014), but significant inequalities remain (Orton et al., 2014)
Family size and structure	Larger families (Bijur et al., 1988), more older siblings (Bijur et al., 1988), second and subsequent children (Orton et al., 2012), overcrowded households (Alwash and McCarthy, 1988), single-parent households (O'Connor et al., 2000; Orton et al., 2012), step-families (O'Connor et al., 2000), and younger mothers (Orton et al., 2012) have increased injury risk
Ethnic group	Some evidence of increased injury risk in black and ethnic minority groups for burns, poisonings, and falls (Pearson et al., 2009), and reduced fracture risk (Tobin et al., 2002)
Child behaviour and supervision	Behavioural problems, hyperactive or aggressive behaviour (Bijur et al., 1986; Pearson et al., 2009), attention deficit hyperactivity disorder, and oppositional defiant disorder (Rowe et al., 2004) increase injury risk. Some evidence effective supervision reduces injury (Morrongiello et al., 2006; Schnitzer et al., 2015), including for children with difficult temperaments (Schwebel et al., 2004)
Parental mental health	Maternal depression (O'Connor et al., 2000; Orton et al., 2012) anxiety (Bradbury et al., 1999), stress (Harris and Kotch, 1994), drug misuse (Braun et al., 2005), and drinking above recommended alcohol levels (Orton et al., 2012) increases injury risk, particularly more severe and long-lasting depression (Schwebel and Brezausek, 2008). Maternal depression is associated with fewer safety behaviours (Conners-Burrow et al., 2013) and less intense supervision (Phelan et al., 2014)

safety gates every time after opening, or putting medicines away after each use), while passive approaches do not (e.g. boiler manufacturers pre-setting thermostat levels or families lowering hot water thermostats). Passive approaches are usually more effective than active ones (Haddon 1980), as are combined approaches, addressing multiple levels of injury prevention than those using a single approach (Dowswell et al., 1996).

The National Institute for Health and Care Excellence (NICE) recommend the following effective behaviour change interventions:

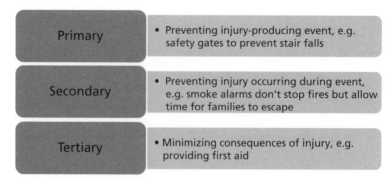

Fig. 14.3 Injury prevention levels.

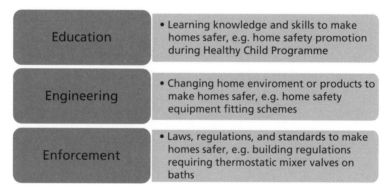

Fig. 14.4 Injury prevention approaches.

Interventions should motivate and support people to:

◆ 'Understand short, medium and longer-term consequences of their health-related behaviours, for themselves and others

◆ Feel positive about benefits of health-enhancing behaviours and changing their behaviour

◆ Plan changes in terms of easy steps over time

◆ Recognise how social contexts and relationships may affect behaviour, and identify and plan for situations that might undermine changes they are trying to make

◆ Plan explicit 'if–then' coping strategies to prevent relapse

◆ Make a personal commitment to adopt health-enhancing behaviours by setting (and recording) goals to undertake clearly defined behaviours, in particular contexts, over a specified time

◆ Share behaviour change goals with others' (NICE, 2007).[5]

---

[5] © NICE (2007) *PH6 Behaviour change: general approaches.* Available from www.nice.org.uk/guidance/ph6. All rights reserved. Subject to notice of rights. NICE guidance is prepared for the National Health Service in England. All NICE guidance is subject to regular review and may be updated or withdrawn. NICE accepts no responsibility for the use of its content in this product/publication.

What works to prevent unintentional injuries in childhood?

Prevention of home injuries in the under-fives

Intensive home visiting programmes

Intensive home visiting programmes aimed at improving a range of mother and child outcomes significantly reduce injury risk in young children. A meta-analysis found children in families receiving these programmes were 13% less likely to have an injury than children in families not receiving these programmes (pooled relative risk 0.87, 95% confidence interval 0.73–0.94) (Kendrick et al., 2013). The UK's home visiting programme (Family Nurse Partnership (FNP)) is based on evidence from trials included in the meta-analysis. A recent FNP evaluation in families with children aged 2 years did not find a reduction in injuries (Robling et al., 2016). This may have resulted from the FNP focusing on less disadvantaged and vulnerable mothers than previous studies and high levels of health visiting contact among non-FNP families (Olds, 2016). The FNP are now investigating targeting the programme towards the most vulnerable groups who may benefit most.

Home safety education and safety equipment

Several meta-analyses show home safety education and provision of safety equipment helps families make homes safer (DiGuiseppi and Roberts, 2000; Kendrick et al., 2012). This includes increasing possession of functional smoke alarms; safety gate use on stairs; fireguard use; safe storage of poisons; having a safe hot tap water temperature, a fire escape plan, and emergency contact numbers; and reducing baby walker use. The most effective interventions combine education with home safety inspections and providing or fitting equipment (Cooper et al., 2012; Achana et al., 2015; Hubbard et al., 2015). NICE guidance (PH29 and PH30) and PHE recommend:

◆ families with children at high risk of injury receive home safety assessments and advice and referral to safety equipment schemes

◆ home safety advice is incorporated into home visits taking place for other reasons

◆ health visitors, school nurses and GPs are informed about families who may benefit from injury prevention advice and home safety assessments

◆ training in injury prevention is provided for healthcare professionals and other practitioners such as early years staff (NICE, 2010a, 2010b; PHE 2014a).

Preventing injuries to primary school-aged children

A recent systematic review found some evidence that school-based educational programmes aimed at preventing a range of different types of injuries improved safety skills, safety behaviour or practices, and knowledge among primary school-aged children. There was a lack of evidence that programmes reduced injury occurrence and the quality of evidence was low (Orton et al., 2016). Further research is required in this area.

Prevention of road injuries

Preventing injuries to pedestrians and cyclists

As motor vehicle speed at the point of impact increases, so does the risk of injury and death. Reducing motor vehicle speed is therefore of paramount importance. NICE guidance on reducing road traffic injuries (PH31) (2010c), PHE (NICE, 2010a, 2010b; PHE, 2014b), and the Welsh Government (2013) make similar recommendations, which include:

◆ reducing speed in streets that are primarily residential or with high numbers of pedestrians and cyclists, through traffic-calming measures on single streets, or 20 mph zones across wider areas, 20 mph limits on single streets or city or town-wide 20 mph limits, with enforcement activities

◆ where 20 mph limits are not introduced, segregate pedestrians and cyclists from motor vehicles

◆ encouraging safer active travel before and after school with school travel plans and engineering measures on routes commonly used by children and young people (e.g. to schools, parks, colleges, and recreational sites), accompanied by law enforcement activities.

Preventing injuries to motor vehicle occupants

The Road Safety Observatory (2017) summarizes evidence about the effectiveness of chid car restraints. In terms of injury risk reduction, properly fitted and used rearward-facing restraints are the most effective in 0–4-year-olds and booster seats in 4–10-year-olds. Injury rates are higher in forward-facing than rearward-facing restraints, but lower than for unrestrained children or those wearing seat belts. Injury risk is lower for children travelling in rear seats than front seats. Overall, the most effective way to prevent injuries to children travelling in cars is to use an appropriate child restraint in the rear of the vehicle.

Child restraints are only effective if they are correctly fitted and used. There is some evidence that restraints using the ISOFIX system are more likely to be correctly fitted than those using seat belts.

Interventions to promote child car restraint use are also effective. Education is effective, but combining education with free restraints or financial incentives (discounts or gift vouchers) is more effective.

Putting injury prevention into practice

For practitioners with contact with children and families

A wide range of practitioners have injury prevention opportunities through contacts with children and families. Injury prevention is one of the six early years high-impact areas for health visiting (PHE, 2014c) and health visiting teams lead delivery of the Healthy Child Programme. Other early years services have important roles to play, particularly children's centres and other health professionals (e.g. general practitioners (GPs) and midwives), other organizations (e.g. fire and rescue services and housing services), and voluntary organizations. Good partnership working and co-ordination of activities is essential for effective injury prevention (PHE, 2014a), and NICE guideline PH29 (2010a) includes recommendations for effective partnership working.

PHE (2014a) recommends focusing home injury prevention for the under-fives on injuries causing the highest number of deaths or hospital admissions:

- Choking, suffocation, and strangling
- Falls
- Poisoning
- Burns and scalds
- Drowning.

They also highlight the importance of not ignoring injuries caused by smoke, fire, and flames and newer hazards such as liquid laundry detergent capsules, e-cigarettes, button batteries, and hair straighteners.

The Healthy Child Programme

The five mandated contacts in the universal Healthy Child Programme provide injury prevention opportunities. The Child Accident Prevention Trust (CAPT) and the University of Nottingham have produced a commissioners guide which recommends the key home safety messages for inclusion in the Healthy Child Programme (Hayes et al., 2016). PHE and CAPT have also produced a guide for staff working with children under 5 years (Public Health England and the Child Accident Prevention Trust, 2017). Table 14.2 incorporates recommendations from these two documents.

For public health practitioners and commissioners

As a result of the Health and Social Care Act 2012, health visiting services, the Healthy Child Programme, the FNP, and school nursing services are commissioned by local authorities. Health and well-being boards were created to improve integration and partnership working between the NHS, local authorities, and public health. These boards produce a joint strategic needs assessment and a health and well-being strategy which should address child injury prevention in their locality.

Several key documents support local authorities in this role. The Kings Fund resource on improving the public's health (Buck and Gregory, 2013) lists nine areas where local authorities can have a significant impact, including preventing child injuries. It recommends implementation of NICE PH29 (2010a) and PH30 (2010b), provision and fitting of home safety equipment, and injury prevention training for staff. PHE's guidance on child home injury prevention highlights the importance of providing strategic leadership and effective partnership working, training and supporting the early years workforce to deliver injury prevention, and implementing NICE guidelines PH29 and PH30 (PHE, 2014a). CAPT and the University of Nottingham's guide for commissioners of child health services recommends key home safety messages for the Healthy Child Programme (Hayes et al., 2016).

Table 14.2 Injury prevention topics for each of the five mandated contacts in the Healthy Child Programme

Injury prevention topic	Antenatal health promotion visit	New baby review	6–8-week review	9–12-month review	2–2.5-year review
Choking, suffocation, and strangling	Put babies to sleep in cot/Moses basket in the same room as you for the first 6 months	Put babies to sleep in cot/Moses basket in the same room as you for the first 6 months	Put babies to sleep in cot/Moses basket in the same room as you for the first 6 months	Put babies to sleep on their back with feet to bottom of the cot	Cut food up into batons, not balls
	Put babies to sleep on their back with feet to bottom of the cot/Moses basket	Put babies to sleep on their back with feet to bottom of the cot/Moses basket	Put babies to sleep on their back with feet to bottom of the cot/Moses basket	Don't sleep with baby on sofas/armchairs or in bed if you smoke, drink alcohol, take drugs, or baby has a low birthweight	Supervise toddlers while they are eating
	Don't sleep with baby on sofas/armchairs or in bed if you smoke, drink alcohol, take drugs, or baby has a low birthweight	Don't sleep with baby on sofas/armchairs or in bed if you smoke, drink alcohol, take drugs, or baby has a low birthweight	Don't sleep with baby on sofas/armchairs or in bed if you smoke, drink alcohol, take drugs, or baby has a low birthweight	Don't cover baby's face or head	Keep small objects out of reach
	Don't cover baby's face or head	Don't cover baby's face or head	Don't cover baby's face or head	Don't use a duvet, pillow, or cot bumper and don't leave toys where baby sleeps	Be aware that older children's toys may have small parts and keep these away from toddlers
	Don't use a duvet, pillow, or cot bumper and don't leave toys where baby sleeps	Don't use a duvet, pillow, or cot bumper and don't leave toys where baby sleeps	Don't use a duvet, pillow, or cot bumper and don't leave toys where baby sleeps	Use blinds without cords, use cord devices or tie cords up to keep away from babies/children	Use blinds without cords, use cord devices or tie cords up to keep away from babies/children
	Use blinds without cords, use cord devices or tie cords up to keep away from babies/children	Use blinds without cords, use cord devices or tie cords up to keep away from babies/children	Use blinds without cords, use cord devices or tie cords up to keep away from babies/children	Keep nappy sacks out of baby's reach	Learn first aid for choking
	Keep nappy sacks out of baby's reach	Keep nappy sacks out of baby's reach	Keep nappy sacks out of baby's reach	Don't prop feed baby	
			Keep small objects out of reach	Cut food up into batons, not balls	
			Don't prop feed baby	Supervise babies while they are eating	
				Keep small objects out of reach	
				Learn first aid for choking	

Falls					
The safest place to change a baby's nappy is on the floor. Baby walkers don't help babies to walk sooner but can lead to falls or babies reaching hazards (hot objects, poisons); think carefully before using a walker	The safest place to change a baby's nappy is on the floor. Don't put car/bouncing seats on raised surfaces Don't leave baby unattended on raised surface (e.g. changing table, bed, sofa) Baby walkers don't help babies to walk sooner but can lead to falls or babies reaching hazards (hot objects, poisons); think carefully before using a walker	The safest place to change a baby's nappy is on the floor. Don't put car/bouncing seats on raised surfaces Don't leave baby unattended on raised surface (e.g. changing table, bed, sofa) Baby walkers don't help babies to walk sooner but can lead to falls or babies reaching hazards (hot objects, poisons); think carefully before using a walker Use harnesses in high chairs Learn first aid for head injuries, broken bones, cuts, and bruises	The safest place to change a baby's nappy is on the floor. Don't put car/bouncing seats on raised surfaces Don't leave baby unattended on raised surface (e.g. changing table, bed, sofa) Baby walkers don't help babies to walk sooner but can lead to falls or babies reaching hazards (hot objects, poisons); think carefully before using a walker Fit a safety gate to prevent babies/toddlers getting to the stairs. Use the gate until child is 24 months old. Always close the gate after use. Babies/toddlers are less likely to be injured on stairs with carpets than those without Use harnesses in high chairs Learn first aid for head injuries, broken bones, cuts, and bruises	Supervise toddlers going up and down stairs and use handrails Toddlers are less likely to be injured on stairs with carpets than those without Use window locks or restrictors Ensure things children could climb on are not left near windows Teach children where not to climb Restrict access to balconies Learn first aid for head injuries, broken bones, cuts, and bruises

(continued)

Table 14.2 Continued

Injury prevention topic	Antenatal health promotion visit	New baby review	6–8-week review	9–12-month review	2–2.5-year review
Poisoning	Fit a carbon monoxide (CO) alarm in rooms with flame-burning appliances	Fit a CO alarm in rooms with flame-burning appliances	Fit a CO alarm in rooms with flame-burning appliances	Fit a CO alarm in rooms with flame-burning appliances	Fit a CO alarm in rooms with flame-burning appliances
	Make sure flame burning appliances are serviced at least annually	Make sure flame burning appliances are serviced at least annually	Make sure flame burning appliances are serviced at least annually	Make sure flame burning appliances are serviced at least annually	Make sure flame burning appliances are serviced at least annually
			Fit cupboard locks where medicines and household chemicals are stored	Fit cupboard locks where medicines and household chemicals are stored	Fit cupboard locks where medicines and household chemicals are stored
			If locks are not possible, store items up high—at or above adult eye level	If locks are not possible, store items up high—at or above adult eye level	If locks are not possible, store items up high—at or above adult eye level
			Put medicines and household chemicals away straight after using them	Put medicines and household chemicals away straight after using them	Put medicines and household chemicals away straight after using them
			If tablets are kept in handbags or other bags, make sure these are out of the baby's reach	If tablets are kept in handbags or other bags, make sure these are out of the baby's reach	If tablets are kept in handbags or other bags, make sure these are out of the baby's reach
			Ask grandparents to make sure they keep their medicines out of the baby's reach	Ask grandparents to make sure they keep their medicines out of the baby's reach	

			Don't leave button batteries within reach of babies and children Learn first aid for poisoning	Don't leave button batteries within reach of babies and children Learn first aid for poisoning	Ask grandparents to make sure they keep their medicines out of the toddler's reach Don't leave button batteries within reach of babies and children Learn first aid for poisoning
Burns and scalds	Don't drink hot drinks while feeding or holding the baby Learn first aid for burns and scalds	Don't drink hot drinks while feeding or holding baby Consider fitting a thermostatic mixer valve (TMV) to prevent bath water scalds If you don't have a TMV, put cold water in the bath first and check the temperature before bathing baby Don't leave baby in the bath with other children Learn first aid for burns and scalds	Don't drink hot drinks while feeding or holding baby Consider fitting a TMV to prevent bath water scalds If you don't have a TMV, put cold water in the bath first and check the temperature before bathing baby Don't leave baby in the bath with other children Learn first aid for burns and scalds	Keep hot drinks out of baby's reach Keep babies away from kettles, cookers, and other hot things in the kitchen and barbeques in the garden Keep babies away from hot hair straighteners and irons Use a fire guard to prevent baby from touching gas, electric, wood-burning, multi-fuel, or open fires Consider fitting a TMV to prevent bath water scalds If you don't have a TMV, put cold water in the bath first and check the temperature before bathing baby	Teach toddlers kitchen safety rules about hot things, not climbing, and what to do/not do when adults are cooking Keep toddlers away from kettles, cookers, and other hot things in the kitchen and barbeques in the garden Keep toddlers away from hot hair straighteners and irons

(continued)

Table 14.2 Continued

Injury prevention topic	Antenatal health promotion visit	New baby review	6–8-week review	9–12-month review	2–2.5-year review
				Don't leave baby in the bath with other children Learn first aid for burns and scalds	Use a fire guard to prevent toddlers from touching gas, electric, wood-burning, multi-fuel, or open fires Consider fitting a TMV to prevent bath water scalds If you don't have a TMV, put cold water in the bath first and check the temperature before toddlers get in the bath Don't leave toddlers alone in the bathroom or alone in the bath Don't leave toddlers alone in the bath or with other children in the bath with other children Learn first aid for burns and scalds

Drowning	Bath seats are not safety devices and children have drowned in them. Think carefully before using a bath seat	Babies need constant adult supervision while in the bath Bath seats are not safety devices and children have drowned in them. Think carefully before using a bath seat	Babies need constant adult supervision while in the bath Bath seats are not safety devices and children have drowned in them. Think carefully before using a bath seat	Babies need constant adult supervision while in the bath Bath seats are not safety devices and children have drowned in them. Think carefully before using a bath seat Always supervise babies/toddlers in paddling pools Restrict access to garden ponds Be aware of risks around swimming pools, including when on holiday when adults are relaxed and children are excited Learn how to resuscitate a baby	Toddlers need constant adult supervision while in the bath Always supervise toddlers in paddling pools Restrict access to garden ponds Be aware of risks around swimming pools, including when on holiday when adults are relaxed and children are excited Learn how to resuscitate a toddler
House fires	Ensure there is a fitted and working smoke alarm on every level of the home Check the alarm is working every month Ensure families know how to test their alarm Make and practise a plan for how to escape from a house fire	Ensure there is a fitted and working smoke alarm on every level of the home Check the alarm is working every month Ensure families know how to test their alarm	Ensure there is a fitted and working smoke alarm on every level of the home Check the alarm is working every month Ensure families know how to test their alarm	Ensure there is a fitted and working smoke alarm on every level of the home Check the alarm is working every month Ensure families know how to test their alarm	Ensure there is a fitted and working smoke alarm on every level of the home Check the alarm is working every month Ensure families know how to test their alarm

(continued)

Table 14.2 Continued

Injury prevention topic	Antenatal health promotion visit	New baby review	6–8-week review	9–12-month review	2–2.5-year review
	Don't put clothes/furnishings near fire	Make and practise a plan for how to escape from a house fire	Make and practise a plan for how to escape from a house fire	Make and practise a plan for how to escape from a house fire	Make and practise a plan for how to escape from a house fire
	Use reputable mobile charging devices and don't leave devices to charge on beds or furniture	Don't put clothes/furnishings near fire	Don't put clothes/furnishings near fire	Don't put clothes/furnishings near fire	Don't put clothes/furnishings near fire
	Ensure cigarettes, candles, and tea lights are put out, especially when going to bed	Use reputable mobile charging devices and don't leave devices to charge on beds or furniture	Use reputable mobile charging devices and don't leave devices to charge on beds or furniture	Use reputable mobile charging devices and don't leave devices to charge on beds or furniture	Use reputable mobile charging devices and don't leave devices to charge on beds or furniture
		Ensure cigarettes, candles, and tea lights are put out, especially when going to bed	Ensure cigarettes, candles, and tea lights are put out, especially when going to bed	Ensure cigarettes, candles, and tea lights are put out, especially when going to bed	Ensure cigarettes, candles, and tea lights are put out, especially when going to bed
		Don't leave pans with hot oil unattended	Keep matches and lighters away from babies	Keep matches and lighters away from babies/toddlers	Keep matches and lighters away from babies/toddlers
		Don't overload plug sockets	Don't leave pans with hot oil unattended	Don't leave pans with hot oil unattended	Keep matches and lighters way from babies/toddlers
		Take extra care around fire when drinking alcohol, using medication or drugs	Don't overload plug sockets	Don't overload plug sockets	Don't leave pans with hot oil unattended
		The fire and rescue service offers free home fire safety checks	Take extra care around fire when drinking alcohol, using medication or drugs	Take extra care around fire when drinking alcohol, using medication or drugs	Don't overload plug sockets
			The fire and rescue service offers free home fire safety checks	The fire and rescue service offers free home fire safety checks	

				Take extra care around fire when drinking alcohol, using medication or drugs The fire and rescue service offers free home fire safety checks
Road traffic injuries	Use a correctly fitted rear-facing child seat in the car on every trip, preferably in the back seat. If you have to use the front seat, turn off the front air bag Use rear facing seat for as long as possible based on manufacturer's height/weight recommendations Avoid distractions including using mobile phones	Use a correctly fitted rear-facing child seat in the car on every trip, preferably in the back seat. If you have to use the front seat, turn off the front air bag Use rear facing seat for as long as possible based on manufacturer's height/weight recommendations Avoid distractions including using mobile phones	Use a correctly fitted rear-facing child seat in the car on every trip, preferably in the back seat until baby is 12–15 months old. If you have to use the front seat, turn off the front air bag Use rear facing seat for as long as possible based on manufacturer's height/weight recommendations Avoid distractions including using mobile phones Never allow a child under five out alone Hold your baby or toddler's hand when near or crossing roads	Never allow a child under five out alone Hold your toddler's hand when near or crossing roads Explain traffic and its dangers to your child Behave safely around roads so your toddler learns from watching you Use a correctly fitted car seat for every journey progressing to a high-backed booster seat

Source: data from Hayes M., Kendrick D, and on behalf of the Keeping Children Safe study team, *A guide for commissioners of child health services on preventing unintentional injuries among the under fives*, Copyright © 2016, available from https://www.nottingham.ac.uk/research/groups/injuryresearch/documents/kcs-guide-for-commissioners.pdf; and Public Health England and The Child Accident Prevention Trust, *Preventing unintentional injuries: A guide for all staff working with children under five years*, © Crown Copyright 2017, available from https://www.gov.uk/government/uploads/system/uploads/attachment_data/file/59501?/Preventing_unintentional_injuries_guide.pdf under the Open Government Licence v.3.0.

PHE's guidance on reducing unintentional injuries on the roads recommends local authorities work with schools to develop school travel plans and introduce 20 mph speed limits in priority areas, with education, road engineering measures, and enforcement of traffic law (PHE, 2014b).

Resources to help prevent child injuries

A range of resources to help practitioners, parents, and commissioners are available online (see 'Learning links').

Learning links

- Module 10 ('Health Promotion') of the Healthy Child Programme outlines vital areas of interest in promoting health from the start in pregnancy through to the first 5 years of life, including injury prevention: https://www.e-lfh.org.uk/programmes/healthy-child-programme/.

Recommendations

- Include a home safety assessment and injury prevention (addressing the topics in Table 14.2) in the Child Health Programme. (*Evidence: moderate.*)
- Provide access to safety equipment schemes and injury prevention and advice to families with children at high risk of injury. (*Evidence: moderate.*)
- Every opportunity between families with young children and health professionals should be used to encourage behaviour change. This includes incorporating injury prevention into home visits taking place for other reasons as this allows an assessment of the context where most injuries in young children occur. (*Evidence: moderate.*)
- Provide appropriate training for health visitors and early help services (on specific topics outlined in Table 14.2). (*Evidence: moderate.*)
- Establish systems for fire and rescue services to act upon referrals from health professionals to undertake home fire risk assessments and provide and fit smoke alarms, especially in the most disadvantaged households. (*Evidence: moderate.*)
- Collaboration between public health commissioners, social housing providers, and landlord organizations to promote installation of thermostatic mixing valves when undertaking major refurbishments and provide scald prevention advice. (*Evidence: moderate.*)

References

Achana, F.A., Sutton, A.J., Kendrick, D., et al. (2015). The effectiveness of different interventions to promote poison prevention behaviours in households with children: a network meta-analysis. *PLoS One*, **10**, e0121122.

Alwash, R. and McCarthy, M. (1988). Accidents in the home among children under 5: ethnic differences or social disadvantage? *British Medical Journal (Clinical Research Edition)*, **296**, 1450–1453.

Bijur, P.E., Golding, J., and Kurzon, M. (1988). Childhood accidents, family size and birth order. *Social Science & Medicine*, **26**, 839–843.

Bijur, P.E., Stewart-Brown, S., and Butler, N. (1986). Child behavior and accidental injury in 11,966 preschool children. *American Journal of Diseases of Children*, **140**, 487–492.

Bradbury, K., Janicke, D.M., Riley, A.W., and Finney, J.W. (1999). Predictors of unintentional injuries to school-age children seen in pediatric primary care. *Journal of Pediatric Psychology*, **24**, 423–433.

Braun, P.A., Beaty, B.L., DiGuiseppi, C., and Steiner, J.F. (2005). Recurrent early childhood injuries among disadvantaged children in primary care settings. *Injury Prevention*, **11**, 251–255.

Buck, D., and Gregory, S. (2013). The King's Fund. Improving the public's health. A resource for local authorities. [online] Available at: http://www.kingsfund.org.uk/projects/improving-publics-health/warmer-and-safer-homes. [Accessed 25 Oct. 2016].

Conners-Burrow, N.A., Fussell, J.J., Johnson, D.L, et al. (2013). Maternal low- and high-depressive symptoms and safety concerns for low-income preschool children. *Clinical Pediatrics*, **52**, 171–177.

Cooper, N.J., Kendrick, D., Achana, F., et al. (2012). Network meta-analysis to evaluate the effectiveness of interventions to increase the uptake of smoke alarms. *Epidemiologic Reviews*, **34**, 32–45.

Currie, E., Williams, J., Wright, P., Beattie, T., and Harel, Y. (1996). Incidence and distribution of injury among schoolchildren aged 11–15. *Injury Prevention*, **2**, 21–25.

Department for Transport (2016). *Reported Road Casualties Great Britain, Annual Report: 2015*. London: Department for Transport.

DiGuiseppi, C., and Roberts, I.G. (2000). Individual-level injury prevention strategies in the clinical setting. *The Future of Children*, **10**, 53–82.

Dowswell, T., Towner, E.M.L., Simpson, T.G., and Jarvis, S.N. (1996). Preventing childhood unintentional injuries – what works? A literature review. *Injury Prevention*, **2**, 140–149.

Fraser, J., Sidebotham, P., Frederick, J., Covington, T., and Mitchell, E.A. (2014). Learning from child death review in the USA, England, Australia, and New Zealand. *The Lancet*, **384**, 894–903.

Haddon, W. (1980). Advances in the epidemiology of injuries as a basis for public policy. *Public Health Reports*, **95**, 411–421.

Hardelid, P., Davey, J., Dattani, N., Gilbert, R., and the Working Group of the Research Policy Directorate of the Royal College of Paediatrics Child Health (2013). Child deaths due to injury in the four UK countries: a time trends study from 1980 to 2010. *PLoS One*, **8**, e68323.

Harris, M.J., and Kotch, J.B. (1994). Unintentional infant injuries: sociodemographic and psychosocial factors. *Public Health Nursing*, **11**, 90–97.

Hayes, M., Kendrick, D., and Keeping Children Safe study team. (2016). A guide for commissioners of child health services on preventing unintentional injuries among the under fives. [online] Available at: http://www.nottingham.ac.uk/research/groups/injuryresearch/projects/kcs/index.aspx [Accessed 27 Oct. 2016].

Hippisley-Cox, J., Groom, L., Kendrick, D., Coupland, C., Webber, E., and Savelyich, B. (2002). Cross sectional survey of socioeconomic variations in severity and mechanism of childhood injuries in Trent 1992-7. *British Medical Journal*, **324**, 1132–1134.

Hubbard, S., Cooper, N., Kendrick, D., et al. (2015). Network meta-analysis to evaluate the effectiveness of interventions to prevent falls in children under age 5 years. *Injury Prevention*, **21**, 98–108.

Kendrick, D., Mulvaney, C.A., Ye, L., Stevens, T., Mytton, J.A., and Stewart-Brown, S. (2013). Parenting interventions for the prevention of unintentional injuries in childhood. *Cochrane Database of Systematic Reviews*, **3**, CD006020.

Kendrick, D., Young, B., Mason-Jones, A.J., et al. (2012). Home safety education and provision of safety equipment for injury prevention. *Cochrane Database of Systematic Reviews*, **9**, CD005014.

Marmot, M., Allen, J., Goldblatt, P., et al. (2010). *Fair Society, Healthy Lives: A Strategic Review of Inequalities in England post-2010*. London: Institute of Health Equity.

Morrongiello, B.A., Corbett, M., McCourt, M., and Johnston, N. (2006). Understanding unintentional injury risk in young children II. The contribution of caregiver supervision, child attributes, and parent attributes. *Journal of Pediatric Psychology*, **31**, 540–551.

National Institute for Health and Care Excellence (NICE) (2007). Behaviour change: general approaches. NICE public health guidance [PH6]. Available at: https://www.nice.org.uk/guidance/ph6 [Accessed 13 Jan. 2017].

National Institute for Health and Care Excellence (NICE) (2010a). Unintentional injuries: prevention strategies for under 15s. NICE public health guidance [PH29]. [online] Available at: https://www.nice.org.uk/guidance/ph30 [Accessed 23 Aug. 2016].

National Institute for Health and Care Excellence (NICE) (2010b). Preventing unintentional injuries in the home among children and young people aged under 15: home safety assessments and providing safety equipment. NICE public health guidance [PH30]. [online] Available at: https://www.nice.org.uk/guidance/ph30 [Accessed 23 Aug. 2016].

National Institute for Health and Care Excellence (NICE) (2010c). Preventing unintentional road injuries among under-15s: road design. NICE public health guidance [PH31]. Available at: https://www.nice.org.uk/guidance/ph31 [Accessed 23 Aug. 2016].

NHS Digital (2015). Hospital Episode Statistics, Admitted Patient Care - England, 2014-15: External causes. [online] Available at: http://content.digital.nhs.uk/searchcatalogue?productid=19420&q=title%3a%22Hospital+Episode+Statistics%2c+Admitted+patient+care+-+England%22&sort=Relevance&size=10&page=1#top [Accessed 3 Jan. 2017].

O'Connor, T.G., Davies, L., Dunn, J., and Golding, J. (2000). Distribution of accidents, injuries, and illnesses by family type. ALSPAC Study Team. Avon Longitudinal Study of Pregnancy and Childhood. *Pediatrics*, **106**, E68.

Office for National Statistics (2015). *Death Registrations Summary Statistics, England and Wales, 2014*. London: Office for National Statistics.

Olds, D. (2016). Building evidence to improve maternal and child health. *The Lancet*, **387**, 105–107.

Orton, E., Kendrick, D., West, J., and Tata, L.J. (2012). Independent risk factors for injury in pre-school children: three population-based nested case-control studies using routine primary care data. *PLoS One*, **7**, e35193.

Orton, E., Kendrick, D., West, J., and Tata, L.J. (2014). Persistence of health inequalities in childhood injury in the UK; a population-based cohort study of children under 5. *PLoS ONE*, **9**, e111631.

Orton, E., Whitehead, J., Mhizha-Murira, J., et al. (2016). School-based education programmes for the prevention of unintentional injuries in children and young people. *Cochrane Database of Systematic Reviews*, **12**, CD010246.

Pearson, M., Hewson, P., Moxham, T., and Taylor, R. (2009). *Review 2: A Systematic Review of Risk Factors for Unintentional Injuries Among Children and Young People Aged Under 15 Years. Quantitative Correlates Review of Unintentional Injury in Children*. Exeter: Peninsula Medical School, Universities of Exeter and Plymouth.

Phelan, K.J., Morrongiello, B.A., Khoury, J.C., Xu, Y., Liddy, S., and Lanphear, B. (2014). Maternal supervision of children during their first 3 years of life: the influence of maternal depression and child gender. *Journal of Pediatric Psychology*, **39**, 349–357.

Public Health England (PHE) (2014a). Reducing unintentional injuries in and around the home among children under five years. [online] Available at: https://www.gov.uk/government/publications/reducing-unintentional-injuries-among-children-and-young-people.

Public Health England (PHE) (2014b). Reducing unintentional injuries on the roads among children and young people under 25 years. [online] Available at: https://www.gov.uk/government/uploads/system/uploads/attachment_data/file/322212/Reducing_unintentional_injuries_on_the_roads_among_children_and_young_people_under_25_years.pdf. [Accessed 23 Aug. 2016].

Public Health England (PHE) (2014c). Overview of the six early years and school aged years high impact areas. [online] Available at: https://www.gov.uk/government/uploads/system/uploads/attachment_data/file/413127/2903110_Early_Years_Impact_GENERAL_V0_2W.pdf [Accessed 3 Nov. 2016].

Public Health England and the Child Accident Prevention Trust. (2017). Preventing unintentional injuries. A guide for all staff working with children under five years. [online] Available at: https://www.gov.uk/government/publications/unintentional-injuries-prevention-in-children-under-5-years [Accessed 20 Mar. 2017].

Robling, M., Bekkers, M.J., Bell, K., et al. (2016). Effectiveness of a nurse-led intensive home-visitation programme for first-time teenage mothers (Building Blocks): a pragmatic randomised controlled trial. *The Lancet*, **387**, 146–155.

Rowe, R., Maughan, B., and Goodman, R. (2004). Childhood psychiatric disorder and unintentional injury: findings from a national cohort study. *Journal of Pediatric Psychology*, **29**, 119–130.

Royal Society for the Prevention of Accidents (2002). Home & Leisure Accident Surveillance System. Annual Report 2000–2002. 2002 data. [online] Available at: http://www.hassandlass.org.uk/reports/2002data.pdf [Accessed 31 Oct. 2016].

Royal Society for the Prevention of Accidents (2012). *Big Book of Accident Prevention*. Birmingham: RoSPA. Available at: https://www.rospa.com/rospaweb/docs/advice-services/public-health/big-book.pdf

Schnitzer, P.G., Dowd, M.D., Kruse, R.L., and Morrongiello, B.A. (2015). Supervision and risk of unintentional injury in young children. *Injury Prevention*, **21**, e63–70.

Schwebel, D.C. and Brezausek, C.M. (2008). Chronic maternal depression and children's injury risk. *Journal of Pediatric Psychology*, **33**, 1108–1116.

Schwebel, D.C. and Brezausek, C.M. (2010). Brief report: unintentional injury risk among children with sensory impairments. *Journal of Pediatric Psychology*, **35**, 45–50.

Schwebel, D.C., Brezausek, C.M., Ramey, S.L., and Ramey, C.T. (2004). Interactions between child behavior patterns and parenting: implications for children's unintentional injury risk. *Journal of Pediatric Psychology*, **29**, 93–104.

Sellar, C., Ferguson, J.A., and **Goldacre, M.J.** (1991). Occurrence and repetition of hospital admissions for accidents in preschool children. *British Medical Journal*, **302**, 16–19.

Sethi, D., Towner, E., Vincenten, J., Segui-Gomez, M., and **Racioppi, F.** (2008). *European Report on Child Injury Prevention*. Geneva: World Health Organization.

Shi, X, Shi, J., Wheeler, K.K., et al. (2015). Unintentional injuries in children with disabilities: a systematic review and meta-analysis. *Injury Epidemiology*, **2**, 21.

The Road Safety Observatory (2017). Child restraints – how effective? [online] Available at: http://www.roadsafetyobservatory.com/HowEffective/vehicles/child-restraints [Accessed 25 Oct. 2016].

Tobin, M.D., Milligan, J., Shukla, R., Crump, B., and **Burton, P.R.** (2002). South Asian ethnicity and risk of childhood accidents: an ecological study at enumeration district level in Leicester. *Journal of Public Health Medicine*, **24**, 313–318.

Walsh, S.S.M., Jarvis, S.N., Towner, E.M.L., and **Aynsley-Green, A.** (1996). Annual incidence of unintentional injury among 54,000 children. *Injury Prevention*, **2**, 16–20.

Warrington, S.A., Wright, C.M., and **ALSPAC Study Team** (2001). Accidents and resulting injuries in premobile infants: data from the ALSPAC study. *Archives of Disease in Childhood*, **85**, 104–107.

Welsh Government (2013). Road Safety Framework for Wales. [online] Available at: http://gov.wales/docs/det/publications/130719delplanen.pdf [Accessed 9 Aug. 2017].

World Health Organization (1998). Health Promotion Glossary. [online] Available at: http://www.who.int/healthpromotion/about/HPR%20Glossary%201998.pdf [Accessed 23 Aug. 2016].

Chapter 15

Prevention of sudden infant death syndrome (SIDS)

Peter S. Blair and Anna Pease

Summary

This chapter:

- describes the epidemiology of sudden infant death syndrome (SIDS)
- summarizes the potential causal mechanisms for SIDS
- reviews the impact of the 'Back to Sleep' campaign, and the current risk reduction messages
- addresses the divergence of opinion over preventative advice surrounding infant bed sharing.

Sudden infant death syndrome and the 1991 'Back to Sleep' campaign

Sudden infant death syndrome (SIDS) is defined as the sudden death of an infant under 1 year old that is unexpected by history and unexplained after a thorough postmortem examination, including a complete autopsy, investigation of the scene of death, and review of the medical history (Willinger et al., 1991). Death often occurs unobserved, during infant sleep, with no discernible signs of a major illness. The diagnosis is reached by exclusion, by failing to demonstrate an adequate cause of death. These deaths have been recognized throughout history but were only given an international classification code in 1969. Subsequent observational studies revealed similar epidemiological characteristics among these infants and families across different cultures. The age distribution is unique to the syndrome, few deaths in the first weeks of life when infants are most vulnerable, a peak around the third and fourth month, and few deaths after 8 months. Like other infant deaths, it is more prevalent in males and the risk, until recently, increased in winter months. SIDS occurs across the social strata but is more prevalent in the socio-economically deprived groups and strongly associated with parental smoking. Lower birthweight and shorter gestation is more prevalent while maternal factors are important: there is a correlation with young maternal age and higher parity and the risk increases with multiple births.

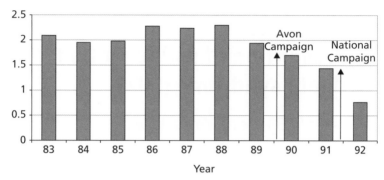

Fig. 15.1 SIDS rate in England and Wales per 1000 livebirths (1983–1992).

Source: data from the Office of National Statistics, *Unexplained Deaths in Infancy,*
England and Wales: 2014, © Crown Copyright, available from https://www.ons.gov.uk/
peoplepopulationandcommunity/birthsdeathsandmarriages/deaths/bulletins/unexplaineddeathsininfa
ncyenglandandwales/2014. Contains public sector information licensed under the Open Government
Licence v3.0.

By the late 1980s, the focus of research was on the infant sleeping environment and
evidence from several different countries suggested SIDS deaths could be related to
infants sleeping in the prone position (Davies, 1985; Saturnus, 1985; De Jonge et al.,
1989; Fleming et al., 1990; Mitchell et al., 1991). In Avon in 1990 and nationally in
1991, the 'Back to Sleep' campaign was initiated to encourage parents to avoid placing
their infants on their front, to use less bedclothes, and discourage smoking. As Figure
15.1 shows, the SIDS rate dramatically fell from a peak of 2.3 deaths in 1988 to 0.77
deaths per 1000 livebirths in 1992. This constitutes a 67% fall from 1597 deaths in
England and Wales in 1988 to just 531 deaths by 1992. Similar reductions in the death
rate were observed in several countries after such a campaign.

Subsequent risk factors and protective factors identified

In England and Wales, the SIDS rate continued to fall at a less dramatic but consistent rate
from 0.77 deaths per 1000 livebirths in 1992 to 0.3 deaths by 2014 (Figure 15.2). This constitutes a further 60% fall from 531 deaths to 212 SIDS deaths by 2014 as well as an overall
87% fall in rate since 1988. There is also evidence that this further fall was not due to any
change in prone positioning but concomitant with changes in other identified risk factors.

Evidence from two population-based, case–control studies conducted 10 years apart
in England between 1993–1996 (Fleming et al., 1996) and 2003–2006 (Blair et al.,
2009) suggests parental behaviour in terms of placing infants prone to sleep did not
change in these populations but behaviour regarding other identified factors did. The
risks associated with certain factors decreased:

♦ Wrapped too warmly
♦ Placed on their side to sleep

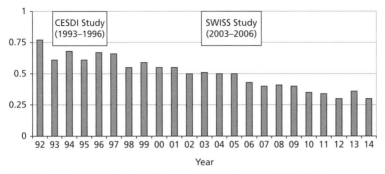

Fig. 15.2 SIDS rate in England and Wales per 1000 livebirths (1992–2014).

Source: data from the Office of National Statistics, *Unexplained Deaths in Infancy, England and Wales: 2014*, © Crown Copyright, available from https://www.ons.gov.uk/peoplepopulationandcommunity/birthsdeathsandmarriages/deaths/bulletins/unexplaineddeathsininfancyenglandandwales/2014. Contains public sector information licensed under the Open Government Licence v3.0.

- Infants exposed to tobacco smoke after the birth
- Infants found with bedding over their heads

while the protective effect of other factors increased:

- Infants being placed 'feet to foot' (with their feet at the foot of the cot to avoid wriggling under the covers)
- Infants being breastfed.

The dramatic fall in SIDS rates over a relatively short period of time has led to changes in the characteristic profile of these deaths. SIDS infants are now almost exclusively from socio-economically deprived families, infant vulnerability in terms of low birthweight and prematurity has become more marked, the peak age of death has fallen from 3 months to 2 months, and the prevalence of co-sleeping deaths has increased from 12% to 50% (Blair et al., 2006). This rather alarming proportional rise in co-sleeping SIDS deaths has led some countries to recommend against bed sharing including the American Academy of Pediatrics (2005). However, on closer inspection of 300 consecutive SIDS cases in Avon over a 20-year period (Blair et al., 2009) the number of co-sleeping SIDS deaths in the parental bed declined, just not as rapidly as solitary sleeping deaths in a cot. This coupled with a numerical increase in co-sleeping deaths on a sofa accounts for the proportional rise of co-sleeping deaths.

The difficulty with the recommendations in the US is partly that bed sharing is strongly associated with breastfeeding (Das et al., 2014; Ward 2015); ironically, the reason why the 'Back to Sleep' campaign was probably less effective at reducing bed-sharing deaths is that mothers were less likely to place infants prone if they intended to breastfeed. The other difficulty is that taking such a direct and simplistic approach does not seem to work (Moon et al., 2017) as higher-risk groups continue to bed share and the SIDS rate in the US has flat-lined since an initial decline in the 1990s. There is also evidence that the risk to infants is not so much co-sleeping but the hazardous environment in which some of these co-sleeping SIDS infants were found: sleeping next to adults who had consumed alcohol, taken illegal drugs, or co-slept on a sofa (Blair et al., 2009, 2014). The National Institute for Health and Care Excellence (NICE, 2015) reviewed the available evidence and suggested health professionals should not advise against bed sharing, but rather acknowledge it occurs both intentionally and unintentionally and discuss hazardous circumstances that can put infants at risk.

Other care practices and associated SIDS risks have also been investigated, including swaddling and dummy use. Swaddling had originally been hypothesized to reduce the risk of SIDS by keeping sleeping babies in the supine position, but a recent meta-analysis (Pease et al., 2016) found this not to be the case, although the risk for being placed on the back and swaddled was low, it was not protective (ISPID Physiology Working Group, 2017). The risk associated with infants being placed on their side or front increased further when the infant was swaddled. Current advice in the UK is that where parents choose to swaddle, babies should always be placed for sleep on their back and swaddling should be discontinued as soon as infants show signs of being able to roll over. Several case–control studies have found a protective effect for using a dummy, although the mechanism for protection is unclear as most dummies fall out or get removed after the initial sleep onset. This, combined with evidence that dummies may inhibit frequency and duration of breastfeeding, make this recommendation less robust. Again, the UK has taken a cautious approach to the evidence and recommends that where parents choose to use a dummy, they should do so after breastfeeding has been established.

Potential causal mechanisms of SIDS

There are characteristic postmortem findings in many cases of SIDS, but they are not diagnostic and do not yield an explanation as to why the infant died. After several decades of research, the hope of finding a single cause for SIDS has proved elusive and current thinking is that several potential causal mechanisms could be involved. The 'triple risk' hypothesis—which envisages SIDS occurring as a result of (i) a final insult (one which is not usually fatal on its own) that affects a baby with (ii) an intrinsic vulnerability (arising from genetic or early developmental factors), at (iii) a potentially vulnerable stage of physiological development (e.g. immunological, respiratory, cardiovascular, thermal)—has been proposed in various forms by a number of authors (Tonkin, 1986; Filiano and Kinney, 1994; Guneroth and Spiers, 2002). This seems to fit with the proposed pathogenesis of established risk factors and known physiology.

In the prone position, babies are potentially more vulnerable to the effects of re-breathing expired gases, particularly if sleeping on soft bedding (Bolton et al., 1993). A further effect of the prone sleeping position is that the arousal threshold is higher (Franco et al., 1998); response to adverse events such as hypoxia may have more profound and lethal effects in the prone position. Blackwell and Weir (1999) have suggested a possible mechanism by which the prone sleeping position, heavy wrapping, and the presence of a viral infection might predispose to the development of a secondary infection leading to the lethal development of shock.

While the final sequence of events leading to death is not known, physiological recordings of some infants prior to death suggest a cardiovascular rather than a respiratory event as the primary trigger for the final collapse (Poets, 2004). One possible physiological explanation for such a pattern might be a catastrophic fall in blood pressure as a consequence of sudden peripheral vasodilatation, for example, in response to toxins or as a consequence of heat stress (Morris, 1999). Head covering may cause death by the effects of thermal imbalance. Thermal modelling of clothed infants over a wide range of environmental temperatures suggests that the most important determinant of heat loss is not the quantity of insulation (unless extreme) but the area of exposed skin, particularly that of the head (Nelson, 1989).

The mechanism by which exposure to tobacco smoke increases the risk of SIDS is not clear, although exposure may contribute to deficient hypoxia responses, may impair the development of the autonomic function, and increase the prevalence of respiratory infections throughout childhood. An intriguing finding currently being investigated is whether differences found in infant hearing test scores is a marker for exposure to tobacco smoke *in utero* or a marker for brainstem dysfunction that could be used to identify families with infants at high risk of SIDS (Rubens, 2008).

The circumstances in which co-sleeping SIDS victims are discovered would suggest that entrapment or accidental overlaying may be the primary mechanism, especially if alcohol or other sleep-inducing drugs are involved, although it would be wrong to assume this for the majority of cases. Cot death is not the preserve of the cot but happens in different sleeping environments. In England on any one particular night, nearly a quarter of parents bring the infant into the parental bed, thus one would expect a certain proportion of SIDS to be discovered during co-sleeping (Blair and Ball, 2004). Apart from possible signs of intrapulmonary haemorrhage, suffocation cannot be detected at postmortem investigation. The diagnosis of overlaying would require supportive evidence from the death scene investigation and parental interview.

Current recommendations and the prevention of SIDS

The debate on the safety, advantages, and disadvantages of infant care practices must be informed not just by epidemiological evidence from one narrow field but from many disciplines from different fields if it is to lead to effective change. The advantages when we get this advice right are evident in the dramatic fall in SIDS deaths; if the SIDS rates had remained unchanged since 1988, a further 30,000 families in England and Wales would have lost an infant to SIDS in the subsequent 25 years.

The current advice in the UK (Box 15.1) tries to strike a balance between a cautious approach to what we have learnt in SIDS research and what we have learnt from other related fields and disciplines. The UNICEF UK Baby Friendly Initiative also provides information on safe infant sleep, aligned with The Lullaby Trust messages with a focus on promoting breastfeeding and infant bonding (UNICEF, 2016). This includes specific advice to parents who choose to share a bed with their babies on how to make the sleeping environment as safe as possible, thus adopting a risk minimization approach.

Box 15.1 Current UK advice on the risk reduction of SIDS

1. Always place your baby on their back to sleep.

2. Keep your baby smoke free during pregnancy and after birth.

3. Place your baby to sleep in a separate cot or Moses basket in the same room as you for the first 6 months.

4. Breastfeed your baby.

5. Use a firm, flat, waterproof mattress in good condition.

6. Never sleep on a sofa or in an armchair with your baby.

7. Don't sleep in the same bed as your baby if you smoke, drink alcohol, have taken drugs or are extremely tired, if your baby was born prematurely, or was of low birth-weight.

8. Avoid letting your baby get too hot.

9. Don't cover your baby's face or head while sleeping or use loose bedding.

Adapted with permission from The Lullaby Trust, *Safer sleep for babies: A guide for parents*, Copyright © 2013 The Lullaby Trust, available from https://www.lullabytrust.org.uk/wp-content/uploads/safer-sleep-for-parents.pdf.

Conclusion

Despite the decline in SIDS, it is still one of the major causes of post-neonatal infant death. It is a complex disorder and continued research and monitoring are needed to fully understand the subtle interactions between different factors. The SIDS rate will decline further if the current recommendations are followed. Community midwives already provide SIDS risk reduction advice for all mothers shortly after the birth along with plenty of helpful information regarding other infant care practices. If a scoring system can be derived to identify a relatively small group of mothers at higher risk of SIDS, they could be targeted for enhanced messaging during this critical period of dependency on the healthcare system. How to disseminate these guidelines, especially among high-risk families, encourage putting them into practice, and increase our understanding of the potential causal mechanisms are the future challenges.

Learning links

◆ Information for professionals can be accessed via The Lullaby Trust: https://www.lullabytrust.org.uk/professionals/.

Recommendations

- Commissioners should ensure that the latest evidence-based recommendations are followed in their local area. (*Evidence: strong.*)

- Practitioners should ensure that all parents are given evidence-based advice antenatally, and that additional time for discussion is given to families with infants at potentially higher risk of SIDS. (*Evidence: strong.*)

- Consistent messages should be given to parents both prenatally from midwives and at the new baby check from health visitors. (*Good practice.*)

- All parents should be provided with the latest advice from UNICEF/The Lullaby Trust/NICE around sleeping habits (co-sleeping), to enable them to make informed choices. (*Evidence: moderate.*)

- Practitioners should ensure that all at-risk, hard-to-reach families are given support in implementing the latest guidance. (*Good practice.*)

References

American Academy of Pediatrics (2005). The changing concept of sudden infant death syndrome: diagnostic coding shifts, controversies regarding the sleeping environment, and new variables to consider in reducing risk. *Pediatrics*, **116**, 1245–1255.

Blackwell, C.C. and **Weir, D.M.** (1999). The role of infection in sudden infant death syndrome. *FEMS Immunology and Medical Microbiology*, **25**, 1–6.

Blair, P.S. and **Ball, H.L.** (2004). The prevalence and characteristics associated with parent-infant bed-sharing in England. *Archives of Disease in Childhood*, **89**, 1106–1110.

Blair, P.S., Sidebotham, P., Berry, P.J., Evans, M., and **Fleming, P.J.** (2006). Major epidemiological changes in sudden infant death syndrome: a 20-year population-based study in the UK. *The Lancet*, **367**, 314–319.

Blair, P.S., Sidebotham, P., Evason-Coombe, C., et al. (2009). Hazardous cosleeping environments and risk factors amenable to change: case-control study of SIDS in south west England. *BMJ*, **339**, b3666.

Blair, P.S., Sidebotham, P., Pease, A., and **Fleming, P.J.** (2014). Bed-sharing in the absence of hazardous circumstances: is there a risk of sudden infant death syndrome? An analysis from two case-control studies conducted in the UK. *PLoS One*, **9**, e107799.

Bolton, D.P., Taylor, B.J., Campbell, A.J., Galland, B.C., and **Cresswell, C.** (1993). Rebreathing expired gases from bedding: a cause of cot death? *Archives of Disease in Childhood*, **69**, 187–190.

Das, R.R., Sankar, M.J., Agarwal, R., and **Paul, V.K.** (2014). Is 'bed sharing' beneficial and safe during infancy? A systematic review. *International Journal of Pediatrics*, **46**, 8538.

Davies, D.P. (1985). Cot death in Hong Kong: a rare problem? *The Lancet*, **2**, 1346–1349.

De Jonge, G.A., Engleberts, A.C., Koomen-Liefting, A.J., and Kostense, P.J. (1989). Cot death and prone sleeping position in The Netherlands. *BMJ*, **298**, 722.

Filiano, J.J. and Kinney, H.C. (1994). A perspective on neuropathologic findings in victims of the sudden infant death syndrome: the triple-risk model. *Biology of the Neonate*, **65**, 194–197.

Fleming, P.J., Blair, P.S., Bacon, C., et al. (1996). Environment of infants during sleep and risk of the sudden infant death syndrome: results of 1993–5 case-control study for confidential inquiry into stillbirths and deaths in infancy. Confidential Enquiry into Stillbirths and Deaths Regional Coordinators and Researchers. *BMJ*, **313**, 191–195.

Fleming, P.J., Gilbert, R., Azaz, Y., et al. (1990). Interaction between bedding and sleeping position in the sudden infant death syndrome: a population based case-control study. *BMJ*, **301**, 85–89.

Franco, P., Pardou, A., Hassid, S., Lurquin, P., Grosswasser, J., and Kahn, A. (1998). Auditory arousal thresholds are higher when infants sleep in the prone position. *Journal of Pediatrics*, **132**, 240–243.

Guneroth, W.G. and Spiers, P.S. (2002). The triple risk hypotheses in sudden infant death syndrome. *Pediatrics*, **110**, e64.

ISPID Physiology Working Group (2017). To Swaddle or Not to Swaddle? [online] Available at: https://www.ispid.org/infantdeath/id-statements/swaddling/.

Mitchell, E.A., Scragg, R., Stewart, A.W., et al. (1991). Results from the first year of the New Zealand cot death study. *New Zealand Medical Journal*, **104**, 71–76.

Moon, R.Y., Mathews, A., Joyner, B.L., Oden, R.P., He, J., and McCarter, R. (2017). Health messaging and African-American infant sleep location: a randomized controlled trial. *Journal of Community Health*. **42**, 1–9.

Morris, J.A. (1999). The common bacterial toxins hypothesis of sudden infant death syndrome. *FEMS Immunology and Medical Microbiology*, **25**, 11–17.

National Institute for Health and Care Excellence (NICE) (2015). Recommendations. In: *Postnatal Care up to 8 Weeks After Birth* [CG37]. London: NICE. Available at: https://www.nice.org.uk/guidance/cg37/chapter/1-Recommendations.

Nelson, E.A., Taylor, B.J., and Weatherall, I.L. (1989). Sleeping position and infant bedding may predispose to hyperthermia and the sudden infant death syndrome. *The Lancet*, **1**, 199–201.

Pease, A.S., Fleming, P.J., Hauck, F.R., et al. (2016). Swaddling and the risk of sudden infant death syndrome: a meta-analysis. *Pediatrics*, **137**, e20153275.

Poets, C.F. (2004). Apparent life-threatening events and sudden infant death on a monitor. *Paediatric Respiratory Reviews*, 5(Suppl A), S383–S386.

Rubens, D.D., Vohr, B.R., Tucker, R., O'Neil, C.A., and Chung, W. (2008). Newborn oto-acoustic emission hearing screening tests: preliminary evidence for a marker of susceptibility to SIDS. *Early Human Development*, **84**, 225–229.

Saturnus, K. (1985). *Plotzicher Kindstod - eine Folge der Bauchlage? Festschrift Professor Leithoff.* Heidelberg: Kriminalstatistik.

Tonkin, S.L. (1986). Epidemiology of cot deaths in Auckland. *New Zealand Medical Journal*, **99**, 324–326.

UNICEF UK Baby Friendly Initiative (2016). Caring for your baby at night: a guide for parents. [online] Available at: https://www.unicef.org.uk/babyfriendly/baby-friendly-resources/leaflets-and-posters/caring-for-your-baby-at-night/.

Ward, T.C. (2015). Reasons for mother-infant bed-sharing: a systematic narrative synthesis of the literature and implications for future research. *Maternal and Child Health Journal*, **19**, 675–690.

Willinger, M., James, L., and Catz, C. (1991). Defining the sudden infant death syndrome (SIDS): deliberations of an expert panel convened by the National Institute of Child Health and Human Development. *Pediatric Pathology*, **11**, 677–684.

Chapter 16

Integrating immunizations into the programme

Helen Bedford and David Elliman

Summary

This chapter:

♦ summarizes how immunization is a highly effective intervention to protect children from serious infectious diseases

♦ describes how pockets of low uptake, and social inequalities compromise herd immunity in the UK

♦ reviews the evidence for strategies to increase and maintain vaccine uptake

♦ concludes that multicomponent strategies tailored to local need are most effective.

Introduction

In the UK, the universal immunization programme extends throughout the life course. From September 2017, with the addition of universal hepatitis B vaccine, children under 7 years are offered protection against 14 diseases. The 2017–2018 schedule is available from https://www.gov.uk/government/uploads/system/uploads/attachment_data/file/633691/Childhood_imm_schedule_2017.pdf.

Changes to the schedule are frequent, and for up-to-date information, the relevant website of the appropriate UK nation should be consulted:

♦ England (Gov.uk, 2017a)

♦ Scotland (Immunisationscotland.org.uk, 2017)

♦ Wales (Wales.nhs.uk, 2017)

♦ Northern Ireland (Publichealth.hscni.net, 2017).

The evidence for the effectiveness of immunization is powerful. In the UK, overall vaccine uptake rates are high and most vaccine-preventable diseases are uncommon. However, there continue to be outbreaks of some diseases, including pertussis, measles, and mumps for a variety of reasons. The focus of this chapter is on ensuring children are as fully protected with available vaccines as possible.

Immunization in the child health programme

The child health programme provides opportunities to introduce immunization to parents, to offer ongoing advice and information, and to review children's immunization status and take action when required. Antenatal vaccines to protect mothers and newborns against influenza and pertussis were introduced in 2010 and 2012 respectively. Health professional contacts antenatally provide opportunities both to discuss vaccines in pregnancy as well as to introduce the childhood vaccination schedule so parents can start considering it early (Ames et al., 2017).

Immunization uptake in the UK

Although overall immunization vaccine coverage rates in the UK are high, pockets of lower coverage and social inequalities in uptake persist. Sustaining and improving vaccine uptake rates remain a high priority: to focus interventions appropriately, the causes of and groups at risk of lower uptake need to be identified. High-quality studies have identified two broad groups of children at risk of under-immunization. The largest group, those with difficulties accessing services for logistical or practical reasons, are often partially immunized with incomplete immunization courses or not done in a timely fashion. A smaller group, comprising about 1–2% of the population, are children whose parents have declined immunization because they consider the vaccines to be unsafe or unnecessary (Samad et al., 2006; Campbell et al., 2017). As these unvaccinated children may cluster in the population, outbreaks may occur. A few children may not be fully immunized because of a false contraindication.

Vaccine acceptance is complex. Although some parents' perspectives divide into pro- or anti-vaccination, others may be selective in the vaccines they accept, delay vaccination, or, more commonly, accept them while still having concerns. The term 'vaccine hesitancy' is generally used to describe individuals who are on a spectrum between automatically accepting or declining vaccines. Parents thus may have differing information requirements, some needing detailed information and others little or none (Leask et al., 2012). The health professional's role is to recommend and encourage immunization, provide information as required, and, where necessary, direct parents to additional sources of reputable information.

Information about immunization

Most parents report receiving and trusting information from health professionals (Campbell et al., 2017), yet a consistent finding from studies of parents' attitudes to and experiences of the immunization process is a lack of information (Ames et al., 2017). This lack of information or an inadequate response to questions or concerns can undermine parents' confidence in the immunization programme, reinforcing the need for health professionals to be well informed and equipped to answer questions. However, simply giving parents leaflets is not adequate—a detailed, tailored discussion may be required and the nature of the communication is fundamental to a successful immunization conversation.

Communicating with parents about immunization

Despite a lack of evidence for effective interventions to reduce vaccine hesitancy or refusal (Sadaf et al., 2013), using the principles of good communication can help to build a trusting relationship with parents; advice from a trusted professional has been found to be the pivotal factor for a parent in changing their mind over immunizations they have previously delayed or declined (Benin et al., 2006; Bedford, 2017).

In immunization discussions, strategies to gain trust include starting from a position of understanding what information parents have accessed and offering the opportunity to ask questions and voice concerns (Leask et al., 2012). Many parents will access the internet where it is easy to locate misinformation which may confirm their concerns (Ruiz and Bell, 2014; Campbell et al., 2017). However ill-founded, parents' concerns should be addressed respectfully and empathetically. Many questions are predictable and resources are available to support professionals in their discussions (see Box 16.1). In view of a reported increase in 'anti-vaccine' sentiment in the US, especially expressed on social media (Hotez, 2017), it is increasingly important that health professionals are equipped and confident to discuss vaccine concerns. NHS Choices provides guidance on interpreting health news articles (Nhs.uk, 2017) and the World Health Organization publishes a list of websites providing credible information on immunization (World Health Organization, 2017a).

Box 16.1 Immunization resources

Public Health England—'Immunisation: Information for immunisation practitioners and other health professionals':*

- Link: https://www.gov.uk/government/collections/immunisation
- Government website with links to 'Immunisation against infectious disease', vaccine uptake statistics, minutes of the Joint Committee on Vaccination and Immunisation, information about immunization programmes, leaflets and guidance for parents, and training slide sets for health professionals.

NHS Choices*:

- Link: http://www.nhs.uk/Conditions/vaccinations/pages/vaccination-schedule-age-checklist.aspx
- Website for the public.

Oxford Vaccine Group—Vaccine Knowledge Project*:

- Link: http://vk.ovg.ox.ac.uk/
- Designed for the general public (and also very useful for health professionals) to aid in their immunization decision-making, a source of independent information about vaccines and vaccine-preventable diseases, includes case studies of people affected by infectious diseases.

* These websites are all included in the World Health Organization's list of credible vaccine safety websites.

Selective immunization programmes

Children at higher risk of severe infection may require additional vaccines or doses. However, coverage of vaccines offered selectively is often poor; for example, uptake of influenza vaccine in children aged 6 months to 2 years in a clinical risk group was 19.5% in 2016/2017 (Gov.uk, 2017b).

Additional doses of hepatitis B vaccine at birth, 4 weeks, and 1 year are indicated for babies born to mothers infected with hepatitis B to prevent chronic carriage and serious liver disease in adulthood, but a significant proportion do not complete the course by 24 months. In one London-based study, fewer than half the high-risk babies received the full vaccine course but high uptake was achieved in areas with good communication between acute and community services and a clear pathway for follow-up immunization (Giraudon et al., 2009).

Improving and maintaining vaccine uptake

The best evidence of effectiveness for reducing inequalities in vaccine uptake in disadvantaged, urban, and ethnically mixed communities is complex, locally designed interventions (Crocker-Buque et al., 2016). However, this is based largely on US, Canadian, and Australian studies, raising issues about the generalizability to the UK health system.

The World Health Organization (2017b) has published guidance for designing strategies to increase uptake of childhood immunization using proven methods and tools. Although designed for national programmes, it provides a useful step-by-step approach that could be considered for use on a local basis.

In 2017, the National Institute for Health and Care Excellence (NICE) published a quality standard on vaccine uptake among under 19-year-olds (NICE, 2017). This was related to guidance issued in 2009 and updated in 2017 (NICE, 2009). The aim is to highlight the priority areas needed to gain measurable improvements in uptake of vaccines. Four of the statements are relevant to children under 7 years. These form the basis for the recommendations at the end of this chapter and are discussed below.

Immunization recall and reminders

High-quality evidence supports the use of call–recall systems to improve vaccine uptake (Jacobson Vann and Szilagyi, 2005). Invitations may be sent by letter, email, or text with an appointment or a reminder to make one. Preferably before the appointment and reinforced at the time of vaccination, parents should be provided with an explanation of the vaccines to be given, what they are for, and their potential side effects, so that they can consider their questions and make a fully informed decision (Ames et al., 2017).

Providing accessible immunization services

Providing family-friendly immunization services, with clinic timings so that parents with older children can attend, improves the accessibility of services for some families who have logistical or practical challenges. Children living in disadvantage, in lone parent families, and larger families are at risk of lower vaccine uptake. Other vulnerable groups, such as looked after children, refugees, mobile populations, and those with a disability, may need particular attention; as well as challenges accessing traditional services, they may need additional or catch-up vaccines if previously missed. Public Health England publishes an algorithm to assist in determining the vaccines needed to bring children up to date (Gov.uk, 2017c).

Special clinics may be arranged by local paediatric services, but with a little flexibility they can often be accommodated within general practice. Hospital-based immunization, for children who have missed vaccines and for long-stay neonates, has proved successful (Shingler et al., 2012; McCrossan et al., 2015). Domiciliary immunization may be required for some families.

Reviewing immunization status

Every contact with a health professional, for example, each of the scheduled health visitor contacts, is an opportunity to check children's immunization status and if necessary to immunize or make arrangements for it to be done. The latter is the second best option as it requires more time and effort for a busy parent. Public Health Wales has published good practice guidelines for the follow-up of preschool children with outstanding immunizations (Wales.nhs.uk, 2017). Entry to nursery and transfer to primary and secondary schools are all important opportunities to check children's immunization status and remind parents about missing vaccines. Attendance at hospital is another important opportunity infrequently made use of.

Data collection

When managing an immunization programme, within a general practice, at school, or nationally, the immunization status of each child should be recorded and kept up to date. As a minimum, this information should be stored on the local Child Health Information System, the general practitioner (GP) records, and patient-held records—the PCHR. Operating an effective call–recall system requires accurate and timely communication between these sources of data. Data can be used locally to manage individual children, aggregated by GP, provider trust, Clinical Commissioning Group, local authority, school, or locality, to monitor and manage pockets of poor uptake, prevent and manage outbreaks, and, nationally, to monitor trends.

Conclusion

Immunization is a highly effective and cost-effective intervention to protect children's health. Despite current high levels of uptake, there is room for improvement—but maintaining high uptake can be challenging as once diseases become less common people may consider vaccination to be no longer necessary. In view of the relationship that health visitors build, they are the key professionals to work with families to ensure that children are immunized fully and in a timely fashion.

Learning links

♦ UK Government—'Immunisation: Information for immunisation practitioners and other health professionals': https://www.gov.uk/government/collections/immunisation.

♦ Module 9 ('Immunisation') of the Healthy Child Programme provides guidance for healthcare professionals working with families, providing advice and support, and addressing parental anxieties around immunization: https://www.e-lfh.org.uk/programmes/healthy-child-programme/.

Recommendations

For improving and maintaining high vaccine uptake:

♦ Target support where uptake is poor by reviewing coverage statistics. (*Evidence: strong.*)

♦ Encourage, train, and support opportunistic immunization, for example, in hospital settings and by health visitors. (*Evidence: strong.*)

♦ Follow up children who do not attend their immunization appointment with a written recall invitation and a phone call or text message. (*Evidence: strong.*)

♦ Children identified as having missed a childhood vaccination should be offered the outstanding vaccination. (*Evidence: strong.*)

♦ Record a child's vaccination in their GP record, the Child Health Information System, and in their Personal Child Health Record. (*Evidence: strong.*)

♦ Check a child's immunization status at school entry and each mandated contact. (*Evidence: strong.*)

♦ Discuss immunization with parents at timely opportunities. (*Evidence: strong.*)

References and further reading

Ames, H.M.R., Glenton, C., and Lewin, S. (2017). Parents' and informal caregivers' views and experiences of communication about routine childhood vaccination: a synthesis of qualitative evidence. *Cochrane Database of Systematic Reviews*, 2, CD011787.

Bedford, H. (2017). Talking with parents about immunisation. *Practice Nursing*, 28, 104–107.

Benin, A.L., Wisler-Scher, D.J., Colson, E., Shapiro, E.D., and Holmboe, E.S. (2006). Qualitative analysis of mothers' decision-making about vaccines for infants: the importance of trust. *Pediatrics*, 117, 1532–1541.

Campbell, H., Edwards, A., Letley, L., Bedford, H., Ramsay, M., and Yarwood, J. (2017). Changing attitudes to childhood immunisation in English parents. *Vaccine*, 35, 2979–2985.

Crocker-Buque, T., Edelstein, M., and Mounier-Jack, S. (2016). Interventions to reduce inequalities in vaccine uptake in children and adolescents aged < 19 years: a systematic review. *Journal of Epidemiology and Community Health*, **71**, 87–97.

Giraudon, I., Permalloo, N., Nixon, G., et al. (2009). Factors associated with incomplete vaccination of babies at risk of perinatal hepatitis B transmission: a London study in 2006. *Vaccine*, **27**, 2016–2022.

Gov.uk (2017a). Immunisation. [online] Available at: https://www.gov.uk/government/collections/immunisation [Accessed 25 Sep. 2017].

Gov.uk (2017b). Seasonal flu vaccine uptake in GP patients in England: winter season 2016 to 2017. [online] Available at: https://www.gov.uk/government/statistics/seasonal-flu-vaccine-uptake-in-gp-patients-in-england-winter-season-2016-to-2017 [Accessed 25 Sep. 2017].

Gov.uk (2017c). Vaccination of individuals with uncertain or incomplete immunisation status. [online] Available at: https://www.gov.uk/government/publications/vaccination-of-individuals-with-uncertain-or-incomplete-immunisation-status [Accessed 25 Sep. 2017].

Hotez, P. (2017). How the anti-vaxxers are winning. *New York Times*, 8 Feb. [online] Available at: https://www.nytimes.com/2017/02/08/opinion/how-the-anti-vaxxers-are-winning.html?_r=0.

Immunisationscotland.org.uk (2017). Immunisation information in Scotland from the NHS. [online] Available at: http://www.immunisationscotland.org.uk/ [Accessed 25 Sep. 2017].

Jacobson Vann, J.C. and Szilagyi, P. (2005). Patient reminder and recall systems to improve immunization rates. *Cochrane Database of Systematic Reviews*, **3**, CD003941.

Leask, J., Kinnersley, P., Jackson, C., Cheater, F., Bedford, H., and Rowles, G. (2012). Communicating with parents about vaccination: a framework for health professionals. *BMC Pediatrics*, **12**, 154.

McCrossan, P., McCafferty, C., Murphy, C., and Murphy, J. (2015). Retrospective review of administration of childhood primary vaccination schedule in an Irish tertiary neonatal intensive care unit. *Public health*, **129**, 896–898.

National Institute for Health and Care Excellence (NICE) (2009). Immunisations: reducing differences in uptake in under 19s. [online] (Last updated Sep. 2017). Available at: https://www.nice.org.uk/guidance/ph21 [Accessed 25 Sep. 2017].

National Institute for Health and Care Excellence (NICE) (2017). Vaccine uptake in under 19s. Quality standard [QS145]. [online] Available at: https://www.nice.org.uk/guidance/qs145 [Accessed 25 Sep. 2017].

Nhs.uk. (2017). How to read articles about health and healthcare. [online] Available at: http://www.nhs.uk/news/Pages/Howtoreadarticlesabouthealthandhealthcare.aspx [Accessed 25 Sep. 2017].

Publichealth.hscni.net (2017). Immunisation/vaccine preventable diseases. [online] HSC Public Health Agency. Available at: http://www.publichealth.hscni.net/directorate-public-health/health-protection/immunisationvaccine-preventable-diseases [Accessed 25 Sep. 2017].

Ruiz, J.B. and Bell, R.A. (2014). Understanding vaccination resistance: vaccine search term selection bias and the valence of retrieved information. *Vaccine*, **32**, 5776–5780.

Sadaf, A., Richards, J.L., Glanz, J., Salmon, D.A., and Omer, S.B. (2013). A systematic review of interventions for reducing parental vaccine refusal and vaccine hesitancy. *Vaccine*, **31**, 4293–4304.

Samad, L., Tate, A.R., Dezateux, C., Peckham, C., Butler, N., and **Bedford, H.** (2006). Differences in risk factors for partial and no immunisation in the first year of life: prospective cohort study. *BMJ*, **332**, 1312–1313.

Shingler, S., Hunter, K., Romano, A., and **Graham, D.** (2012). Opportunities taken: the need for and effectiveness of secondary care opportunistic immunisation. *Journal of Paediatrics and Child Health*, **48**, 242–246.

Wales.nhs.uk (2017). Immunisation and vaccines. [online] Public Health Wales. Available at: http://www.wales.nhs.uk/sitesplus/888/page/43510 [Accessed 25 Sep. 2017].

Wales.nhs.uk (2017). Vaccines for children. [online] Public Health Wales. Available at: http://www.wales.nhs.uk/sitesplus/888/page/59487 [Accessed 25 Sep. 2017].

World Health Organization (2017a). Vaccine safety websites meeting good information practices criteria. [online] Available at: http://www.who.int/vaccine_safety/initiative/communication/network/approved_vaccine_safety_website/en/ [Accessed 25 Sep. 2017].

World Health Organization (2017b). The Guide to Tailoring Immunization Programmes (TIP). [online] Regional Office for Europe. Available at: http://www.euro.who.int/en/health-topics/communicable-diseases/poliomyelitis/publications/2013/guide-to-tailoring-immunization-programmes [Accessed 25 Sep. 2017].

Section 4

Secondary prevention: screening and identification of impairments

Chapter 17

Secondary prevention: principles and good practice/screening tests

David Elliman

Summary

This chapter:

- describes how screening can reduce the morbidity and mortality of conditions that cannot currently be prevented. However, it also has the capacity to do harm by incorrectly labelling people as having a condition, when in reality they do not, thus causing anxiety and sometimes resulting in unnecessary interventions

- outlines how the UK National Screening Committee recommends national policy on screening on the basis of the evidence of the overall effects of a potential programme and its cost-effectiveness.

- emphasizes that, once a programme is introduced, it should be carefully monitored to ensure that it lives up to expectations, coverage is appropriately high, the expected outcomes are delivered, and that it does not increase inequality.

More details can be found on the UK National Screening Committee website (https://www.gov.uk/government/groups/uk-national-screening-committee-uk-nsc).

Principles of screening

Secondary prevention is the early detection of problems with a view to ameliorating any adverse effects. When organized on a systematic basis, this is known as screening. The term is often used loosely and so it is important to have a clear definition. That by Wald includes all the relevant elements: 'The systematic application of a test or inquiry, to identify individuals at sufficient *risk* of a specific disorder to benefit from further investigation or direct preventive action, among persons who have not sought medical attention on account of symptoms of that disorder' (Wald, 1994, p. 76, emphasis added).

The purpose is to separate out those people who are at increased risk of a problem and would profit from intervention at a stage when the problem has not otherwise been recognized. The 'test' can be a blood test or imaging, such as ultrasound, but also a question or series of questions. Usually, it needs to be followed up by a more definitive diagnostic test.

Screening tests are not perfect. Often the test is measuring a continuous variable and there is no cut-off at which one can say all results on one side of a cut-off indicate a problem and all results on the other indicate no problem. This means that there will be some people labelled as having a problem who don't—false positives—and some who will be labelled as not having a problem, but do—false negatives. It is important that this is explained to anyone considering having a screening test. It is also important that professionals are not falsely reassured by a normal screening test. If a child develops symptoms of a condition, the presence of a normal screening test should not stop appropriate investigations being undertaken.

There are a number of parameters that can be applied to a screening test:

Sensitivity (sometimes known as 'detection rate')—this is the proportion of people with the condition who are correctly identified as such. This is very high for screening for inborn errors of metabolism and much lower when screening for physical anomalies, whether this be congenital heart disease antenatally or developmental dysplasia of the hips neonatally.

Specificity—this is the proportion of the population who do not have the condition and are correctly identified as such. It is important that this is very high, otherwise, when screening for rare conditions, there will be many false positives. The false-positive rate is the proportion of those people who don't have the condition who are labelled as higher risk by the screening test.

There is always a balance between sensitivity and specificity—a desire not to miss too many cases versus the need to protect those without the condition from having too many investigations and the inevitable anxiety of being falsely told they, or their child, have a serious condition. Anxiety following a positive screening test, even though not confirmed when the diagnostic test is performed, may persist. This can result in increased health service utilization (Karaceper et al., 2016), although the evidence is mixed (Lipstein et al., 2009). However, the anxiety can be substantially reduced if parents have been provided with the appropriate information prior to the screening test being undertaken (Gurian et al., 2006; Vernooij et al., 2014). Where to set the balance is partly subjective and, to some extent, explains why, with the same evidence, some countries will adopt a screening programme, while others reject it. A culture which considers it of paramount importance to detect people with a condition may be more willing to adopt a screening programme where the test specificity is low and the sensitivity is high, while others may attach more weight to the false labelling of people who do not have the condition. Therrell and colleagues (2015) recently reviewed the status of newborn screening worldwide. They found that, in the US, it is recommended that 32 core conditions and 25 secondary conditions are screened for in the neonatal period, whereas in Europe, the number of conditions sought is much more variable, with some countries screening for almost as many as in the US and others seeking only a handful or less. The UK is towards the more 'conservative' end of the spectrum. Another reason for variations in policy may be different incidences of some conditions in different ethnic groups, for example, sickle cell disease, which is screened for in England, but not in a number of countries where the disease is less common.

Positive predictive value (PPV)—is the percentage of those 'failing' the screening test who actually have the condition in question. This is an important measure as it indicates how many people will have been falsely labelled and caused unnecessary anxiety.

While specificity and sensitivity are dependent only on test performance, PPV is dependent also on the prevalence of the condition. A test which has a sensitivity and specificity of 99%, will have a PPV of 50% with a disease prevalence of 1 in 100. However, with the same test and a prevalence of 1 in 10,000, the PPV is only 1%. This means that 99 of 100 people referred for diagnostic testing would not have had the condition and would have been worried unnecessarily. There is also a financial cost attached in terms of diagnostic testing and clinical referrals. When screening for metabolic disorders, very high specificities and sensitivities are required for the tests as the conditions may occur in less than 1 in 100,000 newborn babies.

The UK National Screening Committee (UKNSC) advises ministers of the four nations on population screening programmes. Under the NHS Constitution for England, the NHS pledges 'to provide screening programmes as recommended by the National Screening Committee'.

Before the UKNSC recommends a screening programme, a number of criteria are considered. These relate to the condition, the test, and the management of the condition as well as cost-effectiveness.

The criteria used are based on those originally set out by Wilson and Jungner (1968), but fleshed out so as to be suitable for current needs (see Box 17.1 for an outline and the UKNSC website for more detail). Although these criteria have been criticized

Box 17.1 Considerations for a good screening programme

The condition is an important health problem, its natural history should be known, and all feasible measures should have been taken to prevent it.

There should be a simple, safe, reliable, and acceptable test, with an agreed cut-off. The diagnostic pathway, once an individual has screened positive, should be agreed.

There should be an effective intervention, with benefit to the individual screened.

The screening programme, as a whole, should be effective in reducing morbidity and/or mortality, as well as being acceptable to the public and professionals. Any harms should be outweighed by the benefits. The opportunity cost of the programme must be acceptable.

Prior to the introduction of the programme, clinical management should be optimized, quality assurance measures agreed, and information for the public and professionals prepared.

When genetic testing is involved, ramifications for the rest of the family should be considered.

Source: data from UK National Screening Committee, available from https://www.gov.uk/government/groups/uk-national-screening-committee-uk-nsc, © Crown Copyright. Contains public sector information licensed under the Open Government Licence v3.0.

as being too rigid (Forman et al., 2013), when the UK criteria were last updated in October 2015, as a result of a review of the UKNSC, little change was needed. All programmes are reviewed at regular intervals to ensure that they are still appropriate and that no change in the present form of screening is necessary. Topics which have been reviewed in the past, but not adopted for screening, are reviewed again, at intervals, to ensure there is no new evidence that might change the previous recommendations and, each year, the UKNSC puts out a call for new suggestions for screening.

Patients who are offered screening should be provided with adequate information so that they can choose whether they wish to take up the offer. Previously known as 'informed consent', this is often referred to as 'informed choice' as they are deciding which course of action to follow. The information offered should include details of the condition and its treatment as well as what the test entails and how accurate it is. Materials should be made available in different languages and forms, so as to be suitable for the individual person. These materials should be made available in advance of any screening, so that an unhurried decision can be made.

UK screening programmes

The UKNSC-approved antenatal and childhood screening programmes in place in England are as follows:

1. Antenatal:

   a. Antenatal sickle cell and thalassaemia (SCT) programme.

   All pregnant women are offered screening for sickle cell disease and thalassaemia, early in pregnancy.

   b. Fetal Anomaly Screening Programme (FASP).

   Using a combination of blood tests and ultrasound, nine structural anomalies and three chromosome disorders, including Down syndrome, can be detected.

   c. Infectious Diseases in Pregnancy Screening (IDPS—HIV, hepatitis B, and syphilis).

   These three treatable infections have important connotations for the mother and fetus. Early detection results in more effective intervention and can reduce, if not eliminate, the risk of the fetus and newborn baby being infected.

2. Newborn:

   a. Newborn bloodspot screening (NBS).

   A sample of blood is taken onto a special card at 5 days old and screened for nine conditions—phenylketonuria, congenital hypothyroidism, sickle cell disease, cystic fibrosis, medium-chain acyl-CoA dehydrogenase deficiency, maple syrup urine disease, isovaleric acidaemia, homocystinuria, and glutaric aciduria type 1. Some of these are very rare, but devastating, disorders with a prevalence of the order of 1 in 100,000 or less at birth.

b. Newborn and infant physical examination (NIPE).

Examinations of the hips, heart, eyes, and testes are considered screening tests and should be carried out before 72 hours of age and again at 6–8 weeks. See Chapter 19 for more details.

c. Newborn Hearing Screening Programme (NHSP).

Semi-automated screening of the hearing of all neonates detects significant hearing loss, allowing early fitting of aids or cochlear implants. See Chapter 20 for more details.

3. Childhood:

a. Vision (4–5 years old).

The UKNSC recommends that all children have their vision checked at 4–5 years of age. Compliance is patchy. See Chapter 21 for further details.

b. Hearing (4–5 years old).

The UKNSC recommends that all children should have their hearing screened at 4–5 years old. The evidence for this is not robust and the programme is to be reviewed. See Chapter 20 for further details.

Screening is not carried out for many conditions. This does not mean they are not important. It may be there is no evidence that screening is effective or that another form of management (i.e. prevention) is more appropriate.

Further details of all the UKNSC screening programmes can be found on the UKNSC website.

Failsafe

Although screening is not compulsory, it is important that all members of the target population are offered the appropriate tests. For inborn errors of metabolism, it is important that samples are taken in a timely fashion, otherwise irreversible harm may take place. To ensure that this happens, a number of programmes have IT failsafe systems in place. For example, NBS has a national database of babies on which is recorded all babies born in England. When the laboratory receives a bloodspot card, it is recorded against the baby's name and later the results are also recorded. If a card is not received within 12 days of birth, the maternity unit is alerted, by the system. They can then check whether a sample has been taken and, if not, ensure one is taken urgently. The NHSP IT system also provides a failsafe system.

Quality assurance

It is extremely important that screening programmes are kept under constant review to ensure that they are performing as they are supposed to. As many of the conditions are uncommon, year-on-year fluctuations in detection rates would be difficult to interpret on a local level. For this reason, most quality assurance relates to processes rather than outcomes. Apart from the two childhood programmes, all programmes have a suite of monitoring measures. Key performance indicators (KPIs) are a limited number of high-level measures reported at provider level. They are designed to drive change and so for each KPI, there are two thresholds—an acceptable level which all providers should achieve and an achievable level to which all should aspire. Each programme has one to three KPIs which are reported quarterly. Apart from FASP, all programmes include coverage and many have a measure of timeliness. Commissioners can use these to monitor programmes locally.

In addition to the limited number of KPIs, programmes also have a set of standards which they measure yearly. These are tailored to the individual programme. Examples include the 'avoidable repeats' where blood samples have to be repeated due to poor technique or incorrect completion of the bloodspot card (NBS), referral rates following first-line testing (NHSP), percentage of cases of serious congenital cardiac anomalies detected (FASP), and timely administration of neonatal hepatitis B vaccine (IDPS). Providers can compare themselves against the threshold levels and against other units. In this way, it is hoped not just to maintain standards, but to push them up.

Learning links

◆ Several e-learning resources are available at e-Learning for Health including modules on antenatal and newborn screening, newborn blood spot, and fetal anomaly screening: https://www.e-lfh.org.uk/programmes/nhs-screening-programmes/.

Recommendations

◆ Commissioners should work with screening programmes to measure clinical outcomes, that is, effect on the child and family. (*Evidence: strong.*)
◆ Where coverage is less than 100% in neonatal programmes, providers should look for reasons and ensure there are no issues of inequality. (*Evidence: strong.*)

References

Forman, J., Coyle, F., Levy-Fisch, J., Roberts, P., Terry, S., and Legge, M. (2013). Screening criteria: the need to deal with new developments and ethical issues in newborn metabolic screening. *Journal of Community Genetics*, **4**, 59–67.

Gurian, E.A., Kinnamon, D.D., Henry, J.J., and Waisbren, S.E. (2006). Expanded newborn screening for biochemical disorders: the effect of a false-positive result. *Pediatrics*, **117**, 1915–1921.

Karaceper, M.D., Chakraborty, P., Coyle, D., et al. (2016). The health system impact of false positive newborn screening results for medium-chain acyl-CoA dehydrogenase deficiency: a cohort study. *Orphanet Journal of Rare Diseases*, **11**, 12.

Lipstein, E.A., Perrin, J.M., Waisbren, S.E., and Prosser, L.A. (2009). Impact of false-positive newborn metabolic screening results on early health care utilization. *Genetics in Medicine*, **11**, 716–721.

Therrell BL, Padilla CD, Loeber JG, et al. (2015). Current status of newborn screening worldwide: 2015. *Seminars in Perinatology*, **39**, 171–187.

UK National Screening Committee. Homepage. [online] https://www.gov.uk/government/groups/uk-national-screening-committee-uk-nsc [Accessed 23 Oct. 2017].

Vernooij-van Langen, A.M., van der Pal, S.M., Reijntjens, A.J., Loeber, J.G., Dompeling, E., and Dankert-Roelse, J.E. (2014). Parental knowledge reduces long term anxiety induced by false-positive test results after newborn screening for cystic fibrosis. *Molecular Genetics and Metabolism Reports*, **1**, 334–344.

Wald, N.J. (1994). Guidance on terminology. *Journal of Medical Screening*, **1**, 76.

Wilson, J.M.G. and **Jungner, G.** (1968). *Principles and practice of screening for disease*. Public Health Paper Number 34. Geneva: World Health Organization. http://apps.who.int/iris/bitstream/10665/37650/17/WHO_PHP_34.pdf [Accessed 20 April 2017].

Chapter 18

Growth monitoring

Charlotte M. Wright

Summary

This chapter:

- outlines best practice in the use and interpretation of growth data and charts, and describes the conditions most likely to be identified as a result
- reviews the evidence supporting growth monitoring
- draws on the experience of developing and implementing the UK-World Health Organization growth charts between 2008 and 2012 (see https://www.rcpch. ac.uk/resources/growth-charts) with recommendations expanded or modified where there is newer relevant evidence

Other useful resources are the National Institute for Health and Care Excellence (NICE) 2008 guidelines on 'Maternal and child nutrition' (PH11) and NICE 2017 guidelines on 'Faltering growth: recognition and management of faltering growth in children' (NG75).

Introduction

The subject of how growth should be monitored and recorded was addressed by the Royal College of Paediatrics and Child Health (RCPCH) Growth Chart working group in the process of developing and implementing the UK-World Health Organization (WHO) growth charts between 2008 and 2012. Chart instructions and supporting educational materials were developed, drawing on the collective views of focus groups, stakeholder meetings, and the considered views of the working group (Wright et al., 2010, 2012; Cole et al., 2012; Sachs et al., 2012; Moy and Wright, 2013). These have been expanded or modified where there is newer relevant evidence and the section is also informed by the 2008 National Institute for Health and Care Excellence (NICE) guideline on 'Maternal and child nutrition' (2008) and the new guideline on 'Faltering growth' (2017).

Growth charts

Growth monitoring has historically been an almost ubiquitous aspect of primary care in childhood. It was originally used to screen for undernutrition as well as disorders of growth and more recently to identify overnutrition. Growth charts allow us to compare a measurement in one child to the normal range of measurements for other children of the same age and sex. All growth charts are constructed using measurements from a large number of children at different ages. The 50th centile represents the average (median) for the population, while the 98th and 2nd centiles are roughly two standard deviations (SDs) above and below the median. In addition, there are 0.4th and 99.6th centiles below which only 1/250 (0.4%) optimally growing children will fall. British growth charts thus consist of nine centile lines (0.4th, 2nd, 9th, 25th, 50th, 75th, 91st, 98th, and 99.4th) with the distance between each centile line being two-thirds of a SD, known as a 'centile space' (Figure 18.1).

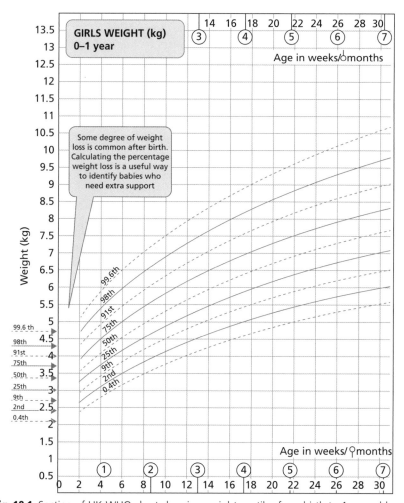

Fig. 18.1 Section of UK-WHO chart showing weight centiles from birth to 1 year old.

Chart developed by RCPCH, and Department of Health. Reproduced with permission of Royal College of Paediatrics and Child Health.

The centile lines show the range of heights and weights for age and the percentage of healthy children in the population expected to fall below a particular line (e.g. 50% below the 50th, 91% below the 91st). Half of all optimally growing children will have measurements between the 25th and 75th centile lines and 99% will be between the two outer lines. There is no single threshold below which a child's weight or height is definitely abnormal, but a weight or height below the 0.4th centile should usually be assessed further.

The WHO Child Growth Standards for infants and children up to the age of 5 years were published in April 2006. They are based on the growth of healthy, breastfed, non-deprived children living in in six different countries: Brazil, Ghana, India, Norway, Oman, and US (WHO MGRSG and de Onis, 2006). These charts provide, for the first time, a standard of how children 'should grow', rather than a traditional growth reference that describes how children 'are growing'. This standard was adopted for children under 4 years by England and Wales in 2009 (2010 in Scotland) and used to construct the new UK-WHO charts.

The UK 1990 growth charts, which are still used at birth and beyond the age of 4 years, are based on measurements from a large number of British children collected in the late 1980s and were the main charts in use until 2009 (Freeman et al., 1995; Cole et al., 1998). They are a description of typical, but not necessarily healthy growth in UK children from 1980 to 1990. They should be used for all children with the exception of children with Down syndrome, who have their own specific charts.

How to measure

Anyone who measures a child, or plots or interprets charts, should be suitably trained. Always remove the child's shoes or other footwear when measuring either weight or height.

Babies should be *weighed*, without any clothes or nappy, on clinical electronic scales (class III) in metric setting. Children older than 2 years can be weighed in vest and pants. If clothes cannot be removed, this should be documented. *Head circumference* should be measured using a narrow plastic (lasoo) or disposable paper tape and the measurement should be taken where the head circumference is widest. It is good practice to take three measurements and use the average. Any head wear should be removed. Head circumference measurements taken in the first 24 hours are unreliable as the head will have been subjected to moulding.

Proper equipment is essential for measuring either length or height. *Length* should be measured using a length board or rollameter with one observer holding the head and one the feet. Extra-long rollameters are available to measure older, non-ambulant children. Measurement of *height* requires a correctly installed stadiometer or appropriate portable measuring device. Shoes must be removed. The child should stand with their heels, bottom, and back of head touching the vertical measuring column. The head should be in the in the Frankfurt plane: looking straight ahead, making sure the chin is not tipped up or down (see Figure 18.2). The height measurement is taken by lowering the measuring arm onto the child's head after asking

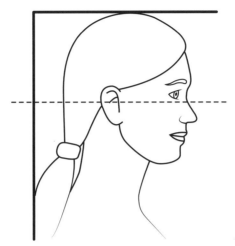

Fig. 18.2 The Frankfurt plane for measuring height.

Reproduced with permission of Royal College of Paediatrics and Child Health.

the child to breathe in and then out. It is good practice to take three measurements and use the average. The measurement should be recorded in centimetres, to the nearest millimetre.

Plotting measurements on the chart

The point on the graph should be marked with a small but noticeable dot • drawn with a pencil, not an ink pen, to allow correction of misplots. Once plotted on a chart, a child's measurement should be described as either being on one major centile line—if the point marked is within one-quarter of a space of the line—or between two if the point is further away (e.g. between the 75th and 91st centile). A centile space is the distance between two of the marked centile lines or equivalent distance if midway between centiles.

Age calculation errors or misplotting of age are the commonest mistakes made when plotting charts. To prevent errors, for at least the first 6 months, age should be calculated in weeks using a calendar or date wheel. After that, calendar months should be used, remembering that there are 13 weeks per 3 calendar month.

Plotting at birth

All babies born between 37 and 42 weeks are considered 'term' and should be plotted at age 0 on the chart. Term infants should not be plotted at their exact gestation, as this can lead to confusion at later ages (Cole et al., 2012). Weight loss and regain in the early days varies a lot from baby to baby, so there are no lines on the chart between 0 and 2 weeks (see Figure 18.1). However, by 2 weeks of age most babies will be on a centile close to their birth centile as the WHO charts allow for neonatal weight loss.

Plotting preterm infants born between 32 and 36 weeks

Weight and head circumference for preterm infants born between 32 and 36 weeks should be plotted in the preterm section on the A4 chart, or the preterm page of the Personal Child Health Records, until 2 weeks after the expected date of delivery. Where there is a concern about length at birth, this should be plotted on the Neonatal and Infant Close Monitoring chart (see 'Plotting preterm infants born before 32 weeks'). Subsequent measurements should be plotted on the 0–1 chart, using gestationally corrected age, which adjusts the plot for the number of weeks before 40 weeks a baby was born. This is easiest using the arrow drawn back method: work out how many weeks early the infant was, mark a dot at the actual postnatal age, then draw a dotted line back for the number of weeks the baby was early and mark this point with an arrow head (Figure 18.3). The point of the arrow shows the baby's centile with adjustment for preterm birth. This is easier and less prone to error than calculating the corrected age and makes it clear to subsequent measurers whether gestational correction has been applied. Gestational correction should be continued until corrected age 1 year for babies born at 32–36 weeks.

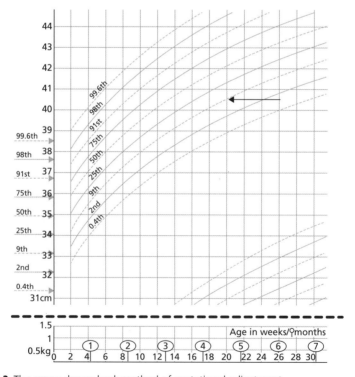

Fig. 18.3 The arrow drawn back method of gestational adjustment.

Plotting preterm infants born before 32 weeks

The Neonatal and Infant Close Monitoring chart should be used for preterm infants of less than 32 weeks of gestation, as this is a fully gestationally corrected chart which has the larger scale. This can be used be used up to the age of 2 years corrected age, after which gestational correction can cease.

Weight monitoring

Historically, we have used regular weighing to monitor the sufficiency of infant feeding and it has long been known that poor weight gain in infancy is associated with high childhood morbidity and mortality. Babies should be weighed in the first week after birth as part of the assessment of feeding and thereafter as needed. Many children lose weight in the early days and then begin to regain at between 3 and 5 days of age. Recovery of birthweight helps to provide assurance that feeding is effective and that the child is well, but recent evidence suggest that only 50% have regained birth weight by the age of 2 weeks, though over 90% have done so by age 4 weeks (Paul et al., 2016). One in 10 children may drop in weight by 10% at the lowest point around age 3–5 days, but this is less common beyond this age (NICE, 2017).

After the neonatal period and once feeding is established, babies usually need only be weighed at the time of routine immunizations or reviews. If there is concern, it may be necessary to weigh more often, but in general, weighing at intervals too close together may be misleading and causes unnecessary anxiety. NICE (2008) recommends that well babies should be weighed no more than once a month before 6 months, once per 2 months aged 6–12 months, and once per 3 months over age 1 year. Weights usually track within one centile line, but individual measurements may show wide variation. Acute illness may be accompanied by weight loss and weight centile fall, but a child's weight usually returns to its normal centile within 2–3 weeks (NICE, 2017).

Weight gain in preterm babies

After birth, an individual preterm baby's growth is not expected to follow the centile lines shown in the 'preterm' section of charts, because these show only birth measurements. Most preterm babies will show slow initial weight gain or weight loss and so will appear to drop on the chart. If there have been neonatal problems, they may fall by as much as two channel widths in the early weeks. However where infants have remained well, their growth patterns should match the centile at their corrected age, while children who have had problems in the neonatal period and dropped away will usually gradually climb back up the centiles during the first year.

Head circumference

Both acceleration and slowing of head growth can be a sign of important underlying developmental or surgical disorders, such as hydrocephalus. Head circumference should be measured shortly after birth, but not in the first 24 hours as the head will have been subjected to moulding. It should then be measured again at the 8-week review, but it does not then need to be measured again unless there are worries about the child's head growth or development.

Compared to the WHO standard, representative British infants heads appear large (median >75th centile) but appear to be stable after a rise in the first 6 months (Wright et al., 2011; Wright and Emond, 2015). The UK 1990 reference in contrast tends to make representative children and adults look quite small (median ~25th centile) and infants show a decline in mean centile over the first 2 years (Wright et al., 2011). The assessment of change in head size over time is thus complicated, both by this poor fit to the standard and the fact that centile shifts seen in routine practice commonly seem to reflect measurement or recording errors (Wright and Emond, 2015).

The WHO standard extends only to age 5 years, so where measurement is needed beyond this age, the UK 1990 head reference is the only option. As there is a two centile space difference at the transition point between the two charts, where there is a need for continued monitoring beyond the age of 2 years, the UK 1990 should be used, with replotting of head measures collected before 2 years of age.

Growth monitoring

Growth in height is a longer-term index of health and well-being. Slow or stunted growth is associated with many disorders of childhood. It is often difficult to get an accurate measurement of length or height in an uncooperative baby or toddler, so length and height are not recommended as routine surveillance measures. However, length should always be measured if there are concerns about a child's weight gain, growth, or general health. Length should be measured up to the age of 2 years and height from then on. Height should also be measured in any child whose weight is above the 99.6th centile or where there is very rapid weight gain.

Successive measurements commonly show wide variation, so it is important not to place too much reliance on single measurements or apparent changes in centile position between just two measurements. If there are worries about growth (or weight gain), it is a good idea to measure on a few occasions, in order to get a sense of the child's average centile; healthy children will generally show a stable average position over time. If after a number of measurements there seems to be a consistent drop downwards in centile position by more than one centile space, the child should usually be assessed in more detail.

Adult height prediction

A child's current height centile is the best predictor of their future height. The Adult Height Prediction scale on the 0–4 charts provides an estimate of the child's predicted adult height based on their current height, but with a regression adjustment to allow for the tendency of very tall and short children to be less extreme in height as adults (see Figure 18.4). Four out of five children will have a final adult height within ±6 cm of the predicted adult height (Cole and Wright, 2011).

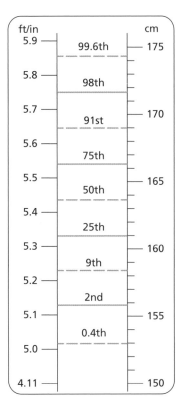

Fig. 18.4 Adult height predictor, using child's height centile. If a girl's height is mid-way between the 50th and the 75th centile, this suggests her adult height will be around 168 cm (plus or minus 6 cm).

Reproduced with permission of Royal College of Paediatrics and Child Health.

Mid-parental centile look-up

Parental heights are not as good a predictor of expected adult height as the child's current centile, but the mid-parental centile look-up on the UK-WHO 2–18 charts can be used to assess the extent to which a child is following their expected genetic trajectory (see Figure 18.5). The 'mid-parental centile' is the average adult height centile to be expected for all children of these parents. It incorporates a regression adjustment to allow for the tendency of very tall and short parents to have children with less extreme heights. This means that children of very short or tall parents will have mid-parental centiles nearer to average than one might expect. This is more accurate than the simple target height calculation (Wright and Cheetham, 1999).

Most children's height centiles (90%) are within ± two centile spaces of the mid-parental centile and only 1% will be more than three centile spaces below. A height centile well below the mid-parental centile should be investigated further, if there are

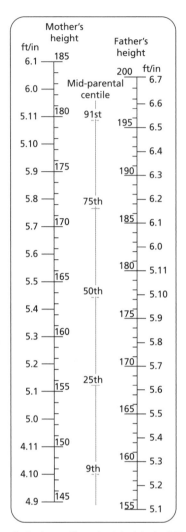

Fig. 18.5 Mid-parental centile look-up. If mother's height is 170 cm and father's 190 cm, the mid parental centile is the 75th centile.

Reproduced with permission of Royal College of Paediatrics and Child Health.

other concerns about the child's growth rate, though most of these children will have no underlying medical condition (Wright and Cheetham, 1999). A child can be growing abnormally while still within their mid-parental height range, so that any child with obviously slow growth should be investigated, whatever their parental heights.

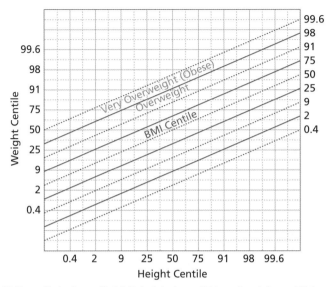

Fig. 18.6 BMI centile look-up. If child's height is on 25th and weight on 75th centile, BMI will be between 91st and 98th centile, in overweight range.

Reproduced with permission of Royal College of Paediatrics and Child Health.

Body mass index

Body mass index (BMI) tells you how heavy a child is relative to their height and is the most practical measure of fatness and thinness from the age of 2, when height can be measured fairly accurately. The BMI centile conversion on the UK-WHO charts chart provides an approximate BMI centile, accurate to a quarter of a centile space (Cole, 2002) (Figure 18.6). Most children will have a BMI between the 25th and 75th centiles, whatever their height centile. BMI is a measure of muscle and bone as well as fat, particularly in children with a BMI within or below the normal range. However, the higher the BMI, the more indicative it is of excess fat (Wright and Garcia, 2012). BMI can vary a lot over time due to measurement error, so where there has been a change, it is important to check whether this reflects a real change, or inaccurate measurements.

Conditions of interest

Neonatal weight loss

Most babies with weight loss greater than 10% will be medically well (Wright and Parkinson, 2004) but many will be having feeding problems of some kind. This may also be the only obvious sign that a baby has an underlying medical problem, such as a cardiac defect or an inherited metabolic disorder. Thus, a sustained weight loss of greater than 10% should trigger a careful health and feeding assessment (NICE, 2017).

Weight faltering after the neonatal period

Less than 2% of infants show a sustained drop through two or more weight centile spaces on the new WHO charts; very large infants are more likely to show weight centile falls, while initially small infants are much less likely to drop away (Wright and Garcia, 2012). If such a drop occurs, the child should be assessed in more detail (Shields et al., 2012; NICE, 2017) including measurement of length to establish whether this reflects thinness (wasting) or slow growth.

Thinness in childhood

A BMI below the second centile is unusual and may reflect undernutrition, but more often simply reflects a small frame or low muscle mass (Wright and Garcia, 2012). It should therefore usually not be a concern, unless there has also been actual weight loss or a more gradual decline in BMI. Advising on diet, or prescribing dietary supplements, without further assessment may be harmful in children who are not actually undereating (Wright and Chillingworth, 2015).

If the BMI is below the 0.4th centile, unless already fully investigated at an earlier age, assessment in secondary care of general health and measurement of skinfolds is reasonable. If low fat stores are confirmed, assessment of diet and feeding behaviour should be undertaken.

Growth disorders and short stature

One of the aims of growth monitoring is to detect reversible forms of short stature. It is thought that around 1 child per 1000 has a potentially treatable form of short stature, with about half of these being growth hormone deficiency and Turner syndrome (Fayter et al., 2008). In addition, children with extreme constitutional short stature may also benefit from growth hormone treatment. Children with underlying medical conditions such as hypothyroidism, inflammatory bowel disease, and coeliac disease may also be short, but these conditions usually present with other symptoms or signs. Children meeting the referral criteria in Box 18.1 should be assessed in secondary care, with further monitoring or investigation as required. Height measurement can be imprecise, so any low reading or large change on height centile should be repeated and the plotting carefully checked.

Hydrocephalus

Hydrocephalus and other intracranial expansive lesions are found in 7 per 10,000 births (Zahl and Wester, 2008). These are associated with rapid head growth and upward centile crossing and this may only be detected once the head size is already above the normal range. However, because of the relatively large size of UK heads compared to the WHO standard, around one in five healthy children will shift upwards though one to two centile spaces and around 10% will have heads consistently above the 98th centile, making the detection of true cases challenging (see Box 18.1). Children with any suggestive neurological symptoms and head centile either increasing through two centile spaces or to above the 99.6th centile should be referred urgently for assessment in secondary care.

Box 18.1 Criteria for extra monitoring or referral

Weight faltering

◆ A baby 10% or more below birth weight after the first 5 days, needs to be carefully assessed in primary care including observed feeding and examination. A sustained drop through two or more weight centile spaces should trigger assessment in primary care of diet and general health, unless below the 9th at birth (one space) or above the 91st centile (three centile spaces).

Underweight

◆ If the BMI is consistently below the 0.4th centile, refer for assessment in secondary care, unless already fully investigated at an earlier age (NICE 2017).

Short stature

◆ Refer for assessment in secondary care unless already fully investigated at an earlier age if:
  • the height is below the 0.4th centile
  • the height centile has shown a sustained fall though more than two centile spaces
  • the height centile has shown a sustained fall though more than one centile space and is more than two centile spaces below the mid-parental centile.
  • the height centile is more than three centile spaces below the mid-parental centile.
◆ If the height centile is two to three centile spaces below the mid-parental centile and there is no previous height measurement, there should be assessment of general health in primary care and re-measurement in 1 year (RCPCH 2–18 Growth Chart).

Box 18.1 Continued

Head circumference

- Asymptomatic children with a head circumference above the 99.6th centile or with a centile rise of more than two centile spaces should be re-measured in 1–3 months; if the head centile is still rising, they should be referred to secondary care. If it is stable or falling, no further action is required.

- Children with any suggestive neurological symptoms and either a head centile increase through two centile spaces or a head circumference above the 99.6th centile should be referred urgently for assessment in secondary care.

- Children with head size consistently below −2 SDs may merit assessment in secondary care. Where there is evidence of developmental delay, the child would usually be referred on that basis, whatever the head size.

Overweight

- If a preschool child aged over 2 years has weight above the 98th centile, or any concerns about possible overweight, their height should be measured in primary care and the BMI centile calculated.

- If the BMI is above the 98th centile, anticipatory guidance should offered in primary care.

- If the BMI is above the 99.6th centile, advice on diet and physical activity should be given, the BMI plotted on the childhood and puberty close monitoring chart, and the child referred to any available treatment programme.

- If the BMI is above +3.33 SDs on the childhood and puberty close monitoring chart, consider referral to secondary care for screening for co-morbidity.

Adapted with permission from Royal College of Paediatric and Child Health (RCPCH), *UK-WHO growth charts-2-18 years*, Copyright © RCPCH, available from https://www.rcpch.ac.uk/resources/uk-who-growth-charts-2-18-years. Source: data from National Institute for Health and Care Excellence (NICE), *Faltering growth: recognition and management of faltering growth in children*, NICE guideline [NG75], Copyright © NICE 2017. All rights reserved. Subject to notice of rights. Available from https://www.nice.org.uk/guidance/ng75.

Microcephaly

While children with small heads are slightly more likely to go on to have developmental problems, most do not, while a small head is not a distinctive feature of most such problems (Wright and Emond, 2015). Slowing of head growth, with a fall down the centiles may rarely be seen where there are evolving problems of brain or skull growth and development (Baxter et al., 2009). Because of the relatively large size of UK heads compared to the WHO standard, only about 1 in 1000 children have heads consistently below −2 SD (Wright and Emond, 2015).

Overweight

Two-thirds of all adults are now overweight and most obese adults were not obese as children, so that anticipatory guidance for all families on a healthy lifestyle is important (see Chapters 11 and 12). One in five English children entering school are overweight, with a BMI above the 91st centile, and just under one in ten are obese with a BMI above the 98th centile. Up to two-thirds of children who were obese in later childhood go on to be obese adults (Power et al., 1997; Venn et al., 2007).

Over a quarter of Scottish toddlers (aged 27–30 months) are overweight or obese and 4% severely obese (>99.6th), but this reflects the use of the more stringent WHO standard and overweight in the preschool years has substantial scope for improvement during childhood. It is widely believed that preschool intervention *should* be beneficial to prevent later obesity, but there is little evidence of efficacy. There are some programmes aimed at preschool children (e.g. HENRY, preschool MEND), but these have not yet been tested in randomized trials. Thus, intervention in this age range should be restricted to the smaller numbers of preschool children with a BMI already well above the normal range (>99.6th centile) as they seem more likely to have obesity persisting into adulthood and are probably at higher risk of co-morbidity in childhood.

Learning links

- Learning materials are available from the RCPCH: http://www.rcpch.ac.uk/growthcharts
- Module 8 ('Growth and Nutrition') of the Healthy Child Programme provides guidance on nutrition, feeding, weaning, growth and growth charts, the social context of food, and obesity in the early years: https://www.e-lfh.org.uk/programmes/healthy-child-programme/.

Recommendations

- Use RCPCH-recommended growth charts for measuring babies and children. (*Evidence: good practice.*)
- Ensure all staff who measure babies and children are competent to assess whether the measurements indicate further action is appropriate and what that action should be. (*Evidence: good practice.*)
- Use approved equipment for measuring babies and children, specifically when measuring height/length, weight, and head circumference. (*Evidence: good practice.*)
- Measure a baby's head circumference at the midwife's 5-day visit or the health visitor's new birth visit at 10–14 days. (*Evidence: good practice.*)
- Appropriate resources should be available in primary care for diagnosis and management of any suspected abnormalities of growth. (*Evidence: good practice.*)

References

Baxter, P.S., Rigby, A.S., Rotsaert, M.H., and Wright, I. (2009). Acquired microcephaly: causes, patterns, motor and IQ effects, and associated growth changes. *Pediatrics*, **124**, 590–595.

Cole, T.J. (2002). A chart to link child centiles of body mass index, weight and height. *European Journal of Clinical Nutrition*, **56**, 1194–1199.

Cole, T.J. and Wright, C.M. (2011). A chart to predict adult height from a child's current height. *Annals of Human Biology*, **38**, 662–668.

Cole, T.J., Freeman, J.V., and Preece, M.A. (1998). British 1990 growth reference centiles for weight, height, body mass index and head circumference fitted by maximum penalized likelihood. *Statistics in Medicine*, **17**, 407–429.

Cole, T.J., Wright, C.M., and Williams, A.F. (2012). Designing the new UK-WHO growth charts to enhance assessment of growth around birth. *Archives of Disease in Childhood. Fetal and Neonatal Edition*, **12**, F219–F222.

Fayter, D., Nixon, J., Hartley, S., et al. (2008). Effectiveness and cost-effectiveness of height-screening programmes during the primary school years: a systematic review. *Archives of Disease in Childhood*, **93**, 278–284.

Freeman, J.V., Cole, T.J., Chinn, S., Jones, P.R., White, E.M., and Preece, M.A. (1995). Cross sectional stature and weight reference curves for the UK, 1990. *Archives of Disease in Childhood*, **73**, 17–24.

Moy, R. and Wright, C. (2013). Using the new UK-WHO growth charts. *Paediatrics and Child Health*, **24**, 6.

National Institute for Health and Care Excellence (NICE) (2008). Maternal and child nutrition. Public health guideline [PH11]. [online] Available at: https://www.nice.org.uk/guidance/ph11.

National Institute for Health and Care Excellence (NICE) (2017). Faltering growth: recognition and management of faltering growth in children. NICE guideline [NG75]. [online] Available at: https://www.nice.org.uk/guidance/ng75.

Paul, I.M., Schaefer, E.W., Miller, J.R., et al. (2016). Weight change nomograms for the first month after birth. *Pediatrics*, **138**, e20162625.

Power, C., Lake, J.K., and Cole, T.J. (1997). Body mass index and height from childhood to adulthood in the 1958 British born cohort. *The American Journal of Clinical Nutrition*, **66**, 1094–1101.

Sachs, M., Sharp, L., Bedford, H., and Wright, C.M. (2012). 'Now I understand': consulting parents on chart design and parental information for the UK-WHO child growth charts. *Child: Care, Health and Development*, **38**, 435–440.

Shields, B., Wacogne, I., and Wright, C.M. (2012). Weight faltering and failure to thrive in infancy and early childhood. *BMJ*, **345**, e5931.

Venn, A.J., Thomson, R.J., Schmidt, M.D., et al. (2007). Overweight and obesity from childhood to adulthood: a follow-up of participants in the 1985 Australian Schools Health and Fitness Survey. *Medical Journal of Australia*, **186**, 458–460.

WHO Multicentre Growth Reference Study Group (MGRSG) and De Onis, M. (2006). WHO Child Growth Standards based on length/height, weight and age. *Acta Paediatrica*, **95**, 76–85.

Wright, C.M. and Cheetham, T.D. (1999). The strengths and limitations of parental heights as a predictor of attained height. *Archives of Disease in Childhood*, **81**, 257–260.

Wright, C.M. and **Chillingworth, A.** (2015). The impact of stopping high-energy oral nutritional supplements on eating behaviour and weight gain. *Archives of Disease in Childhood*, **100**, 1024–1027.

Wright, C.M. and **Emond, A.** (2015). Head growth and neurocognitive outcomes. *Pediatrics*, **135**, e1393–e1398.

Wright, C.M. and **Parkinson, K.N.** (2004). Postnatal weight loss in term infants: what is normal and do growth charts allow for it? *Archives of Disease in Childhood. Fetal and Neonatal Edition*, **89**, F254–F257.

Wright, C.M. and **Garcia, A.L.** (2012). Child undernutrition in affluent societies: what are we talking about? *Proceedings of the Nutrition Society*, **71**, 545–555.

Wright, C.M., **Inskip, H.M., Godfrey, K., Williams, A.F.,** and **Ong, K.K.** (2011). Monitoring head size and growth using the new UK-WHO growth standard. *Archives of Disease in Childhood*, **96**, 386–388.

Wright, C.M., **Sachs, M., Short, J., Sharp, L., Cameron, K.,** and **Moy, R.J.** (2012). Designing new UK-WHO growth charts: implications for health staff use and understanding of charts and growth monitoring. *Maternal & Child Nutrition,* **8**, 371–379.

Wright, C.M., **Williams, A.F., Elliman, D.,** et al. (2010). Using the new UK-WHO growth charts. *BMJ,* **340**, c1140.

Zahl, S.M. and **Wester, K.** (2008). Routine measurement of head circumference as a tool for detecting intracranial expansion in infants: what is the gain? A Nationwide Survey. *Pediatrics,* **121**, e416–e420.

Chapter 19

Physical examination

Alan Emond

Summary

This chapter:

+ summarizes recommended good practice in examining babies and children as part of routine child health surveillance, and reviews the evidence supporting different activities

+ describes routine examinations for conditions which can be screened, and good practice in identifying other common physical abnormalities

+ discusses congenital heart disease, developmental dysplasia of the hip, congenital cataract, undescended testes, cleft lip, tongue tie, and prolonged jaundice in more detail.

Neonatal examination

A thorough physical examination of every newborn infant is accepted as good practice and is expected by parents, who give high satisfaction ratings for the procedure and value the assurance of normality. The precise timing of the examination is not critical, but in the UK it is recommended to be carried out within 72 hours of birth. In most units, it is undertaken in the first 24 hours, and early discharges in maternity services have raised concerns that congenital anomalies are being missed (Lock and Ray, 1999). A large US study showed that discharge on the day of birth was associated with a doubling in rates of readmission for obstructive cardiac defects and low bowel obstruction (Danilesen et al., 2000), although this has not been confirmed in UK studies (Oddie et al., 2005).

The newborn examination (Nhs.uk, 2017) can be undertaken by appropriately trained doctors, midwives, or neonatal nurses. In many centres, the doctors doing these examinations are trainee paediatricians. Advanced neonatal nurse practitioners have been shown to undertake routine examination and care of the newborn to a high standard, offering a service at least as good as doctors (Lee et al., 2001), with more continuity of care and lower staff turnover (Hall and Wilkinson, 2005). A comparative trial (EMREN) showed that the examination by midwives took 50% more time than doctors, because more health promotion topics, such as feeding and sleeping, were discussed, and this was associated with greater maternal satisfaction (Townsend et al., 2004).

The routine examination of the newborn is an opportunity to screen for specific conditions, to identify common physical problems, to reassure parents about their infant's normality, and to offer health promotion. The NHS newborn and infant physical examination (NIPE) screening programme (Gov.uk, 2017a) recommends screening of newborn babies within 72 hours of birth, and then once again between 6 to 8 weeks, for conditions relating to their heart, hips, eyes, and testes. Careful physical examination of the newborn can also identify other common abnormalities which are not part of the newborn screening programme, such as cleft palate and tongue tie, and common problems such as persistent jaundice. These are discussed in more detail below. The National Institute for Health and Care Excellence (NICE) (2015a) gives clear guidance on which aspects of maternal and infant health should be reviewed as part of postnatal care in the first 6 weeks of life. The newborn examination can be a health-promoting contact as well as a process of 'screening' for defects, and any concerns of the parents should be addressed.

New baby visit

An additional opportunity for examination and review of the newborn is provided at the handover from midwife to health visitor between 10 and 14 days. This new birth visit is performed by the health visitor, and should ideally involve both mother and father. The child health programme recommends a review of feeding and a consideration of any parental concerns about the baby, plus promotion of sensitive parenting, child development home safety, and infant sleeping position. Although not recommended as screening by the NIPE, it is good practice to examine the baby naked, weigh (unless a recent weight is available from the midwife), and measure the head circumference, as the newborn examination may have been done only a few hours after birth. Head circumference measurements in the newborn period are not reliable, because of moulding, so a measurement at 10–14 days can act as a 'baseline' for evaluating subsequent measurements. This visit also provides a good opportunity to ask the mother appropriate and sensitive questions to identify depression or other significant mental health problems, such as those recommended by the NICE (2015b) guidelines on antenatal and postnatal mental health. In Wales, the health visitor uses a Family Resilience Assessment Instrument Tool (FRAIT) to identify protective factors within families as well as to identify additional needs and potential safeguarding concerns. The FRAIT is being rolled out across Wales for use on routine health visitor contacts up to the age of 5 years, and is being evaluated.

The 6–8 week examination

This examination is usually undertaken in general practice, and many general practitioners (GPs) combine the review with the first immunization at 8 weeks. The 6–8-week review is usually a combined activity by GP and health visitor, and it is essential that good communication exists to share concerns. The NIPE-recommended screening activities at this examination are heart, hips, eyes, and testes. It is a good time to review the infant's general health, his/her feeding and weight gain, and developmental progress. The appointment also provides an opportunity to deliver key messages about the baby's health, including feeding, sleeping, accident prevention, and play and developmental stimulation. Parents must be given the opportunity to express their concerns about their infant's progress.

The physical examination at 6–8 weeks should start with weight and head circumference measurements. It is important that these are recorded in the Personal Child Health Record Held (PCHR), as they can be useful as 'baseline' measurements if concerns are expressed about the child's growth in the future. The baby should be weighed naked, and the weight plotted on the centile chart in the PCHR. Head circumference should be measured, and those at the extreme ends of the distribution (<2nd centile or >98th centile) may require further investigation. The measurement of occipito-frontal head circumference also provides an opportunity to palpate sutures and fontanelles, and assess head shape. There is no evidence that measuring head circumference routinely after this age is of benefit (Wright and Emond, 2015). However, if a parent or a health professional is concerned about excessive head growth during the first year, the head circumference should be carefully measured and plotted on a monthly basis.

The eyes should be examined for red reflex, or any evidence of a manifest squint. Examination of the mouth with a bright light is necessary to visualize the palate, to exclude a cleft or partial cleft, and the tongue and buccal mucosa. Assessment of the heart includes inspecting and palpating the precordium, listening for a murmur, and palpating femoral pulses. Abdominal examination includes inspecting the umbilical stump, palpation for organomegaly, and looking for umbilical and inguinal hernias. In boys, the presence and position of each testis should be recorded. If a testicle is not fully descended, or is retractile, the infant should be examined again at 3 months. Any asymmetry in the thigh creases, or any differences in leg length or in the position the leg is held, should raise concerns about the hip. When abducting the leg in flexion in the Barlow manoeuvre (see 'Developmental dysplasia of the hip'), differences in the degree of abduction on each side should raise concerns and prompt referral for ultrasound of the hip. Assessment of the baby's resting tone, posture, and spontaneous movement is needed. When held in ventral suspension, the baby should be able to hold their head in line with the rest of their body. The degree of head control can be assessed by pulling to sit from supine.

Routine physical examination after 8 weeks of age

There is little evidence for or against routine physical examinations for screening purposes beyond the age of 8 weeks. The exceptions are screening for growth disorders (Chapter 18) and for hearing and vision problems, which are discussed in Chapters 20 and 21. Opportunistic examination of infants presenting symptomatically unwell to primary or secondary care in the preschool period can identify important conditions such as otitis media, asthma, and hypertension (see Chapter 23).

Rapid weight gain in the first 2 years of life often drives linear growth. After the age of 2 years, any child with weight above the 99.6th centile, or concerns about overweight in primary care, should have length or height measured and body mass index centile plotted (see Chapter 18).

Although widely undertaken in the past, there is insufficient evidence to support a universal physical examination at school entry. A more useful approach to the identification of developmental delay and behavioural difficulties is the concept of school readiness, which is discussed in Chapter 31.

Congenital heart disease

The birth prevalence of congenital heart disease (CHD) in the UK is 7–8 per 1000 live-born infants, and CHD accounts for 3% of all infant deaths and 46% of deaths due to congenital malformations (Knowles et al., 2005). Early detection of CHD is important, as deterioration may be rapid and catastrophic, and the outcome may be better if the infant is treated before this occurs (Brown et al., 2006). If the diagnosis is missed in the first few weeks of life because the infant is asymptomatic, the defect may not present until irreversible changes have occurred (e.g. pulmonary hypertension in children with left-to-right shunt). Even defects that are trivial in haemodynamic terms may predispose to endocarditis and antibiotic prophylaxis should be considered for dental and other procedures. (The recent updated NICE guidelines (2016) stress that the discussion regarding the need for antibiotic prophylaxis should be undertaken with the parent, the dentist and the cardiologist.) Missed diagnoses of heart disease distress parents, even if the delay does not result in any harm to the baby.

Antenatal screening for congenital heart disease

Although the overall detection rate is low, as the quality of scanning improves, an increasing number of cardiac defects are being identified by antenatal ultrasound screening. The Fetal Anomaly Screening Programme (FASP) (Gov.uk, 2017b) recommends all fetuses are screened for CHD at the 18–20 week anomaly scan. Those with a suspected fetal cardiac abnormality on ultrasound should be seen within 5 days a by a specialist cardiologist. Parents who have had CHD themselves or a previous child with CHD have a small but increased risk of a further affected child. They should be offered genetic counselling and fetal echocardiography, preferably at a specialist centre.

Newborn examination for congenital heart disease

The identification of congenital heart defects is one of the important screening tests of the neonatal examination. Ideally the heart should be examined between 6 and 48 hours after birth to allow maximal time for the ductus to close and pulmonary vascular resistance to start to fall, to increase the chances of revealing previously occult congenital heart disease. A Japanese study (Nagasawa et al., 2016) suggested that the median ductal closure time was 27 hours for boys and 45 hours for girls. However, the practical reality is, with early discharge from maternity units the norm, that most newborn examinations are done on day 1 of life. Professionals need to inform parents that normal findings in the newborn infant do not guarantee that the cardiovascular system is normal and that serious heart conditions can present at any time in the first few weeks of life.

Infants with serious CHD may present with tachypnoea (particularly if it interferes with feeding), persistent recession, sweating, cyanosis, or chest infection. Such infants should be urgently referred for specialist cardiac assessment. More commonly, infants with CHD are asymptomatic and identified by the presence of a heart murmur. Murmurs can be heard in 0.5–1.9% of term infants, but only 30–40% of these will have CHD. A prospective audit from a UK centre (Patton and Hey, 2006) showed that a policy of referring every term baby with a murmur at 1 day of age that was still present at 7–10 days resulted in 4.2% requiring cardiac referral, and about one-third of these had an abnormality confirmed.

Knowles et al. (2005) undertook a systematic review of the evidence for screening for CHD and produced a decision analytic model. The model suggested that 122/100,000 infants screened have life-threatening cardiac diseases undetected at the time of the examination, and that just 39 would be identified by examination alone. The pick-up rate could be improved to 82 by the addition of pulse oximetry, at the cost of £4900 per timely diagnosis achieved. The Pulse-Ox study undertaken on 20,000 asymptomatic newborns in six UK maternity units (Ewar et al., 2011) showed that pulse oximetry had a sensitivity of 75.0% for critical cases and 49.1% for all major CHDs. The prevalence of major CHDs in babies with normal pulse oximetry was 1.4/1000. The authors concluded that pulse oximetry is a simple, safe, and feasible test that is acceptable to parents and staff and adds value to existing screening, with the potential to identify cases of critical CHDs that would otherwise go undetected. However, the number that would be identified in addition to antenatal ultrasound and newborn examination is small, and the downside is that using oximetry will pick up infants with low saturations who don't have CHD. Most have other conditions, some of which resolve spontaneously, and some are totally normal.

Pulse oximetry was recommended as a screening tool to detect critical CHD in 2011 by the American Academy of Pediatrics and the American Heart Association, and a pilot of using pulse oximetry in 15 NHS Trusts in England was started in 2015. Until the results of this study are available, it cannot be recommended as a routine addition to the existing newborn physical examination tests within 72 hours of birth.

Loud murmurs in an asymptomatic infant may be due to a small ventricular septal defect, which is benign, but may also be due to valvular stenosis, which needs prompt referral. Patent ductus arteriosus is very common in premature infants. Most close spontaneously or with treatment, but a few persist beyond the neonatal period and may not be detected until later (Tanner et al., 2005).

Specific conditions associated with congenital heart disease

There is also an increased incidence of CHD in a wide variety of other dysmorphic syndromes and in association with malformations, and all such children should be checked with particular care.

Children with Down syndrome are now usually identified antenatally, and if the pregnancy is continued, a cardiac abnormality scan at 17–18 weeks is particularly important as 40–60% have CHD. Whether the diagnosis of Down syndrome is made antenatally or in the neonatal period, referral should be made to a cardiologist soon after birth for expert clinical assessment and echocardiogram. The Down Syndrome Medical Interest Group (http://www.dsmig.org.uk) has a protocol for cardiac investigation of babies with Down syndrome.

Children suspected of having Marfan's syndrome (0.3/1000) need cardiological review, as cardiovascular disease accounts for greater than 90% of premature deaths in patients with the condition (Stuart and Williams, 2007).

Hypertrophic cardiomyopathy is a rare condition (0.2/1000) transmitted by a dominant gene. Decisions about the management of the offspring of people with this condition should be made by a cardiologist with experience of managing the disorder and of counselling affected individuals and their families. Neonatal screening is unlikely to be helpful and is not recommended. Selective screening for hypertrophic cardiomyopathy with a history, examination, and electrocardiogram in any young person embarking on intensive physical activity (such as athletics training) has been suggested, but has not been evaluated.

Developmental dysplasia of the hip

The reported birth prevalence of developmental dysplasia of the hip (DDH) ranges between 1.5/1000 and 20/1000 livebirths, reflecting that DDH is a spectrum condition of hip joint malformation and instability, ranging from mild acetabular dysplasia with a stable hip to a frankly dislocated hip with a dysmorphic femoral head and acetabulum. Early identification of DDH improves outcome, as the early use of dynamic flexion–abduction splints such as the Pavlik harness or static splints such as the Von Rosen splint or the Graf splint may stabilize the hip until the soft tissues tighten (Nakamura et al., 2007). Delayed diagnosis requires more complex treatment and has a less successful outcome than dysplasia diagnosed early. The older the child is at presentation, the more likely it is that an open reduction will be required with the addition of femoral and/or acetabular osteotomies to stabilize the reduction (Sewell et al., 2009).

Traditional screening involves the physical examination in the first 24 hours and at 6–8 weeks of the hips and lower limbs including the Barlow and Ortolani manoeuvres. The sensitivity of this screening test varies from 74% to 99%, and the specificity is greater than 95%, depending on the skill and experience of the examiner. The presence of limited hip abduction (less than 60° in 90° of hip flexion) may be the most sensitive sign for detecting a dislocated hip in young infants (Sewell et al., 2009). After the age of 8 weeks, screening is not recommended, but missed cases of DDH can still be picked up opportunistically when the child is being weighed naked (e.g. at the 9-month review). The signs of unilateral DDH are asymmetry of the inguinal skin creases, any difficulty in abduction of one leg compared to another, or differences in leg lengths. All babies with an abnormality on examination should have an ultrasound examination of the hips performed and be seen by an expert in the management of DDH.

The aim of screening programmes for DDH is to reduce late presentation and the need for surgery. For many years, UK guidelines were based on universal clinical examination at 24 hours and 6 weeks, and in 2008, selective 'at-risk' ultrasound screening (USS) was recommended for infants with a breech presentation at birth and for those with a strong family history of DDH. In a 15-year prospective observational study (Talbot and Paton, 2013), 2984 neonates (46/1000 livebirths) with these risk factors were referred and screened by USS, and 3/1000 males and 25/1000 females were found to have DDH.

Although USS is regarded as the gold standard for detecting DDH in the neonate, with a sensitivity of 100%, (although it can over-diagnose the condition by labelling natural hip immaturity as dysplasia), evidence for its effectiveness in universal screening programmes is mixed. A Cochrane review (Shorter et al., 2013) concluded that there is inconsistent evidence that universal USS results in a significant increase in treatment compared to the use of targeted ultrasound or clinical examination alone. Neither of the ultrasound strategies has been demonstrated to improve clinical outcomes including late diagnosed DDH and surgery. A systematic review for the U.S. Preventive Services Task Force (Shipman et al., 2006) concluded 'Screening with clinical examination or ultrasound can identify newborns at increased risk for DDH, but because of the high rate of spontaneous resolution of neonatal hip instability and dysplasia and the lack of evidence of the effectiveness of intervention on functional outcomes, the net benefits of screening are not clear'.

Congenital cataract

Cataracts in babies and children are rare, affecting 3–4/10,000 children in the UK, but represent an important preventable cause of visual impairment and blindness in childhood. Surgical treatment of dense cataracts is needed within the first 3 months of life to avoid amblyopia, so early identification is important. Infants born with a weight at or below 2500 g have a three- to fourfold increased chance of developing infantile cataract (San Giovanni et al., 2002). The screening test for cataract is inspection of the eyes and evaluation of the pupillary red reflex with a bright light, recommended for all infants during the newborn period and again at 6–8 weeks. However, in a national study (Rahi and Dezateau, 1999), only half (47%) of children newly diagnosed with congenital or infantile cataract were detected through these examinations. Many parents reported concerns about their infant's visual behaviour, (or notice 'white eye' on baby photographs) before the cataract was diagnosed, so these concerns should always be acted upon by clinical staff. If a cataract is suspected, the baby should be referred to an ophthalmologist without delay.

Undescended testes

Careful inspection of the genitalia in the newborn male to detect undescended testes, hypospadias, hydrocoele, and other anomalies is an essential part of the routine neonatal examination. By far the most common problem detectable by screening examination is abnormal descent of the testicle. At birth, 60/1000 males have one or both testes undescended, and the rate is some five times higher in preterm babies than in full-term infants. A high proportion of testes which are undescended at birth have descended normally by 3 months of age, by which age the prevalence drops to 16/1000. If on inspection and palpation a testis is not detectable in the scrotum, the testis should be gently manipulated into the lowest position along the pathway of normal anatomical descent without tension being applied. Bilateral absence of testicles in the scrotal sac, particularly if other abnormalities or minor malformations are present, requires urgent investigation. At the neonatal examination, whether a testis can be identified on each side, and the degree of testicular descent into the scrotum, should be recorded, and the examination should be repeated at the 8-week examination. The second examination is particularly important in those cases where the testis is *not* 'well down' in the scrotum at birth.

Cleft lip and palate

A cleft lip and/or palate is the fourth most common congenital birth defect with a UK birth prevalence of 1/700. A cleft lip is obvious at birth, but an isolated cleft palate is more difficult to recognize, and between 28% and 31% are not being detected on day 1 of life (Habel et al., 2006). Many infants with a cleft palate present symptomatically with milk regurgitating through the nose during feeds. Routine examination for a cleft palate does not meet the criteria for a screening test, but is good practice as early diagnosis can lead to expert help with feeding and referral to a regional multidisciplinary cleft team. The routine examination of the newborn should include assessment of the palate by direct inspection with a bright light. Palpation alone is an unreliable technique, unless the posterior palatal spines can be felt (Merritt, 2005). An assistant depressing the baby's tongue may help the examiner to inspect the whole palate without difficulty. Examination with a laryngoscope is recommended if there are any risk factors such as a family history or other dysmorphic features (Armstrong and Simpson, 2002).

A large cohort study has been set up in the UK to provide more evidence to inform the management of cleft lip and palate. The Cleft Collective (2017) cohort is investigating the biological and environmental causes of cleft, the best treatments for cleft, and the psychological impact of cleft on those affected and their families.

Tongue tie

Ankyloglossia, or tongue tie (TT), is a congenital condition characterized by a short, thickened, or abnormally tight lingual frenulum that affects around 2–5% of newborn babies. It is a spectrum condition, with degrees of functional severity depending on the attachment and mobility of the tongue. Feeding difficulties have been reported in 12–44% of TT babies due to poor latch, nipple damage, and inability to feed continuously. If a TT is identified during the neonatal examination, referral to breastfeeding support or a lactation expert will help ensure that the baby latches on as well as possible during breastfeeding, and the mother is encouraged to continue, and to express if feeding is painful. Many infants with milder forms of TT can successfully breastfeed, and surgical intervention should be reserved for those mother–baby pairs who are having continuing problems with breastfeeding despite expert support and help (Emond et al., 2014). NICE guidance (2005) supports the use of division of TT (frenotomy) in those experiencing breastfeeding difficulties, but suggested that further controlled trials are needed on the effects of this procedure on successful long-term breastfeeding.

A recent Cochrane review (O'Shea et al., 2017) reported that frenotomy results in short-term improvement in self-reported breastfeeding efficacy and maternal pain, but no difference in breastfeeding rates, and concluded: 'Further randomised controlled trials of high methodological quality are necessary to determine the effects of frenotomy'.

Until further trial evidence is available, the best compromise policy may be to consider early frenotomy in infants with severe TT who in spite of expert support cannot feed adequately, and for the milder degrees of TT to wait for 2 weeks, providing support and encouragement with breastfeeding (Power and Murphy, 2015).

Prolonged jaundice

Identification of jaundice is not a screening test on the NIPE programme, but is an essential part of surveillance of the young baby. Any visible jaundice at the newborn check in the first 72 hours is pathological and will need investigation. From day 3 to 7 of life, mild degrees of jaundice are common, especially in breastfed babies, and are due to a 'physiological' unconjugated hyperbilirubinaemia. Jaundiced infants at any age who are unwell (fever, respiratory distress, pallor, and vomiting), have pale stools or dark urine, or have bleeding or bruising should be referred for urgent assessment.

Prolonged jaundice is defined as visible jaundice persisting after 14 days of age in term babies and 21 days in preterm babies. Infants with prolonged jaundice should be referred for a jaundice blood profile, including conjugated and unconjugated bilirubin, liver function tests, haemoglobin and blood group, and thyroid function. The main reason for prolonged jaundice testing is to pick up biliary atresia as early as possible, but there are many other causes of prolonged jaundice, including breast milk jaundice which resolves spontaneously.

Learning links

♦ Training support for NHS staff is available at e-Learning for Healthcare: https://www.e-lfh.org.uk/programmes/nhs-screening-programmes/.

Recommendations

♦ Physical examination of infants should occur within 72 hours of birth and again between 6 and 8 weeks. (*Evidence: strong.*)

♦ Identify common physical problems in the newborn examination, the new baby visit, and the 6–8-week check to reassure parents about their infant's normality and to offer health promotion. (*Evidence: moderate.*)

- At other ages, infants and children should be examined according to parental or professional concerns. (*Good practice.*)

- Children with Down syndrome should have an antenatal cardiac abnormality scan at 17–18 weeks of gestation, and referred to a cardiologist after birth for clinical and echocardiography assessment. (*Evidence: strong.*)

- Good communication is needed between GPs, midwives, health visitors, and other members of the primary care team to ensure that concerns are shared and acted upon. All professionals should work in partnership with parents and record findings in the parent-held Personal Child Health Record. (*Good practice.*)

References

Armstrong, H. and Simpson, R.M. (2002). Examination of the neonatal palate. *Archives of Disease in Childhood. Fetal and Neonatal Edition*, **86**, F210.

Brown, K.L., Ridout, D.A., Hoskote, A., Verhulst, L., Ricci, M., and Bull, C. (2006). Delayed diagnosis of congenital heart disease worsens preoperative condition and outcome of surgery in neonates. *Heart*, **92**, 1298–1302.

Danilesen, B., Castles, A.G., Damberg, C.L., et al. (2000). Newborn discharge timing and readmissions: California 1992–1995. *Pediatrics*, **106**, 34–39.

Emond, A., Ingram, J., Johnson, D., et al. (2014). Randomised controlled trial of early frenotomy in breastfed infants with mild–moderate tongue-tie. *Archives of Disease in Childhood. Fetal and Neonatal Edition*, **99**, F189–F195.

Ewar, A.K., Middleon, L.J., Furmston, A.T., et al. (2011). Pulse oximetry screening for congenital heart defects in newborn infants (PulseOx): a test accuracy study. *The Lancet*, **378**, 785–794.

Gov.uk (2017a). Population screening programmes: NHS newborn and infant physical examination (NIPE) screening programme. [online] Available at: https://www.gov.uk/topic/population-screening-programmes/newborn-infant-physical-examination [Accessed 25 Sep. 2017].

Gov.uk (2017b). Population screening programmes: NHS fetal anomaly screening programme (FASP). [online] Available at: https://www.gov.uk/topic/population-screening-programmes/fetal-anomaly [Accessed 25 Sep. 2017].

Habel, A., Elhadi, N., Sommerlad, B., et al. (2006). Delayed detection of cleft palate: an audit of newborn examination. *Archives of Disease in Childhood*, **91**, 238–240.

Hall, D. and Wilkinson, A.R. (2005). Quality of care by neonatal nurse practitioners: a review of the Ashington experiment. *Archives of Disease in Childhood. Fetal and Neonatal Edition*, **90**, F195–F200.

Knowles, R., Griebsch, I., Dezateux, C., et al. (2005). Newborn screening for congenital heart defects: a systematic review and cost-effectiveness analysis. *Health Technology Assessment*, **9**, 1–152, iii–iv.

Lee, T.W., Skelton, R.E., and Skene, C. (2001). Routine neonatal examination: effectiveness of trainee paediatrician compared with advanced neonatal nurse practitioner. *Archives of Disease in Childhood. Fetal and Neonatal Edition*, **85**, F100–F104.

Lock, M. and Ray, J.G. (1999). Higher neonatal morbidity after routine early hospital discharge: are we sending newborns home too early? *CMAJ: Canadian Medical Association Journal*, **161**, 249–253.

Merritt, L. (2005). Physical assessment of the infant with cleft lip and/or palate. *Advanced Neonatal Care*, **5**, 125–134.

Nagasawa, H., Hamada, C., Wakabayashi, M., et al. (2016). Time to spontaneous ductus arteriosus closure in full-term neonates. *Open Heart*, **3**, e000413.

Nakamura, J., Kamegaya, M., Saisu, T., et al. (2007). Treatment for developmental dysplasia of the hip using the Pavlik harness: long-term results. *Journal of Bone and Joint Surgery*, **89B**, 230–235.

National Institute for Health and Care Excellence (NICE) (2005). Division of ankyloglossia (tongue-tie) for breastfeeding. Interventional procedures guidance [IPG 149]. [online] Available at: http://www.nice.org.uk/Guidance/IPG149

National Institute for Health and Care Excellence (NICE) (2015a). Postnatal care up to 6 weeks after birth. Clinical guideline [CG37]. [online] Available at: https://www.nice.org.uk/guidance/cg37.

National Institute for Health and Care Excellence (NICE) (2015b). Antenatal and postnatal mental health: clinical management and service guidance. Clinical guideline [CG192]. [online] Available at: https://www.nice.org.uk/guidance/cg192.

National Institute for Health and Care Excellence (NICE) (2016). Prophylaxis against infective endocarditis: antimicrobial prophylaxis against infective endocarditis in adults and children undergoing interventional procedures. Clinical guideline [CG37]. [online] Available at: https://www.nice.org.uk/guidance/cg64.

Nhs.uk (2017). Newborn physical examination – pregnancy and baby guide. [online] Available at: http://www.nhs.uk/Conditions/pregnancy-and-baby/Pages/newborn-physical-exam.aspx [Accessed 25 Sep. 2017].

Oddie, S.J., Hammal, D., Richmond, S., et al. (2005). Early discharge and readmission to hospital in the first month of life in the Northern Region of the UK during 1998: a case cohort study. *Archives of Disease in Childhood*, **90**, 119–124.

O'Shea, J.E., Foster, J.P., O'Donnell, C.P.F., et al. (2017). Frenotomy for tongue-tie in newborn infants. *Cochrane Database of Systematic Reviews*, **3**, CD011065.

Patton, C. and Hey, E. (2006). How effectively can clinical examination pick up congenital heart disease at birth? *Archives of Disease in Childhood. Fetal and Neonatal Edition*, **91**, F263–F267

Power, R.F. and Murphy, J.F. (2015). Tongue-tie and frenotomy in infants with breastfeeding difficulties: achieving a balance. *Archives of Disease in Childhood*, **100**, 489–494.

Rahi, J.S. and Dezateau, C. (1999). National cross sectional study of detection of congenital and infantile cataract in the United Kingdom: role of childhood screening and surveillance. *BMJ*, **318**, 362.

San Giovanni, J.P., Chew, E.Y., Reed, G.F., et al. (2002). Infantile cataract in the collaborative perinatal project: prevalence and risk factors. *Archives of Ophthalmology*, **120**, 1559–1565.

Sewell, M.D., Rosendahl, K., and Eastwood, D.M. (2009). Developmental dysplasia of the hip. *BMJ*, **339**, b4454.

Shipman, S.A., Helfand, M., Moyer, V.A., et al. (2006). Screening for developmental dysplasia of the hip: a systematic literature review for the US Preventive Services Task Force. *Pediatrics*, **117**, e557–e576.

Shorter, D., Hong, T., and **Osborn, D.A.** (2013). Cochrane Review: Screening programmes for developmental dysplasia of the hip in newborn infants. *Evidence-Based Child Health*, **8**, 11–54.

Stuart, A.G. and **Williams, A.** (2007). Marfan's syndrome and the heart. *Archives of Disease in Childhood*, **92**, 351–356.

Talbot, C.L. and **Paton, R.W.** (2013). Screening of selected risk factors in developmental dysplasia of the hip: an observational study. *Archives of Disease in Childhood*, **98**, 692–696.

Tanner, K., **Sabrine, N.,** and **Wren, C.** (2005). Cardiovascular malformations among preterm infants. *Pediatrics*, **116**, e833–e838.

The Cleft Collective (2017). University of Bristol: The Cleft Collective. [online] Available at: http://www.bristol.ac.uk/dental/cleft-collective/ [Accessed 25 Sep. 2017].

Townsend, J., **Wolke, D., Hayes, J.,** et al. (2004). Routine examination of the newborn: the EMREN study. Evaluation of an extension of the midwife role including a randomised controlled trial of appropriately trained midwives and paediatric senior house officers. *Health Technology Assessment*, **8**, iii–iv, ix–xi, 1–100.

Wright, C.M. and **Emond, A.M.** (2015). Head growth and neurocognitive outcomes. *Pediatrics*, **135**, e1393–e1398.

Chapter 20

Identification of hearing impairment

David Elliman

Summary

This chapter:

- emphasizes the importance of hearing for optimal development
- describes the newborn hearing screening programme
- reviews the potential uses and limitations of screening at other ages
- provides guidance for practitioners on identifying conductive hearing loss.

Introduction

Normal hearing requires properly functioning outer, middle, and inner ears, auditory nerve, and auditory cortex. A failure in any one of these will reduce the ability to hear. Causes may be divided into congenital or acquired, and sensorineural or conductive. A sensorineural loss is one where the cochlea or auditory nerve is affected, whereas a conductive loss is due to an abnormality of the outer or middle ear. The former is likely to be permanent whereas the latter is usually transient, due to otitis media with effusion, unless there is a congenital malformation or particular predisposition such as Down syndrome. The degree of hearing loss is categorized as mild (21–39 dB), moderate (40–69 dB), severe (70–94 dB), and profound ($\geq$95 dB). Anyone with a hearing loss of 40 dB or greater is likely to have difficulties with spoken conversation, where there is significant background noise.

Each year, in the UK, about 1 in 1000 children are born with a significant degree of bilateral hearing impairment ($\geq$40 dB loss in the better ear) and 0.6 in 1000 have a unilateral loss (Fortnum et al., 2016). These are usually sensorineural in origin and are permanent. A number of children acquire a permanent hearing loss later in life such that, by 9–15 years old, the prevalence of hearing impairment is 2.05 per 1000 (Fortnum et al., 2016). As the ability to hear is an important aid to social, emotional, and cognitive development, if impairment in hearing is not recognized and managed appropriately, children may suffer unnecessarily.

In addition to sensorineural hearing impairment, otitis media with effusion (OME), if prolonged, as well as affecting hearing, can have a significant effect on language development and behaviour (Silva, 1982, 1986). Defined as 'a collection of fluid within the middle ear without signs of acute inflammation', it is commonest at around 2 years of age, with on average 20% of children being affected, and another smaller peak at 5 years of age, before the prevalence declines through childhood (Zielhuis et al., 1990). The effects fluctuate with time and age, so it can be difficult to recognize. Most commonly, the presenting issue is a concern on the part of the child's parent/carer about their hearing.

Prior to the introduction of hearing screening, the evidence for sensorineural hearing loss suggested that the earlier interventions were put in place, the better the outcome for hearing impaired children (e.g. Yoshinaga-Itano et al., 1998). However, studies relying on comparisons of natural history, without a screened population, were open to bias. Therefore, the evidence prior to the introduction of screening was suggestive, but far from conclusive (Davis et al., 1997).

Screening

A school entry screening (SES) programme was in place in many areas for up to a hundred years, but didn't become national until 1955 (Watkin, 1991). Originally described in 1944 (Ewing and Ewing, 1944), from the mid 1950s, an increasing number of areas in the UK instituted a hearing screening programme at 8 months of age. This was conducted by health visitors and involved the use of standardized sound stimuli and the observation of a response by the baby (i.e. turning towards the sound). This was known as the health visitor, or infant, distraction test (IDT). For many decades, the IDT and a SES programme for hearing were the mainstay of screening for hearing impairment in children. This was endorsed by a report (Advisory Committee on Services for Hearing Impaired Children, 1981) recommending they should continue.

Opportunistic recognition by parents or professionals contributed significantly, but meant that diagnosis often did not take place until children were relatively old. Watkin and colleagues (1990) found that only around half of parents of children with a significant hearing loss suspected this to be the case before it was picked up by screening or recognized by a professional. The accuracy of the IDT, as performed, meant that children with a transient hearing loss made up a large proportion of referrals for diagnostic testing and children with a significant sensorineural loss were often missed. Prior to the introduction of neonatal screening, the mean age of referral of cases of moderate to profound hearing loss was 18.8 months, while a quarter had not been referred until after 30.8 months (Davis et al., 1997). This and the fact that the IDT was performed at 8 months, so couldn't pick up young infants, however well performed, prompted the search for methods to screen babies soon after birth.

Newborn hearing screening

Various methods of screening newborn babies have been attempted (Davis et al., 1997). Trials with an auditory response cradle, recording respiratory and body activity responses to auditory stimuli, were reported in the late 1970s and early 1980s, with promising results (Bhattacharya et al., 1984). At the beginning of the 1990s, reports of the potential use of semi-automated screening using otoacoustic emissions (OAEs) appeared (Stevens et al., 1989; Kemp and Ryan, 1993). A small probe is placed in the external auditory meatus with a small microphone and speaker. Regular clicks are produced and the cochlea (outer hair cells) then produces an emission, which is detected by the microphone. It is a relatively quick and easy technique. Automated auditory brainstem responses (AABRs) have also been considered for screening. This technique involves producing an auditory stimulus and noting changes in electrical activity of the brain via three electrical probes. AABR screening is much more time-consuming than that using OAEs. In summarizing the evidence, Davis et al. (1997) pointed out that the tests were measuring slightly different things. The auditory response cradle is dependent on auditory function up to and including the auditory cortex, and the resultant reflex responses; OAE relies on the integrity of the outer, middle, and inner ears; and AABR relies on the integrity of the outer, middle, and inner ears and lower auditory pathways. These differences are not usually of significance in children who only have a hearing problem, but may be important in children with multiple problems and/or those who are or were on a neonatal intensive care unit (NICU) or special care baby unit.

Initial evidence suggested that the performance of the auditory response cradle was not as good as that of the OAE or AABR test and was unlikely to be suitable for those in a high-risk group. Initially, most programmes opted for a two-stage procedure in healthy children—OAE followed by AABR or OEA testing followed by a repeat OAE test for those who failed the first test as it is known that the false-positive rate is higher in the first 24 hours of life, at least in part due to fluid in the external auditory meatus. Comparing the two protocols, Kennedy et al. (2000) found a referral rate of 1.3% with the former and 2.4% with the latter. When reviewed later, they found a sensitivity of 0.92, a specificity of 0.98, and positive predictive value of 6.5% for a bilateral loss of 40 dB or greater, with the OAE/ABR protocol as used in the original trial (Kennedy et al., 2005).

It has been suggested that 'targeted screening' may be a preferable option to universal newborn screening (UNS). By screening what is considered to be a high-risk group only, about 5% of the population, 50% of babies with significant hearing impairment would be identified. In 1997, it was estimated that this would cost £14.1 per child detected as opposed to £19.7 and £81.7 for UNS and IDT respectively (Davis et al., 1997). However the 50% of the cases of hearing impairment in the other 95% of the population would remain undetected until a later age.

From 2006, all babies in the UK have been offered newborn hearing screening. For most babies (non-NICU or 'well babies'), this is an automated OAE test followed by a repeat automated OAE test for those who fail and then a AABR test for those who fail a second time. Babies on neonatal units are screened with both OAE and AABR tests. Babies with unilateral losses, as well as those with bilateral losses, are referred, as there is emerging evidence of its adverse effects on language development (José et al., 2014). Auditory neuropathy spectrum disorder is a neural form of auditory dysfunction that is characterized by evidence of normal cochlear outer hair cell (sensory) function and abnormal inner hair cell or auditory brainstem responses. This has been said to account for about one in ten children with permanent hearing loss (Sininger, 2002), but accurate figures are not available (Feirn et al., 2013). Babies with auditory neuropathy spectrum disorder will pass the OAE, but fail the AABR test. As most of these babies will be on a NICU, the majority should be picked up by screening.

Prior to the screening test, the parents should be given written information, informing them about the test and the possible outcomes. If a baby is confirmed to have a hearing loss, there should be appropriate information explaining this and what to expect in the future.

It is important that the programme is closely monitored, not only to ensure that cases are not missed (i.e. it is sensitive), but also to keep down the number of referrals that are subsequently shown not to have a problem (false positives). Van der Ploeg and colleagues (2008) sent questionnaires to parents 6 months after their baby had had UNS. They compared parents whose babies had passed the first stage of screening with those whose babies had failed at one or other stage, but who were subsequently found to have no hearing loss. Parental anxiety and attitude towards the child were no different between the groups. However, when asked 'How often do you test to see if your child can hear well?' and 'How often do you worry about your child's hearing?' there was a significant difference and this increased with the number of tests failed. This is in keeping with other screening programmes such as that for medium-chain acyl-CoA dehydrogenase deficiency (MCADD) where Karaceper and colleagues (2016) found that babies who had a false-positive result for screening for MCADD were more likely to see their doctor and more likely to be admitted to hospital than those who had a negative screening result. There is evidence that the provision of good quality information prior to screening may reduce anxiety after a false-positive diagnosis of cystic fibrosis (Vernooij-van Langen et al., 2014). This may be so for other screening programmes.

Initially, some programmes were hospital based, while others screened babies after discharge from hospital. The coverage of the former tends to be higher and they are easier to organize. There are few community-based programmes now.

Data from England showed that in the period April 2016 to March 2017, 98.4 of newborn babies were screened and 88.8% of those referred to audiology services were seen within 4 weeks of the screening being completed (Public Health England, 2017a). From April 2016 to March 2017, 2.6% of screened babies were referred to audiology services, of whom 2.8% were confirmed to have a bilateral hearing impairment (Public Health England, 2017b). The rate of bilateral hearing impairment in screened babies was 0.7 per 1000.

Early evidence from screening programmes consistently showed a younger age at detection and, more importantly, at intervention (e.g. Weichnold et al., 2006; Sininger et al., 2009). Follow-up of screened children at 6–10 years old shows good evidence of improved receptive language and reading ability, though still not as good as their hearing peers (Pimperton and Kennedy, 2012). In contrast, at 13–19 years of age, there seemed to be no statistically significant beneficial effect on language of early detection. There are many reasons why this may be so, including selective loss to follow-up and so on. More research is needed on larger cohorts.

Reviewing newborn screening, in general, in 2015, Therrell et al. (2015) found that approximately a quarter of European countries and the majority of US states had newborn screening programmes. Data was not given for other countries. Australia has a universal screening programme, from which the Longitudinal Outcomes of Children with Hearing Impairment (LOCHI) study has confirmed the findings in young children (Ching et al., 2013).

Eight-month infant screening

Because of its limitations, the IDT has no place in screening.

School entry screening

Since the mid 1950s, SES for hearing has been in place in the UK. A review by Bamford et al. (2007) found that it was performed in almost 90% of areas in England, Scotland, and Wales. Although the test used was the pure tone sweep test, the frequencies used, pass criteria, and retest criteria varied. There was no national protocol and no national data collection. There was very little outcome data on the SES, but evidence from an area where UNS had been in place for a number of years showed a reduction in yield of both bilateral and unilateral permanent losses from 1.11 in 1000 to 0.34 in 1000. The authors concluded there was insufficient evidence to assess the value and cost-effectiveness of SES and more research was needed.

In 2016, a further systematic review was reported (Fortnum et al., 2016). The authors reviewed the literature on the programme and found little to support it. They examined the sensitivity of two screening devices, the pure-tone screen (PTS) (Amplivox, Eynsham, UK) and HearCheck (HC) screener (Siemens, Frimley, UK). They had sensitivities of 89% or greater and 83% or greater, respectively, and specificities of 78% or greater and 83% or greater, respectively. Comparing an area in England which had a SES in place, with one that didn't, they found no benefit from the programme. They concluded that a SES programme was unlikely to be cost-effective, but cautioned that this was based on limited evidence and suggested further work including systematic reviews of the accuracy of devices used to measure hearing at school entry; characterization and measurement of the cost-effectiveness of different approaches to the ad hoc referral system; examination of programme specificity as opposed to test specificity; further observational comparative studies of different programmes; and opportunistic trials of withdrawal of SES programmes.

Until a national decision is made, areas should continue as they are, but audit their programme and ensure staff are properly trained and refreshed.

Opportunistic identification

Some children will have a significant hearing loss that is not picked up by screening, either because it was 'missed' or because it was an acquired or progressive loss. Furthermore, there are others who have a temporary fluctuating conductive hearing loss due to OME that can also have significant effect on a child's speech and language and educational development. Parents and professionals need to be aware of this and be sensitive to the indications of hearing impairment. For babies under 1 year old, there are two useful checklists in the Personal Child Health Record (or 'red book') (Harlow Healthcare, 2016). 'Can your baby hear' consists of two checklists—one for

Box 20.1 Features that should raise a suspicion of hearing loss

- Hearing difficulties such as mishearing or requiring information/instructions to be repeated.
- Indistinct or delayed language development.
- Repeated ear infections or earache.
- Behaviour problems, particularly lack of concentration or attention, being withdrawn.
- Poor educational progress.
- Tinnitus and intolerance of load sounds.

© NICE (2008) *CG60 Otitis media with effusion in under 12s: surgery*. Available from www.nice.org.uk/guidance/cg60. All rights reserved. Subject to notice of rights. NICE guidance is prepared for the National Health Service in England. All NICE guidance is subject to regular review and may be updated or withdrawn. NICE accepts no responsibility for the use of its content in this product/publication.

reactions to sounds that one would expect at different ages, and another for sounds one would expect in older children. The National Institute for Health and Care Excellence (2008) lists a number of features, in older children, that should raise a suspicion of hearing loss (see Box 20.1). If any of these are present, referral for a formal assessment of hearing should be seriously considered. It should be remembered that tympanometry can only pick up middle ear problems, not sensorineural deafness.

Children with some identified syndromes/conditions, such as Down syndrome (Down Syndrome Medical Interest Group, 2004) and craniofacial syndromes including cleft palate (Colbert et al., 2015) will need hearing assessment at intervals. Following bacterial meningitis, children should have their hearing assessed as soon as possible in order to detect cochlear ossification early as this may affect insertion of cochlear implant electrodes into the cochlea in cases of severe to profound sensorineural hearing loss.

Management following identification

Screening is of limited value if identification of hearing impairment is not followed by timely diagnosis and management. This requires good audiology services working as a multidisciplinary team with parents, children, and teachers as a minimum.

Hearing impairment is a symptom and not a diagnosis, and therefore timely aetiological investigations should be undertaken, as the results may have an implication for genetic counselling, treatment (e.g. congenital cytomegalovirus infection), minimizing deterioration (e.g. widened vestibular aqueduct), early detection of other medically important abnormalities (e.g. visual, renal, or cardiac disease), and other aspects of management (British Association of Audiovestibular Physicians, 2015a, 2015b). Many children will have additional needs, which will also need attending to, for example, 20–60% of babies with a permanent congenital hearing loss have ophthalmic anomalies.

As well as advice to parents and teachers, interventions may include hearing aids and cochlear implants. The balance between watchful waiting and surgical intervention in OME is still debated, but the National Institute for Health and Care Excellence (2008) guidance is that 'Children with persistent bilateral OME documented over a period of 3 months with a hearing level in the better ear of 25–30 dBHL or worse averaged at 0.5, 1, 2, and 4 kHz (or equivalent dBA where dBHL not available) should be considered for surgical intervention'. In some cases, rather than surgery, the provision of aids should be considered for children with a high risk of recurrence.

Children who appear to be having hearing problems or fail behavioural screening tests, but, on further testing, prove to have normal hearing may have developmental problems (e.g. delay or autism), and so may need further assessment.

Learning links

◆ NHS Newborn Hearing Screening Programme (NHSP): https://www.e-lfh.org.uk/programmes/nhs-screening-programmes/.

Recommendations

◆ SES should be audited at a local level to understand the screening parameters of sensitivity, specificity, and positive protective value. (*Evidence: strong.*)

◆ Raise awareness between healthcare professionals and parents that a child passing the newborn screening is not a guarantee that they do not have hearing impairment, at the time, let alone later in life. (*Evidence: strong.*)

◆ Advise parents of the clues that may indicate a potential hearing loss in a child, this should take place even if no problems were found during the newborn screening. (*Evidence: moderate.*)

◆ Children who fail the screening test should be seen in a timely fashion. (*Evidence: strong.*)

◆ Consider implementation of adequate facilities to fit and manage hearing aids and cochlear implants, with a multidisciplinary team. (*Evidence: moderate.*)

References

Advisory Committee on Services for Hearing Impaired Children (1981). *Final Report.* London: DHSS.

Bamford, J., Fortnum, H., Bristow, K., et al. (2007). Current practice, accuracy, effectiveness and cost-effectiveness of the school entry hearing screen. *Health Technology Assessment,* **11**, 1–168.

Bhattacharya, J., Bennett, M.J., and Tucker, S. (1984). Long term follow-up of newborns tested with the auditory response cradle. *Archives of Disease in Childhood*, **59**, 504–511.

British Association of Audiovestibular Physicians (2015a). Guidelines for aetiological investigation into severe to profound bilateral permanent hearing impairment. April 2015. [online] Available at: http://www.baap.org.uk/Resources/Documents,GuidelinesClinicalSta ndards.aspx [Accessed 25 Sep. 2017].

British Association of Audiovestibular Physicians (2015b). Guidelines for aetiological investigation into mild to moderate bilateral permanent hearing impairment. April 2015. [online] Available at: http://www.baap.org.uk/Resources/Documents,GuidelinesClinicalSta ndards.aspx [Accessed 25 Sep. 2017].

Ching, T.Y.C., Leigh, G., and Dillon, H. (2013). Introduction to the Longitudinal Outcomes of Children with Hearing Impairment (LOCHI) study: background, design, sample characteristics. *International Journal of Audiology*, **52**, S2–S9.

Colbert, S.D., Green, B., Brennan, P.A., and Mercer, N. (2015). Contemporary management of cleft lip and palate in the United Kingdom. Have we reached the turning point? *British Journal of Oral and Maxillofacial Surgery*, **53**, 594–598.

Davis, A., Bamford, J., Wilson, I., Ramkalawan, T., Forshaw, M., and Wright, S. (1997). A critical review of the role of neonatal hearing screening in the detection of congenital hearing impairment. *Health Technology Assessment*, **1**, 1–176.

Down Syndrome Medical Interest Group (2004). Guidance for Essential Medical Surveillance – hearing impairment. [online] Available at: http://www.dsmig.org.uk/ information-resources/guidance-for-essential-medical-surveillance/ [Accessed 25 Sep. 2017].

Ewing, I.R. and Ewing, A.W.C. (1944). The ascertainment of deafness in infancy and early childhood. *The Journal of Laryngology and Otology*, **59**, 309–333.

Fiern, R., Sutton, G., Parker, G., Sirimanna, T., Lightfoot, G., and Wood, S. (2013). Guidelines for the Assessment and Management of Auditory Neuropathy Spectrum Disorder in Young Infants v 2.2. [online] NHSP Clinical Group. Available at: https://www.thebsa.org.uk/ resources/guidelines-assessment-management-auditory-neuropathy-spectrum-disorder-young-infants-v2-2/ [Accessed 25 Sep. 2017].

Fortnum, H., Ukoumunne, O.C., Hyde, C., et al. (2016). A programme of studies including assessment of diagnostic accuracy of school hearing screening tests and a cost-effectiveness model of school entry hearing screening programmes. *Health Technology Assessment*, **20**, 1–178.

Harlow Healthcare (2016). PCHR download. [online] Available at: http://www. healthforallchildren.com/the-pchr/2079-2/ [Accessed 25 Sep. 2017]

José, M.R., Mondelli, M.F.C.G., Feniman, M.R., and Lopes-Herrera, S.P. (2014). Language disorders in children with unilateral hearing loss: a systematic review. *International Archive of Otorhinolaryngology*, **18**, 198–203.

Karaceper, M.D., Chakraborty, P., Coyle, D., et al. (2016). The health system impact of false positive newborn screening results for medium-chain acyl-CoA dehydrogenase deficiency: a cohort study. *Orphanet Journal of Rare Diseases*, **11**, 12.

Kemp, D.T. and Ryan, S. (1993). Use of transiently evoked otoacoustic emissions in neonatal screening programmes. *Seminars in Hearing*, **14**, 33–36.

Kennedy, C.R., Kimm, L., Thornton, A.R.D., and Davis, A. (2000). False positives in universal neonatal screening for permanent childhood hearing impairment. *The Lancet*, **356**, 1903–1904.

Kennedy, C.R., McCann, D., Campbell, M.J., Kimm, L., and Thornton, R. (2005). Universal newborn screening for permanent childhood hearing impairment: an 8-year follow up of a controlled trial. *The Lancet*, **366**, 660–662.

National Institute for Health and Care Excellence (NICE) (2008). *Otitis Media with Effusion in Under 12s: Surgery*. CG60. London: NICE. [Reviewed in 2014 and considered no new evidence requiring updating.] Available at: https://www.nice.org.uk/guidance/cg60/resources/otitis-media-with-effusion-in-under-12s-surgery-pdf-975561238213 [Accessed 25 Sep. 2017].

Pimperton, H. and Kennedy, C.R. (2012). The impact of early identification of permanent childhood hearing impairment on speech and language outcomes. *Archives of Disease in Childhood*, **97**, 648–653.

Public Health England (2017a). NHS screening programmes: KPI reports and briefings 2016 to 2017. [online] Available at: https://www.gov.uk/government/publications/nhs-screening-programmes-kpi-reports-and-briefings-2016-to-2017 [Accessed 25 Sep. 2017].

Public Health England (2017b). NHS screening programmes in England: 2015 to 2016. [online] Available at: https://www.gov.uk/government/publications/nhs-screening-programmes-annual-report [Accessed 25 Sep. 2017].

Silva, P.A. (1982). Some developmental and behavioral problems associated with bilateral otitis media with effusion. *Journal of Learning Disabilities*, **15**, 417–421.

Silva, P.A. (1986). Some audiological, psychological, educational and behavioral characteristics of children with bilateral otitis media with effusion: a longitudinal study. *Journal of Learning Disabilities*, **19**, 165–169.

Sininger, Y.S. (2002). Identification of auditory neuropathy in infants and children. *Seminars in Hearing*, **23**, 193–200.

Sininger, Y.S., Martinez, A., Eisenberg, L., et al. (2009). Newborn hearing screening speeds diagnosis and access to intervention by 20–25 months. *Journal of the American Academy of Audiology*, **20**, 49–57.

Stevens, J.C., Webb, H.D., Hutchinson, J., Connell, J., Smith, M.F., and Buffin, J.T. (1989). Click evoked otoacoustic emissions compared with brain stem electric response. *Archives of Disease in Childhood*, **64**, 1105–1111.

Therrell, B.L., Padilla, C.D., Loeber, J.G., et al. (2015). Current status of newborn screening worldwide: 2015. *Seminars in Perinatology*, **39**, 171–187.

van der Ploeg, C.P., Lanting, C.I., Kauffman-de Boer, M.A., Uilenburg, N.N., de Ridder-Sluiter, J.G., and Verkerk, P.H. (2008). Examination of long-lasting parental concern after false-positive results of neonatal hearing screening. *Archives of Disease in Childhood*, **93**, 508–511.

Vernooij-van Langen, A.M.M., van der Pal, S.M., Reijntjens, A.J.T., Loeber, J.G., Dompeling, E., and Dankert-Roelse, J.E. (2014). Parental knowledge reduces long term anxiety induced by false-positive test results after newborn screening for cystic fibrosis. *Molecular Genetics and Metabolism Reports*, **1**, 334–344.

Watkin, P.M. (1991). The age of identification of childhood deafness – improvements since the 1970s. *Public Health*, **105**, 303–312.

Watkin, P.M., Baldwin, M., and Laoide, S. (1990). Parental suspicion and identification of hearing impairment. *Archives of Disease in Childhood*, **65**, 846–850.

Weichbold, V., Nekahm-Heis, D., and Welzl-Mueller, K. (2006). Ten-year outcome of newborn hearing screening in Austria. *International Journal of Pediatric Otorhinolaryngology*, **70**, 235–240.

Wessex Universal Hearing Screening Trial Group (1998). Controlled trial of universal neonatal screening for early identification of permanent childhood hearing impairment. *The Lancet*, **352**, 1957–1964.

Yoshinaga-Itano, C., Sedey, A.L., Coulter, D.K., and **Mehl, A.L.** (1998). Language of early- and later-identified children with hearing loss. *Pediatrics*, **102**, 1161–1167.

Zielhuis, G.A., Rach, G.H., van den Bosch, A., and **van ben Broek, P.** (1990). The prevalence of otitis media with effusion: a critical review of the literature. *Clinical Otolaryngology*, **15**, 283–288.

Chapter 21

Identification of visual impairments

Ameenat Lola Solebo

Summary

This chapter:

◆ describes how vision develops during childhood, and the measures used to quantify vision in children

◆ describes the common causes of childhood visual defects

◆ summarizes the evidence which underpins the UK's childhood eye and visual disease prevention programmes (neonatal and infant eye examination, and vision screening in 4–5-year-olds).

Introduction

Childhood visual defects can affect one or both eyes, and can range from mild to disabling. While severe impairment of the primary visual function, acuity, can have a significant impact on the affected child's developmental, educational, and socio-economic experiences, there is currently an absence of evidence on the impact of mildly impaired vison, or the impact of defects in the 'secondary' visual functions—colour vision, contrast perception, stereopsis or depth perception, and the higher visual processes (e.g. perception of motion, and object or environment mapping) (Rahi et al., 2009; Solebo et al., 2015).

The visual functions, particularly acuity, rapidly mature during the first few years of life as the anatomy and circuitry of the neural pathways develop (Salomao and Ventura, 1995). There is a sensitive developmental period in early childhood, during which the visual system must be presented with a clear image to enable the child to fulfil their visual potential. Any disorder which affects the presentation of a good image can lead to delayed or abnormal development of the visual system (amblyopia), which is reversible if treatment is undertaken during the window of sensitivity (Lewis and Maurer, 2005). Prevention of permanent amblyopia is therefore dependent on prompt management of the causative disorder, which is the central concern of the management of childhood ophthalmic disease. Many of the blinding diseases, for example, cataract, retinopathy of prematurity, and glaucoma, are treatable if diagnosed promptly. Early detection of visual defects is important for other reasons:

◆ Many ocular disorders have widespread and/or genetic implications. The majority of children with severe visual impairment have multisystem disorders or other impairments (Rahi and Cable, 2003). Early detection enables early diagnosis and management of these disorders.

◆ Childhood visual defects can be the presenting feature of serious systemic disease in the absence of ocular disorders, for example, sudden-onset squint or progressive visual loss may indicate cerebral disease (Rahi and Cable, 2003).

◆ Developmental guidance and early educational advice by specialist teachers for children with visual impairment may reduce the incidence of secondary disabilities such as behavioural problems (Keil et al., 2017).

◆ Many life-threatening childhood visual disorders, for example, retinoblastoma, are treatable if detected early (Rahi and Cable, 2003).

Visual functions in childhood

Acuity

Acuity, the most important visual function, is the ability to discriminate spatial detail and the function which determines the classification of visual impairment as mild, moderate, or severe (Box 21.1), The metric most commonly used within paediatric ophthalmology is the *log*arithm of the *m*inimum *a*ngle of *r*esolution or logMAR. The standardization of logMAR charts, and the logarithmic progression of symbol size within each chart (unlike that of the charts which use the Snellen system) allows for robust comparisons over time as children's vision develops. On the logMAR scale, vision of 0.0 is equivalent to the historical Snellen score of 6/6, that is, ability to discriminate at a distance of 6 metres (m) what the 'normal' individual is able to see at a distance of 6 m. Vision of 1.0 logMAR is equivalent to Snellen 6/60 (needing to be no more than 6 m away to discriminate what the 'normal' individual can see at a distance of 60 m)

Assessing acuity in childhood

Visual acuity rapidly improves in the first 2 years. Newborns have an average acuity of approximately 1.5 logMAR, which improves to 1.0 logMAR at 1 month old, and then an average acuity of 0.5 logMAR by 12 months of age, and 0.35 logMAR by 24 months of age. At 5 years old, children can be expected to have adult levels of resolution (0.0— 0.1 logMAR) (Salomoa, 1995). Alongside this development in acuity comes maturity of motor skills and cognition. The tools used to asses a child's vision are therefore dependent on the child's developmental status.

A normally sighted neonate will have a central, steady gaze which she can maintain for brief periods (abbreviated to CSM), but she will have limited ability to perceive fine detail. Over the first days of life, children develop first the ability to fix their gaze on visual stimuli and then to pursue moving stimuli ('fix and follow' vision). Achievement

Box 21.1 Classifying visual defects: UK taxonomy of sight impairment

Severe sight impairment (blind):

- BACV worse than 3/60 with a full visual field.
- BACV between 3/60 and 6/60 with a severe reduction of field.
- BACV of 6/60 or above with a very reduced field of vision.

Sight impairment (partial sight)

- BACV between 3/60 and 6/60 with a full visual field.
- BACV up to 6/24 with moderate reduction of field.
- BACV of 6/18 or above with a very reduced field of vision.

Best Achievable Corrected Vision (BACV) = vision with both eyes open or in better seeing eye, with correction for refractive error, for example, glasses for short- or long-sightedness.

All other visual defects (e.g. defective colour vision or higher perceptual defects) which are not accompanied by impaired acuity or restricted visual field are not classified as sight or visual impairment.

There is a similar World Health Organization (2006) classification.

Source: data from Department of Health, *Certificate of Vision Impairment: Explanatory Motes for Consultant Ophthalmologists and Hospital Eye Clinic Staff in England,* © Crown Copyright 2007, available from https://www.gov.uk/government/uploads/system/uploads/attachment_data/file/637590/CVI_guidance.pdf. Contains public sector information licensed under the Open Government Licence v3.0.

of CSM gaze and 'fix and follow' visual responses are therefore useful in the qualitative assessment of neonatal acuity.

Beyond the neonatal period, acuity in preverbal or non-verbal children is quantified using high-contrast (black and white) gratings of differing width, or optotypes (shapes or symbols). The preferential gaze pattern of children for 'interesting' visual stimuli versus blank space can be used to determine resolution of the presented image. Verbal children can be asked to resolve and recognize images on optotype charts. A more qualitative measurement of vision is useful when vision is too poor for such assessment, with children described as having perception up to the level of 'counting fingers', 'hand movements perception', or 'perception of light'.

Other signs may be useful to determine the presence of a significant impairment of visual acuity (Lambert and Lyons, 2016):

- The absence of vision-directed behaviour—such as smiling in response to silent parental smiles.
- A strong and prolonged objection to occlusion of one eye over another in pre- or non-verbal children may indicate unilaterally poor vision.
- Strabismus (or squint, with deviation of the poorer seeing eye), is an associated finding in individuals with unilaterally or bilaterally poor vision.

- Nystagmus (constant or cyclical involuntary movements of the eyes) is an associated finding in bilaterally poor vision (but may also occur in those with neurological disease and retained visual acuity).

- 'Roving' eye movements (purposeless, irregular intermittent movements in all directions) may be an indicator of profoundly poor vision.

Electrodiagnostic procedures (only available in a limited number of tertiary centres) may be used to determine retinal function (electroretinogram) and visual pathway potential (visual evoked potentials). While visual electrophysiology can detect, and to some extent quantify, structural and functional abnormalities, it is not yet capable of determining a child's acuity level (Lambert and Lyons, 2016).

The visual field is the sensitivity (or resolution) within the total area of space perceived when the eyes and head are stationary. As such, it is a measure of acuity outside the central area of fixation. Detailed assessment of the sensitivity within different areas of the field requires an individual to keep their eyes stationary for a reasonable duration, and can therefore only be undertaken in a child who has reached a developmental stage which permits compliance with complex instructions. Gross defects of visual field can be indicated by absence of response to visual stimuli silently presented to infants and young children by a second examiner while the first examiner holds the child's attention centrally (Lambert and Lyons, 2016). See Box 21.2.

Box 21.2 Refractive status and strabismus

Refractive state: the optical system of the eye is designed to produce a focused image on the retina. The eye that does this perfectly without refractive correction is known as emmetropic. Few eyes have a perfect optical system, and so most people have some refractive error—ametropia.

Common refractive errors:

- Hypermetropia (long sight), which, if significant, blurs both distance and near vision. The refractive state of the eye changes throughout life, concomitant with eye growth, but particularly in infancy and childhood. Accordingly, hypermetropia is frequent and physiological until at least the age of around 4 years.

- Myopia (short sight) in which distance vision is blurred. This is uncommon in early childhood, but is increasingly common in adolescence.

- Astigmatism, in which there are different degrees of refractive error within an individual eye as measured at separate axes.

- Anisometropia, in which the refraction is significantly different between the two eyes.

Strabismus (squint) is a deviation of the eyes. It can be apparent at the time of examination (manifest squint), or may be detected only when the two eyes are dissociated by testing (latent squint). Latent squints may become manifest under conditions of stress, fatigue, or illness. The prevalence of manifest squint in childhood is between 2% and 5%.

Source: data from Scott R Lambert and Christopher J Lyons, *Taylor and Hoyt's Pediatric Ophthalmology and Strabismus*, Fifth Edition, Elsevier, Copyright © 2016.

Assessing the secondary visual functions in childhood

Quantification of depth perception and the ability to discriminate hue (colour vision) and contrast can be undertaken with specialized charts. These tests require matching or sorting skills, and are not appropriate for children who are unable to comply because of young age, or motor or cognitive impairments. Recently, several tools have been developed to quantify and categorize higher perceptual defects in children, by assessing defects in the detection of movement; the perceptual pathway or ventral visual stream (recognition of objects, people, or orientation), and the action pathway or dorsal visual stream (visual guidance through three-dimensional space) (Good, 2009). There is as yet no consensus on the diagnosis or classification of the higher visual defects.

Summary of the classification of visual impairment and description of some associated findings

Assessment of visual ability or potential in childhood is dependent on the child's development status. Acuity, the most important visual function, can be assessed using qualitative and quantitative methods, and there are other indicators of poor vision in early childhood. Defects in the secondary visual functions are not classified as sight or vision impairment in the presence of retained acuity or visual field. Uniocularly reduced vision is not classified as sight or vision impairment if acuity in the better seeing eye is good.

Causes of visual defects

In the UK, as in other industrialized higher-income countries, the most common causes of childhood severe visual impairment or blindness are cerebral visual impairment and optic nerve disorders (Rahi and Cable, 2003). The most common *treatable* causes are cataract, glaucoma, and retinopathy of prematurity (see Box 21.3).

In the UK, the most common childhood cause of unilaterally poor vision in childhood is amblyopia, which affects between 2% and 4% of children (Cumberland et al., 2010).

Amblyopia

Amblyopia is abnormal development of visual pathways secondary to the failure to present a clear image to the immature pathway during the sensitive developmental window. If the image is not restored prior to the closure of this window, vision will be permanently poor. The image can be affected by the eye's refractive state, the presence of strabismus, or any disorder which disturbs the clarity of the image (e.g. cataract).

Although unilaterally poor vision due to amblyopia is not associated with any impact on general health, socioeconomic, or developmental outcomes (Rahi et al., 2009), it significantly increases the chance of subsequent visual impairment through loss of vision in the non-amblyopic eye. Amblyopes have a two to three times higher lifetime risk of visual impairment when compared to non-amblyopes (Rahi et al., 2002).

There are two phases in the management of amblyopia. First, any obstacle to clear vision (e.g. cataract) is removed and the eye is presented with a focused image by

Box 21.3 Epidemiology of severe visual impairment and blindness in the UK

- The annual incidence of childhood severe visual impairment or blindness (SVI/BL) is 5–6 per 10,000 (children aged under 16 years).

- 77% of SVI/BL children have additional non-ophthalmic disorders or impairments.

- Four of every six affected children will have presented with SVI/BL by their first birthday.

- Almost half will have SVI/BL either wholly or partly due to cerebral visual pathway disorders.

- Low birthweight is a significant risk factor for severe visual impairment, particularly where due to cerebral causes.

- Almost 30% of affected children will have optic nerve disorders.

- Almost 30% will have retinal disorders. Just under half of these children will have inherited retinal dystrophies.

- 10% of affected children will die in the first year following diagnosis of SVI/BL.

There is limited data on the epidemiology of mild or moderate childhood visual impairment in the UK

the correction of any refractive error, usually by spectacles. This is followed by occlusion with patching of the better seeing eye, or penalization with the use of an eyedrop (typically atropine) which defocuses vision in the better eye. Several randomized controlled trials have now demonstrated the benefit of refractive, occlusive, and penalizing therapies for amblyopia (Solebo et al., 2015).

One UK trial reported that following treatment for amblyopia, 4% of children in the treatment group had vision worse than 0.3 logMAR versus 27% in the control group (Clarke et al., 2003). Another two trials reported more modest but significant benefits, with occlusion therapy leading to an average improvement in vision of 0.1 logMAR ('one line of vision') (Taylor et al., 2012; Taylor and Elliott., 2014). In all trials, children with worse amblyopia displayed the greatest response to treatment (Solebo et al., 2015).

There is also evidence that, overall, treatment undertaken before 4 years of age does not confer significantly better vision than treatment started between 4 and 6 years (Solebo et al., 2015). However, a delay in treatment for children over 5 years old may lead to worse outcomes for children with worse amblyopia (Clarke et al., 2003). It is these children who have the greater lifetime risk of disabling bilateral visual impairment should visual loss occur later in the better eye.

There has been some interest in the prevention of amblyopia by detection and treatment in infancy of refractive error and strabismus (squint). However, the natural history of amblyopia and its relationship with these potentially amblyogenic factors is unclear, and currently, neither amblyopia nor strabismus can be reliably predicted or prevented (Solebo et al., 2015).

Vision and eye screening programmes

Two whole-population childhood eye and vision screening programmes are currently recommended by Public Health England (2016, 2017). The aim of these programmes is to prevent preventable blindness due to childhood disorders, thus reducing the burden to the individual and society.

Neonatal and infant examination

As part of the newborn and infant physical examination programme, it is recommended that all children undergo eye examinations in the first day of life, and again at the 6–8-week examination (Public Health England, 2016).

Test

This comprises careful inspection of the eyes and examination for the red reflex. Fundoscopy is not expected, but the ophthalmoscope may be used, focused on infinity from a distance of 20–30 cm (8–12 inches), to detect cataract as an opacity or silhouette against the red reflex. The inspection and the examination should be repeated at 6–8 weeks. Urgent referral is mandatory if there is any suspicion of abnormality.

Target disorders

The target disorders for these tests are as follows:

◆ Cataract: although congenital and infantile cataract is an uncommon disorder, late diagnosis is a common and preventable cause of childhood blindness. Early diagnosis enables early surgical intervention (i.e. within the first 3 months of life), which is essential to prevent profoundly and irreversibly poor vision due to deprivational amblyopia.

◆ Congenital ocular malformations: although these disorders are typically not treatable, early detection allows prompt detection of associated systemic and developmental impairments, and allows early support for the child and family.

◆ Retinoblastoma: the most common ocular childhood cancer, affects 50–60 children in the UK each year. It typically presents after the infantile period; nevertheless, the newborn and infant physical examination eye exam is a vital opportunity to detect the tumour early in life.

Effectiveness of screening

There have been no direct investigations of the effectiveness of this programme. Indirect comparative evidence is provided by the pre-eminence of congenital and infantile cataract as a cause of childhood blindness in nations where early life whole-population screening is not undertaken.

Vision screening at 4–5 years of age

It is recommended that all children undergo testing of acuity in each eye on school entry (i.e. at the age of 4–5 years) (Public Health England, 2016). This recommendation is supported by a recent systematic review of the evidence commissioned by the UK National Screening Committee (Solebo et al., 2015).

Target disorders

As children with bilaterally poor vision will largely present either in the first year of life, in the context of an associated systemic disorder, or following family or health carer detection of poor vision, the target disorder for screening is children with unilaterally poor vision. The majority of these children will have amblyopia.

Test

Each eye should be tested separately with a crowded (lines of letters/shapes rather than a single letter/shape on each line) logMAR chart. Children should be asked to wear any prescribed correction, and to either name images or indicate a match on a separate test card. Several crowded logMAR charts are in use in clinical practice:

- ETDRS (Early Treatment Diabetic Retinopathy Study) charts, which present letter optotypes in linear arrangements. ETDRS charts were designed for use in adults and they are the gold standard measure of visual acuity in adults and in older children (those older than 6 years). There is some limited evidence that these charts underestimate acuity in younger children (Solebo et al., 2015; Anstice et al., 2017; U.S. Preventive Services Task Force, 2017).

- Kay charts, in which separate lines of picture optotypes are presented. Kay pictures are more designed to be recognizable 'real-life' images (cat, duck, windowed house) providing a recognition-based acuity measurement, rather than a pure test of resolution ability. Kay picture cards have consistently been shown to overestimate acuity in preschool children (Anstice et al., 2017).

- Lea charts/cards, in which linear arrangements or separate cards with symbol optotypes are presented. Unlike Kay pictures, all Lea optotypes exhibit internal vertical symmetry (i.e. symbols such as 'H' and 'A' rather than 'R') and standardization of stroke size. There is some limited evidence that internal symmetry aids recognition acuity, resulting in overestimation of acuity (Anstice et al., 2017).

- HOTV charts, in which separate lines of letters or picture optotypes are presented. HOTV optotypes also exhibit internal vertical symmetry and stroke size standardization. The Lea and HOTV charts have been shown to have good levels of agreement, and there is a large body of evidence on reliability within the normal population. Both are recommended by the United States Prevention Service Task Force as the most appropriate tests for vision screening in children aged under 5 years (Solebo et al., 2015; Anstice et al., 2017; U.S. Preventive Services Task Force 2017).

♦ Crowded Keeler cards, in which separate lines of letters or picture optotypes are presented. Keeler card optotypes do not exhibit internal vertical symmetry, but do have standardized stroke sizes. Keeler cards were used to determine acuity in the UK randomized controlled trials on the impact of amblyopia treatment, and are the most commonly used acuity chart within published studies on the management of amblyopia (Taylor et al., 2012; Taylor and Elliott, 2014). They are the acuity test recommended by the British and Irish Orthoptic Society for screening in children aged 4–5 years. However, there is no robust evidence on the comparable precision of the different crowded logMAR tests (Keeler, Lea, and HOTV) available for testing for reduced vision in children aged 4–5 years.

Mean visual acuity at 4–5 years old is between 0.08 and −0.075 using crowded logMAR testing (Solebo et al., 2015; Anstice et al., 2017; U.S. Preventive Services Task Force, 2017). It is difficult to determine a 'cut-off' level of vision to define significantly reduced vision for amblyopia. However, since adult vision of worse than 0.2 is classified as mild impairment, and also in the UK precludes driving, children with vision worse than 0.2 logMAR in either eye on the screening test should be referred for further ophthalmological assessment.

All children who 'fail' screening or who cannot be screened should undergo cycloplegic refraction (a test to determine refractive status), orthoptic assessment (to establish the presence of strabismus), and dilated fundoscopy (examination of ocular media and retinal/optic nerve health).

Effectiveness of screening

Due to a lack of data collection and audit, there is, as yet, no evidence of the effectiveness of the programme in England; however, there is reason to believe it may be so (Solebo et al., 2015).

Opportunistic detection

Primary healthcare team staff should be familiar with the visual development of the normal baby, and should be alert to the various symptoms and signs which first warn parents that there may be a visual defect (e.g. abnormal appearance of the eyes, roving eye movements, poor fixation, and visual following).

Parents should be directed towards the age-related check lists in the Personal Child Health Record, some of which indicate problems with visual function (Healthforallchildren.com, 2017). For example, they can be asked if the baby looks at the parents, follows moving objects with the eyes, and fixates on small objects.

Every parent with concerns about their child's vision should be able to enter a planned referral pathway from first suspicion to diagnosis and management. In the case of concerns about possible serious visual impairment, the referral process should bypass routine waiting lists. Since many causes of visual impairment are part of a multisystem disorder, the referral and assessment process is likely to involve a developmental paediatric clinic working with an ophthalmologist and the eye care team. Management should take account of good practice guidance, for example, the Royal

National Institute of Blind People (RNIB) report 'Taking the time: telling parents their child is blind or partially sighted' (Cole-Hamilton, 1996).

In other circumstances, children can be seen by community optometrists. The following recommendations are targeted at children at particular risk of eye and vision problems.

Retinopathy of prematurity

Babies with a birth weight of less than 1500 g, or born at less than 32 weeks gestation age, should be screened for retinopathy of prematurity, according to current recommendations (Royal College of Ophthalmologists, 2017). The increased risk of other eye problems including myopia, squint, and cerebral visual impairment should also be remembered, and parents should be advised to seek medical attention should they have concerns.

Family history

Parents should be asked if there is a family history of visual disorders. Children at risk of having a genetically determined disabling visual disorder should be examined with extra care, preferably by an ophthalmologist. This is important, even if the usual age of presentation is much later.

Children with other impairments

Approximately 40% of children with sensorineural hearing impairments have eye problems, some very severe (Armitage et al., 1995). All children with sensorineural hearing problems should undergo a specialist eye examination.

All children with dysmorphic syndromes or neurodevelopmental problems should undergo a specialist eye examination as some may have serious defects of vision.

Colour vision defects

Colour vision defects have not been found to affect educational attainment or occupational choice (Cumberland et al., 2004). Whole-population screening for colour vision defects cannot currently be justified.

Children found to have a colour vision defect should be told that they have a difficulty in discriminating colours which may be important with regard to certain career choices. In cases where such a defect could have important career implications, expert advice should be obtained from an optometrist, an ophthalmologist, a special clinic, or a careers adviser.

Vision and 'dyslexia'

There has been much interest in the relationship between visual deficits, such as eye movement disorders and delay in establishment of dominance, and dyslexia or reading problems (Stein, 2014). There is no dispute that any child with reading or other learning problems needs a vision assessment, but this should be in the context of a specialized development programme, rather than a screening programme.

Learning links

- Certificate of Vision Impairment Explanatory Notes for Consultant Ophthalmologists and Hospital Eye Clinic Staff in England: https://www.gov.uk/government/uploads/system/uploads/attachment_data/file/637590/CVI_guidance.pdf
- Resources can be found at Gov.uk with information on child vision screening: https://www.gov.uk/government/publications/child-vision-screening
- The RNIB is also a good resource with a webpage on children's eye conditions: https://www.rnib.org.uk/sites/default/files/Childrens eye conditions.pdf.

Recommendations

- Examination of all babies' eyes for the red reflex should take place in the newborn examination. (*Evidence: strong.*)
- Assess visual acuity in all 4–5-year-olds as recommended by the UK National Screening Committee. (*Evidence: strong.*)
- Use evidence-based tests as part of the 4–5-year-old screening programme. (*Evidence: strong.*)
- Alert parents to the signs of visual dysfunction, per the Personal Child Health Record. (*Good practice.*)
- Carry out specialist eye examinations at appropriate intervals in high-risk groups. (*Evidence: strong.*)

References

Anstice, N., Jacobs, R.J., Simkin, S.K., et al. (2017). Do picture-based charts overestimate visual acuity? Comparison of Kay Pictures, Lea Symbols, HOTV and Keeler logMAR charts with Sloan letters in adults and children. *PLoS One*, **12**, e0170839.

Armitage, I.M., Burke, J.P., and Buffin, J.T. (1995). Visual impairment in severe and profound sensorineural deafness. *Archives of Disease in Childhood*, **73**, 53–56.

Clarke, M.P., Wright, C.M., Hrisos, S., Anderson, J.D., Henderson, J., and Richardson, S.R. (2003). Randomised controlled trial of treatment of unilateral visual impairment detected at preschool vision screening. *BMJ*, **327**, 1251.

Cole-Hamilton, I. (1996). *Taking the Time: Telling Parents their Child is Blind or Partially Sighted*. London: RNIB.

Cumberland, P., Pathai, S., and Rahi, J. (2010). Prevalence of eye disease in early childhood and associated factors: findings from the Millennium cohort study. *Ophthalmology*, **117**, 2184–2190.

Cumberland, P., Rahi, J.S., and Peckham, C.S. (2004). Impact of congenital colour vision deficiency on education and unintentional injuries: findings from the 1958 British birth cohort. *BMJ*, **329**, 1074–1075.

Good, W.V. (2009). Cortical visual impairment: new directions. *Optomotry and Vision Science*, **86**, 663–665.

Healthforallchildren.com. (2017). PCHR download. [online] Available at: http://www. healthforallchildren.com/the-pchr/2079-2/ [Accessed 25 Sep. 2017].

Keil, S., Fielder, A., and Sargent, J. (2017). Management of children and young people with vision impairment: diagnosis, developmental challenges and outcomes. *Archives of Disease in Childhood*, **102**, 566–571.

Lambert, S.R. and Lyons, C.J. (Eds.) (2016). *Taylor and Hoyt's Pediatric Ophthalmology and Strabismus* (5th edn.). Philadelphia, PA: Elsevier.

Lewis, T.L. and Maurer, D. (2005). Multiple sensitive periods in human visual development: evidence from visually deprived children. *Developmental Psychobiology*, **46**, 163–183.

Public Health England (2016). Newborn and infant physical examination: programme handbook. [online] (Last updated April 2018). Available at: https://www.gov.uk/government/ publications/newborn-and-infant-physical-examination-programme-handbook.

Public Health England (2017). Child vision screening. [online] (Last updated Jan. 2018). Available at: https://www.gov.uk/government/publications/child-vision-screening.

Rahi, J. and Cable, N. (2003). Severe visual impairment and blindness in children in the UK. *The Lancet*, **362**, 1359–1365.

Rahi, J., Cumberland, P., and Peckham, C. (2009). Visual function in working-age adults: early life influences and associations with health and social outcomes. *Ophthalmology*, **10**, 1866–1871.

Rahi, J., Logan, S., Timms, C., et al. (2002). Risk, causes, and outcomes of visual impairment after loss of vision in the non-amblyopic eye: a population-based study. *The Lancet*, **360**, 597–602.

Royal College of Ophthalmologists (2017). Clinical guidelines. [online] Available at: https://www. rcophth.ac.uk/standards-publications-research/clinical-guidelines/ [Accessed 25 Sep. 2017].

Salomao, S.R. and Ventura, D.F. (1995). Large sample population age norms for visual acuities obtained with Vistech-Teller Acuity Cards. *Investigative Ophthalmology and Visual Science*, **36**, 657–670.

Solebo, A.L., Cumberland, P.M., and Rahi, J.S. (2015). Whole-population vision screening in children aged 4-5 years to detect amblyopia. *The Lancet*, **385**, 2308–2319.

Stein, J. (2014). Dyslexia: the role of vision and visual attention. *Current Developmental Disorders Reports*, **1**, 267–280.

Taylor, K. and Elliott, S. (2014). Interventions for strabismic amblyopia. *Cochrane Database of Systematic Reviews*, **7**, CD006461.

Taylor, K., Powell, C., Hatt, S.R., and Stewart, C. (2012). Interventions for unilateral and bilateral refractive amblyopia. *Cochrane Database of Systematic Reviews*, **4**, CD005137.

U.S. Preventive Services Task Force (2017). Screening for visual impairment in children ages 1–5 years. [online] Available at: https://www.uspreventiveservicestaskforce.org/Page/Document/ RecommendationStatementFinal/vision-in-children-ages-6-months-to-5-years-screening#table2.

World Health Organization (2006). *International Statistical Classification of Diseases and Related Health Problems, Tenth Revision*. Geneva: World Health Organization Available at: http://apps.who.int/classifications/apps/icd/icd10online/.

Chapter 22

Developmental reviews and the identification of impairments/disorders

Philip Wilson and James Law

Summary

This chapter:

+ focuses on child development from the perspective of the primary care clinician, the health visitor, and the general practitioner

+ discusses the importance of social background and family perceptions of child development

+ considers that many developmental problems are on continua which border on typical development, but also overlap and interact with one another.

The target populations

In this chapter, we review early child development and the identification of children with 'impairments' or 'disorders', that is, levels of difficulty that are thought to warrant targeted or specialist intervention. By 'child development' we mean speech, language, and communication; socio-emotional development and behaviour; fine motor skills; and self-regulation or executive function. We shall use 'neurodevelopment' as a shorthand way to refer to these functions. These skills develop incrementally and, while they continue to become more sophisticated throughout childhood, it is possible to assume a level of mastery in most children by the time they reach school. It also may be possible to identify those children that are not likely to reach this mastery earlier on in their development and to intervene to improve those skills. Underpinning this argument is an assumption that, while all children are programmed to acquire skills, environmental factors may affect how rapidly they are acquired.

The skills are often represented in terms of developmental milestones and those falling outside the range achieved by typically developing children may represent a problem to be addressed by the healthcare and educational systems (Sharma and Cockerill, 2007). In some cases (e.g. with language development), it is assumed that there are sensitive periods or windows of developmental opportunity for the promotion of these skills and that it becomes less easy to modify these skills once the window in question is deemed to have closed (Bailey et al., 2001; West and Williams, 2011). For most practitioners, early identification is seen to be a goal, although there remains a question as to whether 'early' in this context simply means 'young' or at a pre-symptomatic stage at any point in a child's development.

Services should cover the whole population, not just a subsample who routinely make use of services. An audit of over 80,000 children in Scotland (Wood et al., 2012) concluded that although the proportion of parents attending such reviews fell from 99% for the 10-day review to 86% for the 39–42-month reviews, the drop was associated disproportionately with social disadvantage leading the authors to conclude that 'The inverse care law continues to operate in relation to "universal" child health reviews'. It is important that any system of child development reviews must include mechanisms for ensuring equity of provision and commissioners of services should produce statistics on uptake of reviews across all demographic groups on a routine basis.

The perspective in the remainder of this chapter will be that of the primary care clinician—the general practitioner (GP), the health visitor, and their respective teams. The underlying assumption in most primary care developmental reviews is that of normality: definitive diagnostic formulations are more likely to be made in secondary care where the assumption is that some pathology will be identified. The role of the primary care clinician in developmental assessments will, in general, be to differentiate typical and atypical development. There may also be a need to differentiate between general and specific problems when referral to other agencies (audiology, speech and language therapy, physiotherapy, etc.) is being considered, but our focus in this chapter is less on 'diagnosable' conditions than on atypical development. The role of diagnosis will be discussed in more detail below but it is important to bear in mind that the interpretation of examination findings and tests may differ in primary care and secondary care (Mathers and Hodgkin, 1989).

Child development surveillance: an international perspective

Programmes of preventive child healthcare vary enormously between countries and regions. National policies are not necessarily closely reflected in the preventive care that is delivered in all areas, but in general, the national policy represents a minimum programme offered on a universal basis. Among high-income countries with state-funded health services, scheduled contacts with a component involving some assessment of neurodevelopment vary in number from three currently in Scotland to 14–18 in Sweden, Norway, and Denmark between birth and the age of 7 years. Some differences between countries reflect the organization and funding of healthcare: recommended surveillance programmes are substantially less likely to be taken up by poor families in purely private healthcare systems (Chung et al., 2006), but uptake of child health surveillance programmes varies even in countries where attendance is free of charge (Wood et al., 2012).

The wide international variation in child health surveillance policy suggests that the evidence base underlying these policies is generally relatively weak.

Which professionals should offer developmental assessments and what skills are needed?

In countries dominated by private healthcare provision, developmental reviews are generally offered by doctors (paediatricians or family doctors) responsible for children's primary healthcare. Elsewhere, delivery of reviews is usually nurse led or shared between doctors and nurses (Wood and Blair, 2014). Provision can be aligned to primary care and delivered to registered children within general practices (e.g. in parts of Canada), entirely separate to provision of primary medical care and delivered from stand-alone community clinics (e.g. Australia, Finland, Sweden, and Norway), or a mixed model (Denmark).

The professional background of individuals offering developmental assessments is less important than the set of skills that they have to offer. First and foremost, the clinician needs to have a good working knowledge of normal child development and its variations. While an in-depth knowledge of specific syndromes is not required, clinicians must be aware that identification of one potential developmental problem increases the risk of problems in other developmental domains (Gillberg, 2010; Sim et al., 2013)—so assessments need to be flexible rather than formulaic.

Finally, while it is tempting to focus on the accuracy of the assessments employed for the identification of difficulties, it is important to stress that the conversations between professional and parent or carer about a child's development should, if possible, be founded on an existing trusting relationship between the two parties. If the professional knows the family's circumstances, is familiar, for example, with the histories of other children in the family and has had regular discussions about the well-being of the child in question, it is much easier for them to share in the decision-making about what is best for the child. This issue is likely to be especially important where the professional and the parent do not share cultural expectations about child development. 'Culture influences every aspect of human development and is reflected in child rearing beliefs and practices designed to promote healthy adaptation' (Shonkoff and Phillips, 2000). It is also important to recognize that, with modern working practices, care may need to be taken to ensure that contacts and clinics are offered at a time which is acceptable to families.

Diagnosis and co-morbidity

Diagnostic categories are invaluable in communication with parents and professionals about the problem that a child may have and his or her prognosis, and are near essential in the construction of an evidence base for treatments through clinical trials. Furthermore, parents generally find diagnoses helpful. However, almost all neurodevelopmental problems lie on one continuum or another. Most diagnoses involve the creation of a more or less arbitrary threshold of severity: children above the threshold are given the diagnosis, and those below it are not. In some conditions this is generally understood: for example, a clinical diagnosis of intellectual disability (learning difficulties) requires an intelligence quotient (IQ) of less than 70, so a child with an IQ of 71 cannot have this diagnosis even though he or she may have significant problems with cognitive capacity. We routinely refer to 'autism spectrum disorders' but it is important to remember that one end of this diagnostic spectrum has a border with normality. It is less commonly acknowledged, but no less true, that other conditions such as attention deficit hyperactivity disorder (ADHD), language disorders, and conduct disorder are also characterized by continua.

Diagnoses can nevertheless have indirect value to families. At the most basic level, a diagnosis might be the key to obtaining financial benefits. In the UK, it has been the experience of many families that eligibility for Disability Living Allowance and access to charitable support is very difficult without a diagnosis. Furthermore, nurseries and schools may be more flexible in dealing with children and families where there is an easily understood label giving insight into the child's difficulties.

Diagnoses can also cause problems. Labelling a child with a neuropsychiatric condition such as autism or ADHD may lead to stigma and later difficulties in education and work. Many people with ADHD and autism have lamented the fact that others cannot 'see beyond the diagnosis'. Furthermore, diagnoses of conditions with a known genetic basis can have serious implications for the whole family, bringing real challenges in many cases to parents and the broader family (Board of American Society of Human Genetics Board and American College of Medical Genetics, 1995).

Diagnoses, by their nature, categorize and thus appear to simplify problems, but the challenges children face often do not always correspond in a simple way to their diagnosis. Each child will have his or her unique set of strengths and weaknesses. Most neurodevelopmental problems lie on continua, but they also overlap and manifestations may change over time. Gillberg (2010) makes the point that co-morbidity is the rule, rather than the exception in the field of neurodevelopment, and proposes that problems in general development, communication and language, social interrelatedness, motor coordination, attention, activity, behaviour, mood, and sleep should prompt a wide-ranging assessment of a child's abilities. For example, significant language delay at 30 months may greatly increase the chances that a child will have problems with attention, social communication, behaviour, motor function, and general intellectual ability (Miniscalco et al., 2006; Sim et al., 2013, 2015). Gillberg makes the valuable point that it is not good enough to 'wait and see' how developmental problems will unfold: around two-thirds of children with significant language delay at 30 months will manifest a range of significant associated neuropsychiatric problems as they grow older (Miniscalco et al., 2006; Sim et al., 2015) and many of these problems are likely to benefit from early intervention.

An additional difficulty posed by neurodevelopmental diagnoses relates to equity of service provision. The use of certain diagnoses (such as autism) varies according to the local services available as well as with demographic factors such as family income and rurality (Mandell et al., 2005). Historically, autism may have been more likely to be diagnosed among the children of wealthier families, while children in poorer families with similar difficulties may have been more likely to be categorized as having more generic intellectual disabilities (Wing, 1980). Perhaps most importantly, children who narrowly fail to meet diagnostic criteria for several conditions can be at least as disabled as children with a diagnosis: it can be very difficult to get services to support children without a diagnosis.

Screening, thresholds, and risk

To date, no neurodevelopmental assessment beyond the neonatal period has been generally acknowledged to meet the World Health Organization/Wilson and Jungner criteria (Wilson and Jungner, 1968) for screening programmes. Screening approaches have been examined in relation to autism (Fernell et al., 2014), language disorders (Law et al., 1998), and conduct disorder (Wilson et al., 2009), but key criteria have not been met: in particular, the requirements for a sensitive and specific screening test, for cost-effectiveness, and for evidence that early intervention produces better outcomes than waiting until problems manifest themselves before intervening. This lack of evidence for early intervention may appear counterintuitive in the context of knowledge that brain plasticity and thus potential gains are greater in younger children.

In general, neurodevelopmental screening has failed to meet the World Health Organization screening criteria because of lack of evidence of effectiveness, rather than evidence of lack of effectiveness. While it is possible to evaluate how well a screening test functions in a relatively small constrained population, it is much more difficult to carry out gold standard tests in large populations and it can also be challenging to follow up large groups of children to establish the productivity of a screening procedure over time. Such a trial would need to recruit pre-symptomatic children, identify those at high risk of a disorder (thus using a reliable screening tool), offer an intervention that is very likely to be effective, and then follow up intervention and control groups for several years in order to establish cost-effectiveness (Fernell et al., 2014). Trials using this design are extremely costly and are likely to suffer from a variety of methodological challenges including 'contamination' of the control group due to raised awareness of the screening programme. There is nevertheless a need for trials such as these. One review which specifically sought to identify studies which had included screening procedures for children in the 0–4 years age range and interventions designed to improve the cognitive skills of the children identified only found two published papers presenting weak to moderate quality evidence that specifically addressed this issue, one from the US and one from the Netherlands (Warren et al., 2016).

One area where screening is recommended by some authors is universal screening for speech and language followed by appropriate targeted intervention. The problem is that there is still insufficient evidence to support the recommendation of screening (Law et al., 1998; Nelson et al., 2006; Kasper et al., 2011; Siu, 2015; Wallace et al., 2015). There are a number of reasons for this including the variability of the gold standard measures against which screening tests are evaluated, the tendency for such measures to both under-refer (low sensitivity) and over-refer (low specificity), and the difficulty of establishing predictive validity when the trajectory of language development can be so variable especially in the early years—exactly when such measures are commonly recommended.

The most recent review of procedures for identifying developmental impairment (Warren et al., 2016) has adopted some of the strictest inclusion criteria and in doing so sought to answer the following questions:

♦ 'What is the effectiveness of screening children aged 1–4 years without suspected developmental delay to improve their outcomes?

- What is the optimal interval for screening for developmental delay?
- What is the incidence of harms resulting from screening children aged 1–4 years without suspected developmental delay?' (Warren et al., 2016).

Thus their questions go beyond more straightforward questions about whether a given screening test can be shown to 'work' in the sense that it has adequate productivity characteristics (specificity and sensitivity, positive and negative predictive values, etc.).

An alternative approach is to adopt a risk model where key markers of potential difficulties are added into the observations of the child and the report of the parent. 'Recent research emphasises the importance of these risks, strengthens the evidence for other risk factors including intrauterine growth restriction, malaria, lead exposure, HIV infection, maternal depression, institutionalisation, and exposure to societal violence, and identifies protective factors such as breastfeeding and maternal education' (Walker et al., 2011; see also Maggi et al., 2010; Marmot et al., 2010), to which it would be important to add the home learning environment and early book reading (Farrant and Zubrick, 2012). Very few studies have attempted to compare risk models with screening procedures but one which has compared a very early screening procedure with a series of risk factors predicting language development at 4 years suggested that a 'combined risk model' which identified a shortlist of the most powerfully predictive questions about social communication skills at 1 year plus, family characteristics, and parental behaviours, provided 'fair' levels of diagnostic accuracy (McKean et al., 2016). Recent approaches using novel techniques in life course epidemiology may improve the predictive value of early risk models (see, e.g. Caspi et al., 2016).

An alternative approach to developmental assessment uses the results to develop community resources, rather than to help individual children or families. The Early Development Instrument (Hertzman and Williams, 2009; Janus et al., 2016) has been used as a tool, with data on several developmental domains collected on an anonymized basis, to report on the prevalence of potentially remediable developmental problems within small geographical areas. There is some evidence that use of this tool (which is not suitable for clinical use) has led to useful local initiatives and policy changes, but, to date, there is relatively little clear evidence that these initiatives have improved developmental outcomes.

Timelines and life course considerations

One of the critical issues in routine developmental assessment is their timing. Superficially, it would seem to be best *as early as possible*, on the grounds that the environmental modifications necessary to promote optimal development can be started early. But, care has to be taken to distinguish between interventions that target an early point in the child's development and those that target an early stage in the diagnostic process. Either way, late intervention may be costly (Chowdry and Oppenheim, 2015).

While it appears uncontentious that, at the level of primary prevention we need to provide messages about how to promote children's development to all parents, consideration has to be given to the different views that parents have about their role in child rearing and the impact that this may have on a child's development (Miller, 1988; Rowe, 2008). When it comes to secondary prevention, the issue is made more complex by the fact that development is not clearly linear. Children whose skills appear to be underdeveloped at one point do not necessarily appear 'behind' later on. A good example of this can be seen with language delays seen in the development of 18,000 children aged between three and five years in the UK's Millennium Cohort Study (Law et al., 2012). In the cross-classification presentation (Table 22.1), we see the characteristic pattern of high specificity (0.95) and low sensitivity (0.53), where prevalence rates are relatively low, suggesting that the 3-year score was very good at determining who was not likely to have a subsequent difficulty but less accurate in predicting who was. Similar results (high negative predictive values and low positive predictive values for the screening test) were obtained for a combination of language and social, emotional, and behavioural outcomes in a population screened at 30 months (Sim et al., 2015). The key parameters of the process are the measures used, the age they are carried out at, and the outcome or 'gold standard' that we are trying to predict. While it is relatively simple to establish a measure of a specific outcome, such as fine motor skills, language, executive function, and so on, we have to ask whether it is this that we are trying to predict and thus which we are trying to prevent. This raises the question of whether it is the target domain or broader societal characteristics which need to be the focus. A good example of such a societal measure is *school readiness* although there are disagreements as to what this actually represents. Evidently preparing children so that they can cope in the classroom is important. Equally for many parents the key issues are not academic skills but well-being, happiness, and mental health (Roulstone et al., 2012), and the ability to live independent lives and to flourish in the workplace and elsewhere.

One area which has attracted considerable attention has been bilingualism or multilingualism and how this should be seen by those delivering services: half the world's population is functionally bilingual (Wölck, 1988). Bilingual children may, on average, perform more poorly in screening tests, but that does not mean that they necessarily have a 'problem' for which additional services are warranted (Peña et al., 2011). Nonetheless, it is true that many children learning English as an additional language in England are given the label of having 'Speech, Language, and Communication Needs', allowing extra resources to be allocated to meeting their needs (Meschi et al., 2012). A recent systematic review has nevertheless concluded that there was no evidence to suggest that, although the number of studies was relatively small, multilingualism is detrimental to linguistic or social development (Uljarevic et al., 2016).

What should developmental assessments include?

In the following sections, we identify the domains of child development that need to be checked. Key to this process is good observation skills and knowledge of child development. Specific measures to be used to identify problems in the different domains are described in more detail in the later section entitled 'What tools should be used for identifying children with neurodevelopmental difficulties?'

Table 22.1 An outline of what to expect of normal communication development and some potential areas of concern

Normal development			Potential areas of concern		
Speech	**Expression**	**Comprehension**	**Speech**	**Expression**	**Comprehension**
0–1 years					
Cooing after 6 weeks, babbling from 6 months, increasing feeling of child experimenting with sounds	Gradually begins to use specific sounds in specific contexts e.g. 'woof' for all animals	By 9 months understands 'no', 'bye'. By 1 year recognizes names of some objects and responds to simple requests, e.g. 'clap your hands' with a gesture	Very limited parental reaction to the child. Evidence of neuromuscular feeding difficulties. Little evidence of non-verbal communication from the child, e.g. referential pointing. No sounds	Little or no attempt to communicate	Little or no awareness of others
1–2 years					
Initially uses strings of intonation ('jargon') which clearly includes speech sounds. These gradually become assimilated into recognizable words	Words appear slowly at first but child often has a substantial vocabulary by 2 years. May be beginning to combine words by this stage	Almost always in advance of expression. Will hand over familiar objects on request. Begins to understand verbs and simple attributes	Very little intention to communicate on the part of the child Little variation in sounds used. No meaningful intonation	No words by 18 months	No recognition of the words for simple household objects
2–3 years					
A good range of sounds though may have difficulties with fricatives /f/sh/s/ etc.	2- and 3-word utterances. Language used for a variety of purposes—possession/assertion/refusal/attribution etc.	Able to find two or three objects on request	Single sounds only, e.g. /d/. Poor control of facial muscles. Others do not understand much of what is said	No word combinations reported by 2½. Very restricted vocabulary	Unable to find two items on request by 2½

(continued)

Table 22.1 Continued

Normal development			Potential areas of concern		
Speech	**Expression**	**Comprehension**	**Speech**	**Expression**	**Comprehension**
3–4 years					
Most speech sounds correct. May have difficulties with /ch/ or /j/. Intelligibility may decline when excited	Talks increasingly fluently. Able to refer to past and future events. Marks tense with -ed etc. but may be some confusion, e.g. 'I goed to the park'	Able to understand concepts such as colour/size etc. Will understand most of what a parent is saying	Very limited repertoire of sounds—much of what is said is unintelligible. Normal non-fluency, common in younger children may persist	Little feeling of interaction either because the child says very little or because the child continues to echo what is said. Restricted use of verbs/attributes	Comprehension outside everyday context very limited. May still not be aware of the function of objects
4–5 years					
Completely intelligible except for occasional errors	Grammatical errors may persist but rarely affect the meaning. 4–6 word sentences used consistently. Question forms, e.g. 'why?', now common. Is able to construct own stories	Can now understand abstract words, e.g. 'always'. Understands and can reconstruct a story sequence from a book	Much of what is said is still unintelligible. Pattern of stammering may be emerging—especially if beginning to 'block' on certain words/sounds. Increasing awareness and frustration	Child avoiding verbal demands, e.g. in nursery. Continues to respond in single words or using very simple grammatical structures. Little idea of tense. Cannot retell a story	May be able to understand enough to cope with familiar routines but cannot cope if structure changes. Child often isolated because cannot deal with the verbal level of peers

General points to look out for
Family history of speech or language difficulties.
Any history of hearing difficulties.
Concerns about parent/child interaction—your own or those of the parent.
Associated difficulties with behaviour or attention
IF IN DOUBT, ASK A SPEECH AND LANGUAGE THERAPIST

Reproduced from Law J and Harris F, *Promoting Language Development in Sure Start Areas*, DFES, Sure Start, Nottingham, UK, Copyright © 2001, with permission of the authors.

Speech and language disorders

There are a number of useful guides to early communication development and the reader is referred to the UK's 4Children (2015) guide 'What to expect, when?' (Foundationyears. org.uk, 2017), The Communication Trust's 'Universally Speaking' ages and stages from 0 to 5 years (https://www.thecommunicationtrust.org.uk/resources/resources/resources-for-practitioners/universally-speaking.aspx), and ICAN's ages and stages. (http://www.talkingpoint.org.uk/sites/talkingpoint.org.uk/files/stages-speech-language-development-chart001.pdf). Further details of the sequence of different aspects of speech and language (Law et al., 2017a) and other aspects of development (Law et al., 2017b) are summarized elsewhere.

In the first year of life, the infant should be turning to the human voice and to familiar sounds as soon as they have control over their trunk and neck. Obviously this is not a speech and language-related indicator as such but it does make it possible to identify children with severe hearing difficulties. By 6 months, the child should be engaging in active, social play and regularly using babble to indicate that engagement and to copy elements of what they hear. By this age some infants begin to show sensitivity to the meaning of common words (Bergelson and Swingley, 2012).

Vihman (1996) suggests the following sequence of acquisition of sounds, indicating the variability present in the age at which typically developing children reach each substage:

1. 2–4 months: cooing and laughter;

2. 4–7 months: onset of vocal play sounds (squeals, yells, growls). Some babies may start some very simple babbling;

3. 7+ months: start of 'canonical' babbling—strings of repeated syllables (ba-ba-ba, da-da-da) or mixture of syllables (ba-da-ga)' (Vihman, 1996).

A key point is reached when the child reaches 10–12 months when they start to point at objects outside their reach, often accompanied by a sound and in some cases the word itself (Liszkowski et al., 2012). The key issue here is exactly what the point signifies. Initially it is just an observation—'there's the toy'—but soon it becomes an interaction where the child looks at the object, then at the adult, and then perhaps back at the object in an excited way as if to say 'I know that you know what that is'. This is sometimes known as the proto-declarative point: the early stages of a shared reference, the first stages of symbolic communication. Another useful indicator is whether, or not, a child turns towards a person saying his or her name by 12 months (Nadig et al., 2007): failure to respond is highly suggestive of developmental abnormality (particularly autism) but does not identify all children at risk for developmental problems. Thus, this window is a key opportunity for making a professional contact with the child's caregiver, not just to identify children who may not be doing this but also to give parents advice on how they can promote their child's communication development.

The age range for children starting to use their first words varies considerably (Fenson et al., 1994) and there are plenty of examples in the literature of very young children appearing to use long and complicated words. There then follows a relatively long period as children acquire new words and the speed at which they do so varies considerably as does the pattern of acquisition. Some children appear to learn lots of nouns while others seem to start putting words together but don't appear to have such a large vocabulary. Although some studies have attempted to define a key number of words that children need to have by a certain age, in practice, late talking and limited vocabulary should not *in themselves* be used as a means of identifying children with difficulties although they indicate risk. It is important to be careful about asking parents about how many words that the child uses (Law and Roy, 2008). This may work as a question in the early stages of vocabulary development—perhaps up to 50 words—but it becomes meaningless after that point because parents cannot keep track of all the new words that the child is saying. We would be expecting children to start to put words together by 24–30 months of age and again this is a good time to be tapping into how well the child is doing and making suggestions for widening the child's experience and communicative opportunities. Failure to make two-word utterances or having a total vocabulary of fewer than around 20 words at 30 months is likely to indicate a substantial risk of a range of neurodevelopmental problems (Miniscalco et al., 2006; Sim et al., 2015).

Although the focus is commonly on what the child has said and how 'clear' the child's speech is, how much the child *understands* by what is said to them is equally important (Tomasello, 2009). But considerable care needs to be taken to avoid unconscious parental bias in reporting. For example, if asked 'Does she/he understand what you say?' the primary carer may answer this in the affirmative by 24–36 months. However, this may be a sign that the parent and child are just familiar with one another and rituals are well established. Thus a parent might say 'Well she understands when I say go and put your hat and coat on, we're going outside'. But this may simply be part of a familiar routine that she has been exposed to at regular intervals and she may be able to watch the parent doing exactly the same thing themselves.

By the age of 3 years, most children are combining words into short sentences and are starting to make up novel sentences that they would not have heard before, and in some cases new words. The key characteristics are the child's creativity and their interest in language and in wanting to communicate their ideas to others. By this age it is usually possible to assess the child's ability directly rather than relying on parental report. Thereafter, we see a steady increase in the child's language skills and for most children they become increasingly clear in this speech, so that family members and then others in their immediate environment, such as teachers, can now understand them. As they move into early years settings and nurseries they are exposed to a wide range of other speakers and have to learn to communicate effectively and to understand what others are saying. We also see them starting to develop what are sometimes termed *preliteracy* skills, for example, phonological awareness, as they start to identify letters and their corresponding sounds and to combine sounds together in sequence (Every Child Ready to Read, 2010). It is important to stress that the range of skills in children can vary considerably and it is often difficult to be clear that there is one age by which time children should have reached a given milestone on a specific skill. It is the pattern of skills which matters.

Autism spectrum disorders and other types of social communication difficulty

Language is only one form of social communication: a wide range of interactional behaviours can be observed in children at all ages. The best-known set of problems in social communication is the autism spectrum disorders. Many theories have been proposed to explain the development of autism (Coleman and Gillberg, 2011), but a lack of 'social instinct' described by Wing et al. (2011) is perhaps the description with most face validity and simplicity. Autism is commonly combined with other neurodevelopmental problems such as learning difficulties, language delay, epilepsy, motor stereotypies, and attention problems but when occurring alone it is most likely to manifest itself in lack of eye contact or other forms of social engagement. Parents will often first express concern to GPs or health visitors about their child's vision or hearing, or about distress caused by noise or touch. Recent evidence of long-term effectiveness of early intervention through promotion of parental social communication with children has strengthened the arguments for early identification of autism (Pickles et al., 2016).

Attachment problems

Attachment describes a pattern of social behaviours that develops over the first year of life, and which persists to a varying degree as an 'internal working model' of social relationship into adulthood (Bowlby, 1969). The normal development of separation anxiety and stranger anxiety crystallizes into a set of behaviours that can be observed reproducibly under situations of stress (Ainsworth et al., 1978). A securely attached preschool child will show mild and brief distress if separated from a familiar attachment figure such as a parent, but will rapidly return to explore the environment and play when the attachment figure returns. In addition, the securely attached child will show an appropriate degree of caution in the presence of a stranger, but this will be reduced when an attachment figure is present. In contrast, insecurely attached children will show a range of attachment patterns ranging from 'avoidant' (showing little signs of distress on separation or reunion with a familiar caregiver) to 'resistant' (showing distress on separation but ambivalence on reunion). A child with severe ('disorganized') attachment problems will show a range of abnormal behaviours, perhaps the most notable of which has been termed 'indiscriminate friendliness' (Chisholm, 1998). This marked loss of normal social inhibition exemplified by behaviours such as hugging a complete stranger can be seen in the consulting room in cases of severe emotional neglect (Wilson and Mullin, 2010). Indiscriminate friendliness is an adaptive behaviour in the context of extreme neglect or abuse, but it poses dangers to the child in other circumstances and as such should be taken seriously, including consideration of any current safeguarding needs.

Emotional disorders

A range of problems including anxiety, depression, and phobias might be raised by parents and carers during developmental reviews. Anxiety is a normal human emotional response which in most cases is developmentally normal and adaptive. Stranger anxiety and separation anxiety are near-universal phenomena in the first and second years of life, and these tend to reduce in intensity by the age of 2 years. Fear of the dark or of animals is also expressed by most children in the preschool years. Nevertheless, if anxieties or phobias appear to be extreme or persistent beyond the expected age at which they normally resolve, they should be taken seriously. The clinician should be open to possible underlying conditions such as autism or problems associated with insecure attachment.

Major depression among preschool children is relatively uncommon: the best prevalence estimate is around 2% (Egger and Angold, 2006) so a typical GP or health visitor might see one new case every 1–4 years assuming an average full-time health visitor caseload of 250 or average full-time GP patient list of 1500. Around half of children with major depressive disorder in the preschool years will have problems that persist for at least 6 months and these children tend to be those with the most severe symptoms at baseline (Luby et al., 2009).

There is relatively little research on the natural history of emotional problems in the preschool years and even less research on the effectiveness of therapies but any child with persisting or severe presentations should be referred for expert assessment.

Attention deficit hyperactivity disorders

ADHD is generally diagnosed around the time a child starts school, but the more severe cases can present earlier than this. Motor restlessness, impulsivity, and lack of ability to concentrate are the key diagnostic features. Although ADHD has a significant genetic basis (Faraone et al., 2005), identification in infancy through observation of the child may be difficult (Allely et al., 2012; Johnson et al., 2014), although lack of positive parental engagement with the child may indicate increased risk (Allely et al., 2013a, 2013b; Marwick et al., 2013; Puckering et al., 2014).

Although there are many studies demonstrating the long-term stability of ADHD symptoms, in many cases into adulthood (Shaw et al., 2012), there is relatively little high-quality information on the natural history of hyperactivity and inattention in the preschool years, or on the responsiveness of symptoms to psychosocial or pharmacological intervention. The studies that have been published (Price et al., 2005) suggest that symptoms tend to be moderately stable from age 2 to 5 years, and that much of this stability is genetically determined. Current National Institute for Health and Care Excellence guidelines suggest that parents of children with preschool ADHD should be offered structured parenting support, but the evidence that parent training programmes produce objective (as opposed to subjective) benefit on ADHD symptoms is weak (Rimestad et al., 2016). Drug treatments are not currently recommended for preschool children with ADHD.

Conduct problems

Most parents struggle with their preschool children's behaviour at some time, but oppositional or aggressive behaviour sometimes becomes unmanageable. Since some behavioural interventions can be beneficial in reducing the impact of such conduct problems (Edwards et al., 2007; Bywater et al., 2009), and since the natural history of significant early-onset disruptive behaviour problems tends to be one of increasing social difficulties (Moffitt et al., 2002), it is sensible to enquire about aggressive and oppositional behaviour during developmental assessments (Wilson et al., 2009). If problems appear to be severe or persistent, referral for psychological input may be valuable.

Disorders of executive function and self-regulation

Executive function has attracted considerable attention in recent years as a skill or more accurately a set of skills which underpin the child's capacity to attend and focus and ultimately to regulate their own behaviour. The three most commonly cited core elements are working memory, response inhibition, and attention shifting (Garon et al., 2008) but other investigators include mental flexibility, as well as the initiation and self-monitoring of actions (Chan et al., 2008). Whatever the combination of included skills, they feed into the child's readiness for school when a child needs to be able to recall what is said to them efficiently, and control their attention and their behaviour to allow them to learn effectively in groups of other children. These skills may be less apparent at home and except in the most extreme cases (e.g. in children with ADHD or autism spectrum disorder), are rarely the focus of parental concern. Although many have assumed that executive function is closely associated with intelligence, more generally this is not necessarily the case (Friedman et al., 2006). These skills are not routinely 'screened' in the population although they are the subject of identification in groups that have already been targeted. Nonetheless, they are part of the overall profile of the developing child, for example, in the ability to control the attention while looking at picture books at 18 months and to retain and understand requests expressed verbally.

Parental judgement versus direct observation in the various domains: does the parent give reliable answers and in which context?

The accuracy of different approaches to identification is rarely taken into consideration. It is often assumed that simply asking about parental observations is the same as specifically assessing the child. In fact, there is some early evidence that this is indeed the case. Parents' concerns can be elicited quickly and 92% of parents can answer questions in writing while in waiting rooms (Glascoe, 2000) and more recent work with premature 2-year-olds using the Ages and Stages questionnaire has indicated the same (Flamant et al., 2011), although use of the Infant/Child Monitoring Questionnaire did not (Dixon et al., 2009). The answer to this is that it probably depends on the populations being studied and whether they are being asked to observe their children and report on those current observations, report on historical milestones, or express concern about a specific aspect of their child's behaviour or performance.

What tools should be used for identifying children with neurodevelopmental difficulties?

General assessment tools

It is not possible to use a single screening measure to identify all children with neurodevelopmental difficulties reliably. Nevertheless, there is a variety of measures which have some utility which are worth considering. Here we draw extensively on a review carried out by Bedford et al. (2013) of whole population assessment measures at 2 years of age covering physical, social and emotional, cognitive, and speech and language development. They identified three types of measure: those completed by parents, those completed by health professionals with involvement of parents, and those completed by professionals only. All those considered were generic measures covering all aspects of development. A fourth category which this review does not address includes screens of single domains. They used systematic methods to search the literature for papers citing measures of child development. Other sources were also used including a search of the internet, gathering review papers, and consulting experts. The instruments which seemed most suitable for the stated purpose were assessed against predetermined requirements set out by the Department of Health in England. These were that the measure:

- 'can be updated on a regular basis (e.g. annually) and enables population level child development at age 2–2½ years to be tracked over time
- is a valid and reliable measure of the aspects of child development we wish to measure
- is applicable to different groups of the population with differing levels of development and needs
- has standardised norms for an appropriate population that can be used to benchmark progress in England
- can be aggregated at the national and local (local authority) level
- is sensitive to changes at a population level
- reflects influences on child development during pregnancy and first two years of life as well as being predictive of later life outcomes, especially school readiness
- is simple to apply and is acceptable to families and professionals
- minimises burdens on professionals and families
- can be integrated with existing clinical contacts with all families around this age' (Bedford et al., 2013).

Thirty five measures met the inclusion criteria, with 13 of these covering all the domains of interest and, of these, two measures (Ages and Stages Questionnaires (ASQ-3™), and Parents' Evaluation of Developmental Status (PEDS)) emerged as the most suitable to be included in the Healthy Child Programme 2-year review as a *population* measure of children's development.

Ages and Stages Questionnaires (2009)

The aim of the ASQ-3 (Squires, 2009), which covers ages 1–66 months is to identify children at risk of developmental delay. It is made up of 21 age-specific questionnaires (for 2, 4, 6, 8, 9, 10, 12, 14, 16, 18, 20, 22, 24, 27, 30, 33, 36, 42, 48, 54, and 60 months) which can be given to the parent in person, mailed, or completed online. Each questionnaire includes 30 questions about the child's development divided into five domains (communication, gross motor, fine motor, problem-solving, and personal-social) with response options of 'yes', 'sometimes', and 'not yet'. Bedford et al., reporting on the evidence underpinning the ASQ, said: 'The ASQ-3 was standardised on 15,138 children (1,443 aged 24 months) whose parents completed 18,232 questionnaires. Families were educationally and economically diverse, and their ethnicities roughly matched estimates from the 2007 U.S. Census. Sensitivity was .86 and specificity was .85 overall' (Bedford et al., 2013).

Parents' Evaluation of Developmental Status (1997)

The aims of the PEDS, which covers 0–96 months, is to elicit parents' concerns about their child's development and health (PEDSTest.com).

PEDS includes a single general question: 'Please list any concerns about your child's learning, development, and behaviour' and is followed by eight short questions to elicit parents' concerns about each developmental domain. It can be conducted as an interview or parents can complete the 'PEDS Response Form' at home or in a waiting room prior to a consultation. In their summary of the evidence, Bedford and colleagues said: 'Sensitivity was 70% or greater (average 83%) and specificity 77% to 93% (average 84%) across ages and developmental domains. For the ages 23 to 33 months, sensitivity ranged between 80% and 93% and specificity 82% to 93%' (Bedford et al., 2013). They warn that these figures are derived from a gold standard test from which the PEDS was originally derived, potentially inflating the accuracy of the measure.

Tools for use when concerns arise during general assessments

Whenever any concern about neurodevelopment arises during a developmental assessment, it is wise to consider whether problems might exist in other developmental domains (Gillberg, 2010). In this situation, there are some useful tools that are simple and quick to administer in routine clinical practice if the questionnaires are completed in advance by parents, and which cover a range of difficulties. The following tools can be used as paper questionnaires without any cost:

- The Strengths and Difficulties Questionnaire (SDQ—http://www.sdqinfo.org (Goodman, 1997, 2001)) can be used from age 2 years. It is a very well-validated screening questionnaire consisting of 25 questions covering conduct problems, hyperactivity/inattention problems, social communication problems, and emotional problems including depression and anxiety as well as prosocial behaviours.

- The ESSENCE-Q (http://gnc.gu.se/english/research/screening-questionnaires/essence-q). This is a questionnaire aiming to help clinicians and researchers to locate children (at any age, but particularly young children) who might have a disorder subsumed under the ESSENCE umbrella (including, among others, autism, ADHD, developmental disorder, language delay, and tic disorders). It can be used as a brief interview or as a questionnaire to be completed by parents. It is currently undergoing psychometric studies in several different settings, including in specialized and non-specialized clinics and in the general population. It is not a diagnostic instrument.

- The M-CHAT-R™ (Modified Checklist for Autism in Toddlers Revised—https://www.m-chat.org/) can be used between ages 16 and 30 months when autism is suspected. It is a two-stage parent-report screening instrument involving responses to 20 questions. If concerns are raised in the initial parent-report screen, additional questions to be asked by the clinician are indicated.
- The 50-word version of the Sure-Start Language Measure (SSLM—http://www.maternal-and-early-years.org.uk/file/03a0a61d-289a-4e4d-8d40-a07400b0af97). This is a simple word list that can be used to assess expressive language between 15 and 30 months of age. Its use at 30 months is strongly correlated with formally assessed language function 1–2 years later and is also highly correlated with global cognitive functioning (Sim et al., 2015).

Alternative approaches to developmental assessment (e.g. web-based systems)

The key to effective child health surveillance is a well-informed consumer—principally the parent or carer. Where, in the past, information about child development was provided by the health visitor in the form of leaflets or verbal advice and a small minority of parents accessed information through readily available books, the picture has changed dramatically since most parents have internet access (see further discussion in Chapter 9 of this volume). A review of information from 44 different websites designed for access by parents concluded: 'Overall, information available for parents about child development is accurate but much of it is incomplete, unclear, or difficult to access' (Williams et al., 2008). In many ways, such a rich source of information will only add to the information parents have at their disposal, but in the event that it is contradictory or overly dramatic, the role of the health provider sometimes shifts from being the provider of information to that of the mediator of the most useful information.

Key messages

There are a number of key messages about the risks associated with restricted child development (Walker et al., 2011). These are not specific to particular aspects of child development and those engaging in the discussion about programmes of screening or surveillance need to hold them in mind. See Box 22.1.

In conclusion, evidence in support of screening for developmental difficulties is generally weak and there may be a temptation to conclude that there really is not sufficient evidence. But the formal analysis of outcomes from screening is not the same as monitoring children's development and encouraging parents to seek support. Indeed, there is a risk that in responding to the lack of good quality evidence we 'throw the baby out with the bath water' and conclude that there is nothing that we can or should do (Scottish Executive Health Department, 2005; Coury, 2015) on a whole-population basis. There is evidence for the effectiveness of interventions for children with developmental difficulties (see Chapter 24), and there is also evidence that without formal identification procedures services may be tipped in favour of better educated parents from the mainstream culture. Formal early identification may thus have the potential to reduce disparities in age at diagnosis (e.g. in the case of autism) and to reduce socio-demographic disparities in access to services (Herlihy et al., 2014).

Box 22.1 Key messages on risks of restricted child development

♦ Formal screening remains problematic in many respects but there is a need for monitoring child development, for engaging with parents about their child's development, for ensuring that they have access to universal services, and where deemed appropriate, referral to secondary care services.

♦ With cumulative exposure to developmental risks, disparities widen and trajectories become more firmly established.

♦ Identification of any developmental problem should prompt a broader evaluation of a child's developmental status.

♦ Reducing inequalities requires early integrated interventions that target the many risks to which children in a particular setting are exposed.

♦ The most effective and cost-efficient time to prevent inequalities is early in life before trajectories have been firmly established.

♦ Action or lack of action may have lifetime consequences for adult functioning, for the care of the next generation, and for the well-being of society more generally.

Text extracts reprinted from *The Lancet*, Volume 378, Issue 97, Susan P Walker et al., Inequality in early childhood: risk and protective factors for early child development, pp. 1325–1338, Copyright © 2011 Elsevier Ltd, with permission from Elsevier, https://www.sciencedirect.com/journal/the-lancet.

Learning links

♦ E-learning for healthcare—'Healthy Child Programme': https://www.e-lfh.org.uk/programmes/healthy-child-programme/

♦ Communication Trust website: http://www.thecommunicationtrust.org.uk/resources/resources.

Recommendations

♦ Healthcare professionals in contact with children should be knowledgeable about normal development and its variations and take any opportunity to establish whether a child is developing normally. (*Evidence: moderate.*)

- Practitioners should consider establishing whether the parent has concerns about their development whenever a child is seen. (*Evidence: moderate.*)
- When concerns are raised, appropriate tools should be used to aid assessment. (*Evidence: strong.*)
- Continuity of care helps in any assessment and should be maintained wherever possible. (*Good practice.*)
- Data on social patterning of uptake of developmental assessments, and of referrals made, should be collected by commissioners. (*Evidence: strong.*)

Acknowledgement

Text extracts from Bedford H et al. *Measures of Child Development: A review*, London Policy Research Unit in the Health of Children, Young People and Families, University College London, UK, Copyright © 2013, reproduced with permission from the author.

References

Ainsworth, M.D.S., Blehar, M.C., Wathen, C.N., and Wall, S. (1978). *Patterns of Attachment: A Psychological Study of the Strange Situation*. New York: Lawrence Erlbaum Associates.

Allely, C.S., Doolin, O., Gillberg, C., et al. (2012). Can psychopathology at age 7 be predicted from clinical observation at one year? Evidence from the ALSPAC cohort. *Research in Developmental Disabilities*, **33**, 2292–2300.

Allely, C.S., Johnson, P., Marwick, H., et al. (2013a). Prediction of 7-year psychopathology from mother-infant joint attention behaviours: a nested case-control study. *BMC Pediatrics*, **13**, 147.

Allely, C.S., Purves, D., and McConnachie, A. (2013b). Parent-infant vocalisations at 12 months predict psychopathology at 7 years. *Research in Developmental Disabilities*, **34**, 985–993.

Bailey, D.B.J., Bruer, J.T., Symons, F.J., and Lichtman, J.W. (Eds.) (2001). *Critical Thinking about Critical Periods*. Baltimore, MD: Paul H Brookes Publishing Co.

Board of American Society of Human Genetics, and Board of American College of Medical Genetics (1995). Points to consider: ethical, legal, and psychosocial implications of genetic testing in children and adolescents. *American Journal of Human Genetics*, **57**, 1233–1241

Bedford, H., Walton, S., and Ahn, J. (2013). *Measures of Child Development: A Review*. London: Policy Research Unit in the Health of Children, Young People and Families.

Bergelson, E. and Swingley, D. (2012). At 6-9 months, human infants know the meanings of many common nouns. *Proceedings of the National Academy of Sciences of the United States of America*, **109**, 3253–3258.

Bowlby, J. (1969). *Attachment and Loss, Volume 1: Attachment*. London: Hogarth Press.

Bywater, T., Hutchings, J., Daley, D., et al. (2009). Long-term effectiveness of a parenting intervention for children at risk of developing conduct disorder. *British Journal of Psychiatry*, **195**, 318–324.

Caspi, A., Houts, R.M., Belsky, D.W., et al. (2016). Childhood forecasting of a small segment of the population with large economic burden. *Nature Human Behaviour*, **1**, 0005.

Chan, R.C., Shum, D., Toulopoulou, T., and Chen, E.Y. (2008). Assessment of executive functions: review of instruments and identification of critical issues. *Archives of Clinical Neuropsychology*, **23**, 201–216.

Chisholm, K. (1998). A three year follow-up of attachment and indiscriminate friendliness in children adopted from Romanian orphanages. *Child Development*, **69**, 1092–1106.

Chowdry, H. and Oppenheim, C.E. (2015). *Spending on Late Intervention: How We Can Do Better for Less*. London: Early Intervention Foundation.

Chung, P.J., Lee, T.C., Morrison, J.L., and Schuster, M.A. (2006). Preventive care for children in the United States: quality and barriers. *Annual Reviews of Public Health and Social Care in the Community*, **27**, 491–515.

Coleman, M. and Gillberg, C. (2011). *The Autisms*. Oxford: Oxford University Press.

Coury, D.L. (2015). Babies, bathwater, and screening for autism spectrum disorder: comments on the USPSTF recommendations for autism spectrum disorder screening. *Journal of Developmental and Behavioral Pediatrics*, **36**, 661–663.

Dixon, G., Badawi, N., French, D., and Kurinczuk, J.J. (2009). Can parents accurately screen children at risk of developmental delay? *Journal of Paediatrics and Child Health*, **45**, 268–273.

Edwards, R.T., Ceilleachair, A., Bywater, T., Hughes, D.A., and Hutchings, J. (2007). Parenting programme for parents of children at risk of developing conduct disorder: cost effectiveness analysis. *BMJ*, **334**, 682.

Egger, H.L. and Angold, A. (2006). Common emotional and behavioral disorders in preschool children: presentation, nosology, and epidemiology. *Journal of Child Psychology and Psychiatry and Allied Disciplines*, **47**, 313–337.

Every Child Ready to Read (2010). Literature review. [online] Available at: http://www.everychildreadytoread.org/project-history%09/literature-review-2010.

Faraone, S.V., Perlis, R.H., Doyle, A.E., et al. (2005). Molecular genetics of attention-deficit/hyperactivity disorder. *Biological Psychiatry*, **57**, 1313–1323.

Farrant, B.M. and Zubrick, S.R. (2012). Early vocabulary development: the importance of joint attention and parent-child book reading. *First Language*, **32**, 343–364.

Fenson, L., Dale, P.S., Reznick, J.S., et al. (1994). Variability in early communicative development. *Monographs of the Society for Research in Child Development*, **59**, 1–185.

Fernell, E., Wilson, P., Hadjikhani, N., et al. (2014). Screening, intervention and outcome in autism and other developmental disorders: the role of randomized controlled trials. *Journal of Autism and Developmental Disorders*, **44**, 2074–2076.

Flamant, C., Branger, B., Nguyen The Tich, S., et al. (2011). Parent-completed developmental screening in premature children: a valid tool for follow-up programs. *PLoS One*, **6**, e20004.

Foundationyears.org.uk (2017). What to expect, when? A parents' guide. From pregnancy to children aged 5. [online] Available at: https://www.foundationyears.org.uk/2015/03/what-to-expect-when-a-parents-guide/ [Accessed 25 Sep. 2017].

Friedman, N.P., Miyake, A., Corley, R.P., Young, S.E., Defries, J.C., and Hewitt, J.K. (2006). Not all executive functions are related to intelligence. *Psychological Science*, **17**, 172–179.

Garon, N., Bryson, S.E., and Smith, I.M. (2008). Executive function in preschoolers: a review using an integrative framework. *Psychological Bulletin*, **134**, 31–60.

Gillberg, C. (2010). The ESSENCE in child psychiatry: Early Symptomatic Syndromes Eliciting Neurodevelopmental Clinical Examinations. *Research in Developmental Disabilities*, **31**, 1543–1551.

Glascoe, F.P. (2000). Evidence-based approach to developmental and behavioural surveillance using parents' concerns. *Child: Care, Health and Development*, **26**, 137–149.

Goodman, R. (1997). The Strengths and Difficulties Questionnaire: a research note. *Journal of Child Psychology and Psychiatry*, **38**, 581–586.

Goodman, R. (2001). Psychometric properties of the Strengths and Difficulties Questionnaire. *Journal of the American Academy of Child and Adolescent Psychiatry*, **40**, 1337–1345.

Herlihy, L.E., Brooks, B., Dumont-Mathieu, T., et al. (2014). Standardized screening facilitates timely diagnosis of autism spectrum disorders in a diverse sample of low-risk toddlers. *Journal of Developmental and Behavioral Pediatrics*, **35**, 85–92.

Hertzman, C. and Williams, R. (2009). Making early childhood count. *Canadian Medical Association Journal*, **180**, 68–71.

Janus, M., Harrison, L.J., Goldfeld, S., Guhn, M., and Brinkman, S. (2016). International research utilizing the Early Development Instrument (EDI) as a measure of early child development: Introduction to the Special Issue. *Early Childhood Research Quarterly*, **35**, 1–5.

Johnson, P., Ahamat, B., McConnachie, A., et al. (2014). Motor activity at age one year does not predict ADHD at seven years. *International Journal of Methods in Psychiatric Research*, **23**, 9–18.

Kasper, J., Kreis, J., Scheibler, F., et al. (2011). Population-based screening of children for specific speech and language impairment in Germany: a systematic review. *Folia Phoniatrica et Logopaedica*, **63**, 247–263.

Law, J. and Harris, F. (2001). *Promoting Language Development in Sure Start Areas*. Nottingham: DFES, Sure Start.

Law, J. and Roy, P. (2008). Parental report of infant language skills - a review of the development and application of the Communicative Development Inventories *Child and Adolescent Mental Health*, **13**, 198–206.

Law, J., Boyle, J., Harris, F., Harkness, A., and Nye, C. (1998). Screening for speech and language delay: a systematic review of the literature. *Health Technology Assessment (Winchester, England)*, **2**, 1–184.

Law, J., Charlton, J., Dockrell, J., et al. (2017a). *Early Language Development: Needs, Provision and Intervention for Preschool Children from Socio-Economically Disadvantage Backgrounds*. London: Education Endowment Foundation.

Law, J., Charlton, J., Dockrell, J., McKean, C., and Boyle, J. (2017b). *Patterns of Competence and Signals of Risk*. London: Early Intervention Foundation

Law, J., Rush, R., Anandan, C., Cox, M., and Wood, R. (2012). Predicting language change between 3 and 5 years and its implications for early identification. *Pediatrics*, **130**, e132–e137.

Liszkowski, U., Brown, P., Callaghan, T., Takada, A., and De Vos, C. (2012). A prelinguistic gestural universal of human communication. *Cognitive Science*, **36**, 698–713.

Luby, J.L., Si, X., Belden, A.C., Tandon, M., and Spitznagel, E. (2009). Preschool depression: homotypic continuity and course over 24 months. *Archives of General Psychiatry*, **66**, 897–905.

Maggi, S., Irwin, L.J., Siddiqi, A., and Hertzman, C. (2010). The social determinants of early child development: an overview. *Journal of Paediatrics and Child Health*, **46**, 627–635.

Mandell, D.S., Novak, M.M., and Zubritsky, C.D. (2005). Factors associated with age of diagnosis among children with autism spectrum disorders. *Pediatrics*, **116**, 1480–1486.

Marmot, M., Allen, J., Goldblatt, P., et al. (2010). *Fair Society, Healthy Lives: The Strategic Review of Health Inequalities in England post-2010.* London: Institute of Health Equity. Available at: http://www.instituteofhealthequity.org/resources-reports/fair-society-healthy-lives-the-marmot-review/fair-society-healthy-lives-full-report-pdf.pdf.

Marwick, H., Doolin, O., Allely, C.S., et al. (2013). Predictors of diagnosis of child psychiatric disorder in adult/infant social-communicative interaction at 12 months. *Research in Developmental Disabilities*, **34**, 562–572.

Mathers, N. and Hodgkin, P. (1989). The gatekeeper and the wizard: a fairy tale. *British Medical Journal*, **298**, 172–174.

McKean, C., Law, J., Mensah, F., et al. (2016). Predicting meaningful differences in school-entry language skills from child and family factors measured at 12 months of age. *International Journal of Early Childhood*, **48**, 329–351.

Meschi, E., Mickelwright, J., Vignoles, A., and Lindsay, G. (2012). *The Transition Between Categories of Special Educational Needs of Pupils with Speech, Language and Communication Needs (SLCN) and Autism Spectrum Disorder (ASD) as they Progress Through the Education System.* Research Report DFE-RR247-BCRP11. London: Department for Education.

Miller, S.A. (1988). Parents' beliefs about children's cognitive development. *Child Development*, **59**, 259–285.

Miniscalco, C., Nygren, G., Hagberg, B., et al. (2006). Neuropsychiatric and neurodevelopmental outcome of children at age 6 and 7 years who screened positive for language problems at 30 months. *Developmental Medicine and Child Neurology*, **48**, 361–366.

Moffitt, T.E., Caspi, A., Harrington, H., and Milne, B. J. (2002). Males on the life-course-persistent and adolescence-limited antisocial pathways: follow-up at age 26 years. *Development and Psychopathology*, **14**, 179–207.

Nadig, A.S., Ozonoff, S., Young, G.S., Rozga, A., Sigman, M., and Rogers, S.J. (2007). A prospective study of response to name in infants at risk for autism. *Archives of Pediatrics Adolescent Medicine*, **161**, 378–383.

Nelson, H.D., Nygren, P., Walker, M., and Panoscha, R. (2006). Screening for speech and language delay in preschool children: systematic evidence review for the US Preventive Services Task Force. *Pediatrics*, **117**, e298–e319.

PEDStest.com. Tools for developmental-behavioral screening and surveillance. [online] Available at: http://www.pedstest.com/Home.aspx.

Peña, E.D., Gillam, R.B., Bedore, L.M., and Bohman, T.M. (2011). Risk for poor performance on a language screening measure for bilingual preschoolers and kindergarteners. *American Journal of Speech-Language Pathology*, **20**, 302–314.

Pickles, A., Le Couteur, A., Leadbitter, K., et al. (2016). Parent-mediated social communication therapy for young children with autism (PACT): long-term follow-up of a randomised controlled trial. *The Lancet*, **388**, 2501–2509.

Price, T.S., Simonoff, E., Asherson, P., et al. (2005). Continuity and change in preschool ADHD symptoms: longitudinal genetic analysis with contrast effects. *Behavior Genetics*, **35**, 121–132.

Puckering, C., Allely, C., Doolin, O., et al. (2014). Association between parent-infant interactions in infancy and disruptive behaviour disorders at age seven: a nested, case-control ALSPAC study. *BMC Pediatrics*, **14**, 223.

Rimestad, M.L., Lambek, R., Zacher Christiansen, H., and Hougaard, E. (2016). Short- and long-term effects of parent training for preschool children with or at risk of ADHD: a systematic review and meta-analysis. *Journal of Attention Disorders*, **14** May [Epub ahead of print].

Roulstone, S., Coad, J., Ayre, A., Hambly, H., and Lindsay, G. (2012). *The Preferred Outcomes of Children with Speech, Language and Communication Needs and their Parents*. Research Report DFE-RR247-BCRP12. London: Department for Education.

Rowe, M.L. (2008). Child-directed speech: relation to socioeconomic status, knowledge of child development and child vocabulary skill. *Journal of Child Language*, **35**, 185–205.

Scottish Executive Health Department (2005). *Health for all Children 4 – Guidance to Implementation in Scotland 2005*. Edinburgh: HMSO. Available at: http://www.scotland.gov. uk/Publications/2005/04/15161325/13269.

Sharma, A. and Cockerill, H. (2007). *From Birth to Five Years: Children's Developmental Progress* (3rd edn.). London: Routledge and Kegan Paul.

Shaw, M., Hodgkins, P., Caci, H., et al. (2012). A systematic review and analysis of long-term outcomes in attention deficit hyperactivity disorder: effects of treatment and non-treatment. *BMC Medicine*, **10**, 99.

Shonkoff, J.P. and Phillips, D.A. (Eds.) (2000). *From Neurons to Neighbourhoods: The Science of Early Childhood Development*. Washington, DC: National Academy Press.

Sim, F., Haig, C., O'Dowd, J., et al. (2015). Development of a triage tool for neurodevelopmental risk in children aged 30 months. *Research in Developmental Disabilities*, **45–46**, 69–82

Sim, F., O'Dowd, J., Thompson, L., et al. (2013). Language and social/emotional problems identified at a universal developmental assessment at 30 months. *BMC Pediatrics*, **13**, 206.

Siu, A.L. (2015). Screening for speech and language delay and disorders in children aged 5 years or younger: US Preventive Services Task Force Recommendation Statement. *Pediatrics*, **136**, e474–e481.

Squires, J. (2009). *ASQ-3 User's Guide* (3rd edn.). Baltimore, MD: Brookes.

Tomasello, M. (2009). *Constructing a Language*. Cambridge. MA: Harvard University Press.

Uljarevic, M., Katsos, N., Hudry, K., and Gibson, J.L. (2016). Practitioner review: multilingualism and neurodevelopmental disorders – an overview of recent research and discussion of clinical implications. *Journal of Child Psychology and Psychiatry*, **57**, 1205–1217.

Vihman, M. (1996). *Phonological Development: The Origins of Language in the Child*. Oxford: Basil Blackwell.

Walker, S.P., Wachs, T.D., Grantham-McGregor, S., et al. (2011). Inequality in early childhood: risk and protective factors for early child development. *The Lancet*, **378**, 1325–1338.

Wallace, I.F., Berkman, N.D., Watson, L.R., et al. (2015). Screening for speech and language delay in children 5 years old and younger: a systematic review. *Pediatrics*, **136**, e448–e462.

Warren, R., Kenny, M., Bennett, T., et al. (2016). Screening for developmental delay among children aged 1–4 years: a systematic review. *CMAJ Open*, **4**, E20–E27.

West, S. and Williams, C. (2011). Amblyopia. *BMJ Clinical Evidence*, **2011**, 0709.

Williams, N., Mughal, S., and Blair, M. (2008). 'Is my child developing normally?': a critical review of web-based resources for parents. *Developmental Medicine and Child Neurology*, **50**, 893–897.

Wilson, J.M.G. and Jungner, G. (1968). Principios y metodos del examen colectivo para identificar enfermedades. *Boletin de la Oficina Sanitaria Panamericana*, **65**, 281–393.

Wilson, P. and Mullin, A. (2010). Child neglect: what has it to do with general practice? *British Journal of General Practice*, **60**, 5–6.

Wilson, P., Minnis, H., Puckering, C., and **Gillberg, C.** (2009). Should we aspire to screen preschool children for conduct disorder? *Archives of Disease in Childhood*, **94**, 812–816.

Wing, L. (1980). Childhood autism and social class: a question of selection? *The British Journal of Psychiatry*, **137**, 410–417.

Wing, L., **Gould, J.,** and **Gillberg, C.** (2011). Autism spectrum disorders in the DSM-V: Better or worse than the DSM-IV? *Research in Developmental Disabilities*, **32**, 768–773.

Wölck, W. (1988). Types of natural bilingual behavior: a review and revision. *Bilingual Review*, **14**, 3–16.

Wood, R. and **Blair, M.** (2014). A comparison of Child Health Programmes recommended for preschool children in selected high-income countries. *Child: Care, Health and Development*, **40**, 640–653.

Wood, R., **Stirling, A., Nolan, C., Chalmers, J.,** and **Blair, M.** (2012). Trends in the coverage of 'universal' child health reviews: observational study using routinely available data. *BMJ Open*, **2**, e000759.

Chapter 23

Opportunistic surveillance in primary care

Philip Wilson and Jackie Kirkham

Summary

This chapter:

♦ looks at the opportunities that clinicians in the primary care team have to identify and assess problems in child development in contexts other than scheduled assessments, when parents may not themselves have identified a developmental concern

♦ describes the domains of child development in which clinicians might identify problems opportunistically, how opportunities for identification can be maximized, and how common problems might be picked up and confirmed

♦ considers how practitioners need to be aware of, and alert to, concerns about physical and social/emotional development, as well as signs of maltreatment and neglect and the quality of parenting.

What does opportunistic surveillance mean?

We define opportunistic surveillance as the process by which a primary care clinician or other team member identifies problems in child development outside the context of scheduled developmental assessments and when children are not brought specifically because of a developmental concern. Opportunistic surveillance can occur, for example, in immunization clinics, 'drop-in' sessions with a health visitor, routine general practice surgeries or home visits, as well as in contacts with dental and pharmacy services. Effective opportunistic surveillance needs an alert practitioner with a sound understanding of normal child development and of 'good enough' (Winnicott, 1973) parenting behaviours.

Is opportunistic surveillance an important part of the work of doctors and nurses?

A typical preschool child will be seen between three and four times per year by a general practitioner (GP) (Wood and Wilson, 2012) and the vast majority are seen at least once. There is greater regional variation in routine health visiting practice, but data from Scotland indicate that 62% of children aged 1–2 and 36% of children aged 3–4 years had seen a health visitor in the previous year (Growing Up in Scotland, 2010). Practice nurses and other practitioners will also see preschool children at the time of scheduled immunizations if they are involved in these clinics, during triage for minor illnesses, or if the child has a chronic disease such as asthma. Scottish data suggest that consultations with GPs are more likely for children living in poorer areas (C. Wilson et al., 2013) and among families with younger mothers and fewer children (McConnachie et al., 2004). Consultation rates for information on children's health are higher in more affluent areas, whereas consultations may be more frequent in more deprived areas for information on behaviour (C. Wilson et al., 2013). Around 6% of families report using a family doctor and 18% a health visitor for information about children's behaviour in the third year of life (Growing Up in Scotland cohort, unpublished data).

The primary healthcare team (GP, health visitor, and practice nurse, as well as other staff working within primary care) therefore have opportunities in their daily work to identify previously unsuspected childhood problems with important prognostic implications. Although we can identify risk factors, the prediction of many conditions is a very inexact science. For example, although we know that language delay is more common among boys, among those from poorer families, and those from families with known developmental problems, scoring systems are very inadequate for predicting which children will have important language delays (P. Wilson et al., 2013). Furthermore, many parents do not know what normal language development is like, so many children will not be brought to their GP or health visitor with parental concerns about poor language abilities. Many children with language delay therefore 'fall through the net' of professional risk assessment and parental concern. To detect children with significant language delay we must therefore either have a robust population-based system for language assessment with near 100% take-up (see Chapter 24), or we need to be alert to the possibility of language delay in our day-to-day clinical contacts. This latter approach is what we shall call opportunistic surveillance, and it may have most value for those children who fall through the net of scheduled assessments.

It is reasonable to assume that at least 10% of children have a hitherto-unrecognized developmental problem (e.g. language delay, growth problems, autism, or attention difficulties—see Thompson et al., 2012; Sim et al., 2013), some of which may be more amenable to early intervention than to later intervention (P. Wilson et al., 2009; Pickles et al., 2016). This proportion may be greater if we include problems in parent–child interaction. In addition, other issues separate to the presenting concern, such as missed immunizations, medication reviews, or chronic disease monitoring, might also present opportunities for intervention. Assuming that a typical GP sees at least two preschool children on a typical day, and a health visitor sees at least as many again outside scheduled developmental assessments, then we would expect that at least one child per week attending these clinicians might benefit from opportunistic surveillance. Attendances with other primary care professionals will provide additional surveillance opportunities.

Maximizing the opportunities for identification: knowledge gathering and assessment

As described in the previous section, using the example of language delay, the use of risk-based systems, in and of themselves, are not sufficient to predict which individual children may need further help or support. Wright et al. (2009) found in a deprived population with very regular health visiting input that only around half of the children who required further intervention or support were identified by the age of 1 year. Some new family problems emerge over time and some issues such as language delay can only be identified reliably when maturation allows it, thus there is a need for ongoing clinical contact with families where such issues can be identified over time (C. Wilson et al., 2012; P. Wilson et al., 2013).

The benefits of continuity of care are rarely mentioned in policy documents, but there is little doubt that continuity increases the potential for good relationships within which parental concerns can be aired (Jack et al., 2005; Hogg and Worth, 2009; Condon, 2011; Bidmead, 2013; Donetto et al., 2013; King, 2013; Cowley et al., 2015). Equally, professionals are more likely in this context to feel confident in raising concerns about issues that the parents may not have necessarily noticed.

When making judgements about children's development, about the parent–child relationship, or about the home environment, it is important to acknowledge the 'lens' through which the clinician sees and assesses need and risk. Factors such as gender, ethnicity, and social class are important, but rarely acknowledged, when assessing the family environment. For example, it is easy to forget the contribution of fathers if we make tacit assumptions about the central caregiving role of mothers (Peckover, 2002a, 2002b; Pritchard, 2005). Similarly, while we know that socio-economic status may be relevant when considering child development, there are dangers in the commonly held assumption that economic deprivation or membership of a particular social or ethnic group equates with developmental vulnerability (C. Wilson et al., 2012; Barry et al., 2015; King, 2016a). Such stigmatizing assumptions can themselves act as a deterrent to families engaging with services or practitioners, and seeking/accepting support (Cortis, 2012; Duvnjak and Fraser, 2013).

Much of the literature on engaging 'harder-to-reach' families focuses on particular defined socio-demographic groups and on barriers to attending targeted services such as parenting classes (Barlow et al., 2005; Axford et al., 2012; Whittaker and Cowley, 2012). These groups tend to include people with lower educational attainment, lower socio-economic status, parents with addictions, teenage parents, or those from some minority ethnic groups. Commonly identified barriers include logistical issues (accessibility, child care, transport), perceptual issues (stigma, no perception of the need for intervention, intervention seen as culturally inappropriate/irrelevant), and issues with the practitioner (lack of trust or identification). Solutions recommended in these accounts include improving accessibility and taking the time to develop ongoing trusting relationships with clients, as well as being more flexible with the type and availability of support offered.

The role of 'intuition' or 'gut instinct' as part of the knowledge-gathering and assessment process is acknowledged (Ling and Luker, 2000; Greenhalgh, 2002; P. Wilson et al., 2008a, 2008b; Shepherd, 2011) but often downplayed (Ling and Luker, 2000). There is some evidence that this may be particularly important in relation to assessments of the parent–child relationship (P. Wilson et al., 2008b). This phenomenon has important implications for record-keeping (Ling and Luker, 2000). Clinicians may be reluctant to include important subjective, 'interpretative' information in the record of a consultation and inclusion of 'third-party' information in a child's records can be problematic. Furthermore, the use of standardized assessment tools, while potentially beneficial in ensuring consistency and equity (and sometimes medico-legal robustness (King, 2016a)) of assessment, can sometimes inhibit free discussion or voicing of concerns (Mitcheson and Cowley, 2003; Cowley et al., 2004; King, 2016b).

If practitioners are to identify developmental problems accurately, they need to be familiar with and confident in assessing 'normal' development. Health visitors should have extensive knowledge in this domain, and their basic and ongoing professional training should prepare them to be confident and accurate in their assessments. Therefore, health visitors have a responsibility to help other primary care professionals to develop skills and knowledge in this area. GPs and other members of the primary care team who work with children should have a good knowledge of basic development, as well as some understanding of parenting and attachment behaviours.

How common problems might be picked up

Clinicians should focus on three distinct components during assessment, namely, the child, the parent(s), and the parent–child relationship. Opportunities to observe and assess arise in the consultation room, the waiting room (McLaughlin et al., 2010), home visits, drop-in clinics, immunization clinics (Pritchett et al., 2012), or opportunistic meetings in the street. Of paramount importance is the professional's observation skills and ability to identify non-verbal cues—much information which is not necessarily the focus of a consultation can be assimilated rapidly. Examples might include attachment behaviour, how a child plays (or not) with available toys, or social communication. Such skills can be improved with experience and observation of more experienced colleagues, but may also need more formal training opportunities. Optimizing the clinical environment for such observations is also important. Unfortunately, infection control constraints have led to the removal of toy boxes from many waiting rooms and consulting rooms but reasonable compromise is necessary as attachment security, fine motor function, and imaginative play can all be observed in seconds when interesting toys are available during a clinical encounter.

In general practice, most consultations are conducted with adults who may present on behalf of themselves or the child. There are, however, times when a parent or carer themselves may have major health and/or social issues which might distract attention from the child. In such cases, the practitioner must also consider the impact of the presenting issues on the child (Hølge-Hazelton and Tulinius, 2010).

Physical problems

There should be opportunities to detect problems through intercurrent contacts with children and their families, as well as through scheduled developmental reviews. This is particularly important when universal developmental assessments are infrequent (Scottish Executive Health Department, 2005): both quantitative and qualitative studies have generated evidence (some of it strong) that it is not sufficient to rely solely on prior risk assessment or parental concern (Hogg et al., 2013; P. Wilson et al., 2013; King, 2015).

Clinical appointments may allow an assessment of a child's physical development in addition to the presenting issue. Ritual or 'embodied' practices, in particular the weighing of babies by health visitors both at home and in the clinic setting (Shepherd, 2011; King, 2016a), can have the advantage of being acceptable to large numbers of parents, and can act as an entry point to assessment and ongoing discussion and relationship with the family. However frequent weighing can cause unnecessary anxiety.

There is considerable variation in the skills of clinicians in relation to assessment of physical development, but we consider that there are minimum standards that should reasonably be expected. Regular contacts between GPs, health visitors, and practice nurses to discuss cases where there is developmental concern would help to nurture these skills. As a minimum, all members of the primary care team dealing with children should be expected to have familiarity with gross (head control, sitting, rolling, walking, etc.) and fine (reaching, grip) motor development, as well as with the use of growth charts.

Social and emotional development

As well as problems in physical development, clinicians should be familiar with the range of normal language and social development as well as attachment-related behaviours. These are discussed in more detail in Chapter 22.

There is strong evidence that identification of any developmental problem should prompt enquiries about problems in other domains (Gillberg, 2010).

Identification of maltreatment

Maltreatment takes many forms, and its severity can range from carelessness to frank abuse. Both reactive and proactive skills are employed by clinicians in identifying and working with children where there are child protection concerns (Ling and Luker, 2000; Peckover, 2013). These skills can be utilized, consciously or otherwise, during every interaction with a child and family.

The key physical signs of child abuse are well known, and all areas have policies for its management. As well as a pattern of suspicious injuries or fearful behaviour, consultation patterns can raise suspicion: examples might include erratic attendance, frequent late attendance, frequent use of emergency departments, and patterns of avoidance at home visits and developmental assessments. These should all raise concern about risk.

Neglect is a more difficult form of maltreatment to identify. Both GPs and health visitors have almost universal (albeit sporadic) longitudinal contact with children and families, and thus are well placed with their complementary knowledge of families to identify and support children at risk of neglect (P. Wilson and Mullin, 2010). The possibility of neglect should be considered in children whose families have problem substance use or other conditions likely to affect caring ability, or who are failing to thrive. Unusual behaviours such as toddlers showing indiscriminate friendliness towards strangers (Zeanah et al., 2002) should also alert the practitioner to the possibility of neglect.

While the management of suspected physical abuse is likely to be determined by clear local guidelines, the management of suspected neglect is much more challenging. These difficulties are inevitably compounded by the fact that there can be no hard and fast threshold for the ascertainment of neglect. Good communication between all primary care professionals should usually be the first step since each of these professionals is likely to have specific insights into the family and the home environment. The Safeguarding Children and Young People Toolkit produced by the Royal College of General Practitioners and the National Society for the Prevention of Cruelty to Children (2014) is a useful resource and a range of tools is available for other community-based practitioners. In identifying future significant risk with families, standardized assessment tools can prove counterproductive in that they can inhibit trust and not necessarily accurately identify risk (Daniel, 2010; Cowley et al., 2013). However, such structured tools (see, e.g. Calder et al., 2012) are increasingly being used at an interagency level, and more research is required to assess their effectiveness.

The management of neglect is almost always challenging. In the more severe cases, action is likely to be mandated by social work services or the courts. In less severe cases, management may be led by primary care. In many cases the parent will not be aware of the impact of their unavailability on the child, and in these circumstances a good deal of work with the family over time is likely to be required.

Problems in parenting

There is strong and high-quality evidence that the quality of parenting received by children is one of the strongest predictors of future mental and physical health (Marmot et al., 2010; Kelly et al., 2011; Allely et al., 2013; Marwick et al., 2013; Puckering et al., 2014). Furthermore, several options for parenting interventions with moderate- to high-quality strength of evidence are available to health professionals to support parents in providing more sensitive and consistent care, leading to better outcomes for their children (Olds et al., 1998; Bakermans-Kranenburg, 2003; Hutchings et al., 2007). It would therefore be useful for clinicians to develop the skills to evaluate the quality of parenting, although it is notable that health professionals have demonstrated some reluctance to commit themselves in writing to an assessment that there is a problem in the parent–child relationship (C. Wilson et al., 2012). At present there are few structured methods for assessing parenting that lend themselves to use in routine practice, although several methods with low to moderate quality and strength of evidence can be used to assess parenting behaviours in video recordings (Crittenden, 2001; Puckering et al., 2014). In general, there is moderately strong evidence that untrained, but experienced, professionals make judgements about parent–child interactions that have a degree of consistency (P. Wilson et al., 2008b, 2010) but this is an area that requires further development. A possibly under-exploited environment in which to observe parent and child in a routinely stressful situation—and thus observe attachment behaviours—is the immunization clinic (Pritchett et al., 2012). One particular problem with current practice is that assumptions about vulnerability and risk among more middle-class parents (particularly mothers) can lead to lost opportunities to build a trusting therapeutic relationship with their health visitor, when an assumption of 'good enough parenting' may act as a barrier to offers of appropriate support (King, 2016a).

Primary care clinicians tend to be more confident in assessing parental mental health (often using structured tools as an aid) than parenting behaviours. In the few moderate-quality studies that have been conducted, parenting behaviours are more strongly predictive of outcomes than maternal depression (Murray et al., 1996). A trusting relationship between a mother and health professional is likely to improve the quality of surveillance in postnatal depression (Davies and Allen, 2007), and there is moderately strong and high-quality evidence of positive health outcomes, particularly in the short and medium term, when clinicians provide psychologically oriented support to women with postnatal depression (Cooper et al., 2003; Murray et al., 2003; Cowley et al., 2013).

How to confirm suspicions

When clinicians are confident that they have identified a developmental problem or problem in parenting, and that they lack the ability to offer appropriate investigations or interventions, they should make appropriate referrals. In many cases, however, there is simply a suspicion that a problem exists. In general, the first step in triangulating such suspicions should be for the clinicians involved to share the different information they have about the family: GPs are more likely to know, for example, about issues in the wider family including fathers, and possibly about parental substance use or mental illness, while health visitors will usually know more about the child's development and home environment. When a child is in school, the school nurse may have useful information. Such discussions can lead to an escalation or a de-escalation of concern. Sometimes discussions with specialist colleagues can be helpful before considering referral. This approach is particularly useful, because it can add to the level of knowledge among primary care clinicians. Finally, sometimes a decision might be made to use structured instruments such as those described in Chapter 22 to explore neurodevelopmental domains or to quantify parental mental health problems (King, 2013).

If the clinician is reasonably confident about identifying a developmental disorder (e.g. language delay), care should be taken to evaluate other potential problems (Gillberg, 2010) before referral. There are dangers, particularly if long waiting lists exist, that children with other important issues may miss opportunities for effective interventions: language delay, for example, is often associated with coordination or neuropsychiatric disorders and referral to a purely speech and language-based service might be inappropriate (Eriksson and Miniscalco, 2010; Gillberg, 2010).

Conclusion

Raising concerns with parents is undoubtedly easiest when there is a pre-existing clinical relationship, and engagement in ongoing work is much easier when a clinician has already earned the trust of the family. In cases where families or particular groups have seemed resistant to engaging with services, the onus should be on the practitioner and their service to offer non-stigmatizing and culturally appropriate support (Almond and Lathlean, 2011), and to evaluate the reasons why services are not being taken up equally by all families. This work is difficult given the daily challenges of limited clinical time and service resources, but early opportunistic detection of remediable problems and sensitive discussion between clinician and families will lead to later benefits for both families and service providers, as well as to reduced health inequalities.

Learning links

♦ Safeguarding Children Toolkit for General Practice: http://www.rcgp.org.uk/clinical-and-research/toolkits/the-rcgp-nspcc-safeguarding-children-toolkit-for-general-practice.aspx.

Recommendations

♦ Consider inclusion of knowledge of basic developmental milestones, attachment and parenting behaviours, and of use of common assessment tools as well as refinement of observational skills for assessing parent–child interaction in training of primary care professionals. (*Evidence: moderate.*)

♦ Consider putting systems in place to monitor professional continuity of care for families with young children, as well as the amount of time available for clinical encounters. (*Evidence: moderate.*)

♦ Ensure timely communication between all primary care healthcare professionals where there is any concern about a child's well-being. Regular primary care team meetings, to include at least a GP, health visitor, and practice nurse and/or nurse practitioner, should take place to facilitate this communication and formulate plans for ongoing work with children. (*Evidence: strong.*)

References

Allely, C., Johnson, P., Marwick, H., et al. (2013). Prediction of 7-year psychopathology from mother-infant joint attention behaviours: a nested case-control study. *BMC Pediatrics*, **13**, 147.

Almond, J. and Lathlean, J. (2011). Inequity in provision of and access to health visiting postnatal depression services. *Journal of Advanced Nursing*, **67**, 2350–2362.

Axford, N., Lehtonen, M., Kaoukji, D., Tobin, K., and Berry, V. (2012). Engaging parents in parenting programs: lessons from research and practice. *Children and Youth Services Review*, **34**, 2061–2071.

Bakermans-Kranenburg, M.J. (2003). Less is more: meta-analyses of sensitivity and attachment interventions in early childhood. *Psychological Bulletin*, **129**, 195–215.

Barlow, J., Kirkpatrick, S., Stewart-Brown, S., and Davis, H. (2005). Hard-to-reach or out-of-reach? Reasons why women refuse to take part in early interventions. *Children & Society*, **19**, 199–210.

Barry, S.J.E., Marryat, L., Thompson, L., et al. (2015). Mapping area variability in social and behavioural difficulties among Glasgow pre-schoolers: linkage of a survey of pre-school staff with routine monitoring data. *Child: Care, Health and Development*, **41**, 853–864.

Bidmead, C. (2013). Health visitor/parent relationships: a qualitative analysis. In: Cowley, S., Whittaker, K., Grigulis, A., et al. (Eds.), *Why Health Visiting? A Review of the Literature about Key Health Visitor Interventions, Processes and Outcomes for Children and Families*, Appendix. London: National Nursing Research Unit, King's College London.

Calder, M.C., McKinnon, M., and Sneddon, R. (2012). *National Risk Framework to Support the Assessment of Children and Young People*. Edinburgh: Scottish Government. Available at: http://www.gov.scot/resource/0040/00408604.pdf.

Condon, L. (2011). Health visitors' experiences of child health promotion policy reform in England. *Community Practice*, **84**, 25–28.

Cooper, P.J., Murray, L., Wilson, A., and Romaniuk, H. (2003). Controlled trial of the short- and long-term effect of psychological treatment of post-partum depression. I. Impact on maternal mood. *British Journal of Psychiatry*, **182**, 412–419.

Cortis, N. (2012). Overlooked and under-served? Promoting service use and engagement among 'hard-to-reach' populations. *International Journal of Social Welfare*, **21**, 351–360.

Cowley, S., Mitcheson, J., and Houston, A.M. (2004). Structuring health needs assessments: the medicalisation of health visiting. *Sociology of Health and Illness*, **26**, 503–526.

Cowley, S., Whittaker, K., Grigulis, A., et al. (2013). *Why Health Visiting? A Review of the Literature about Key Health Visitor Interventions, Processes and Outcomes for Children and Families*. Department of Health Policy Research Programme, ref. 016 0058. London: National Nursing Research Unit, Kings College London. Available at: http://www.kcl.ac.uk/nursing/research/nnru/publications/Reports/Why-Health-Visiting-NNRU-report-12-02-2013.pdf.

Cowley, S., Whittaker, K., Malone, M., Donetto, S., Grigulis, A., and Maben, J. (2015). Why health visiting? Examining the potential public health benefits from health visiting practice within a universal service: a narrative review of the literature. *International Journal of Nursing Studies*, **52**, 465–480.

Crittenden, P. (2001). *CARE-Index Infant and Toddlers. Coding Manual*. Miami, FL: Family Relations Institute.

Daniel, B. (2010). Concepts of adversity, risk, vulnerability and resilience: a discussion in the context of the 'child protection system'. *Social Policy & Society*, **9**, 231–241.

Davies, B. and Allen, D. (2007). Integrating 'mental illness' and 'motherhood': the positive use of surveillance by health professionals. A qualitative study. *International Journal of Nursing Studies*, **44**, 365–376.

Donetto, S., Malone, M., Hughes, J., Morrow, E., Cowley, S., and Maben, J. (2013). *Health Visiting: The Voice of Service Users – Learning from Service Users' Experiences to Inform the Development of UK Health Visiting Practice and Services.* London: National Nursing Research Unit, King's College London. Available at: http://www.kcl.ac.uk/nursing/research/ nnru/publications/Reports/Voice-of-service-user-report-July-2013-FINAL.pdf.

Duvnjak, A. and Fraser, H. (2013). Targeting the 'hard to reach': re/producing stigma? *Critical and Radical Social Work*, **12**, 167–182.

Eriksson, M.W., Westerlund, M, and Miniscalco, C. (2010). Problems and limitations in studies on screening for language delay. *Research in Developmental Disabilities*, **31**, 943–950.

Gillberg, C. (2010). The ESSENCE in child psychiatry: Early Symptomatic Syndromes Eliciting Neurodevelopmental Clinical Examinations. *Research in Developmental Disabilities*, **31**, 1543–1551.

Greenhalgh, T. (2002). Intuition and evidence – uneasy bedfellows? *British Journal of General Practice*, **52**, 395–400.

Growing Up in Scotland (2010). What parents say about children's health and professional support findings from Growing Up in Scotland. [online] Scottish Government. Available at: http:// growingupinscotland.org.uk/wp-content/uploads/2013/04/GUSforHealthVisitors.pdf.

Hogg, R. and Worth, A. (2009). What support do parents of young children need? A user-focused study. *Community Practice*, **82**, 31–34.

Hogg, R., Kennedy, C., Gray, C., and Hanley, J. (2013). Supporting the case for 'progressive universalism' in health visiting: Scottish mothers and health visitors' perspectives on targeting and rationing health visiting services, with a focus on the Lothian Child Concern Model. *Journal of Clinical Nursing*, **22**, 240–250.

Hølge-Hazelton, B. and Tulinius, C. (2010). Beyond the specific child What is 'a child's case' in general practice? *British Journal of General Practice*, **60**, e4–e9.

Hutchings, J., Gardner, F., Bywater, T., et al. (2007). Parenting intervention in Sure Start services for children at risk of developing conduct disorder: pragmatic randomised controlled trial. *BMJ*, **334**, 678–685.

Jack, S.M., Dicenso, A., and Lohfeld, L. (2005). A theory of maternal engagement with public health nurses and family visitors. *Journal of Advanced Nursing*, **49**, 182–190.

Kelly, Y., Sacker, A., Del Bono, E., Francesconi, M., and Marmot, M. (2011). What role for the home learning environment and parenting in reducing the socioeconomic gradient in child development? Findings from the Millennium Cohort Study. *Archives of Disease in Childhood*, **96**, 832–837.

King, C. (2013). From normality to risk: a qualitative exploration of health visiting and mothering practices following the implementation of Health for all Children. [online] Edinburgh Research Archive. Available at: https://www.era.lib.ed.ac.uk/handle/1842/8198.

King, C. (2015). Health visitors' accounts of the impacts of 'Hall 4' on their practice and profession: a qualitative study. *Community Practice*, **88**, 24–27.

King, C. (2016a). 'It depends what you class as vulnerable': risk discourse and the framing of vulnerability in health visiting policy and practice. *Families, Relationships and Societies*, **7**, 39–54.

King, C. (2016b). 'Sticking to carpets' – assessment and judgement in health visiting practice in an era of risk: a qualitative study. *Journal of Clinical Nursing*, **25**, 1901–1911.

Ling, M.S. and Luker, K.A. (2000). Protecting children: intuition and awareness in the work of health visitors. *Journal of Advanced Nursing*, **32**, 572–579.

Marmot, M., Allen, J., Goldblatt, P., et al. (2010). *Fair Society, Healthy Lives: The Strategic Review of Health Inequalities in England post-2010.* London: Institute of Health Equity.

Marwick, H., Doolin, O., Allely, C.S., et al. (2013). Predictors of diagnosis of child psychiatric disorder in adult/infant social-communicative interaction at 12 months. *Research in Developmental Disabilities*, **34**, 562–572.

McConnachie, A., Wilson, P., Thomson, H., et al. (2004). Modelling consultation rates in infancy: influence of maternal and infant characteristics, feeding type and consultation history. *British Journal of General Practice*, **54**, 598–603.

McLaughlin, A., Espie, C., and Minnis, H. (2010). Development of a brief waiting room observation for behaviours typical of reactive attachment disorder. *Child and Adolescent Mental Health*, **15**, 73–79.

Mitcheson, J. and Cowley, S. (2003). Empowerment or control? An analysis of the extent to which client participation is enabled during health visitor/client interactions using a structured health needs assessment tool. *International Journal of Nursing Studies*, **40**, 413–426.

Murray, L., Cooper, P.J., Wilson, A., and Romaniuk, H. (2003). Controlled trial of the short- and long-term effect of psychological treatment of post-partum depression: 2. Impact on the mother-child relationship and child outcome. *British Journal of Psychiatry*, **182**, 420–427.

Murray, L., Hipwell, A., Hooper, R., Stein, A., and Cooper, P. (1996). The cognitive development of 5-year-old children of postnatally depressed mothers. *Journal of Child Psychology & Psychiatry & Allied Disciplines*, **37**, 927–935.

Olds, D., Henderson, C.R., Jr., Cole, R., et al. (1998). Long-term effects of nurse home visitation on children's criminal and antisocial behavior: 15-year follow-up of a randomized controlled trial. *JAMA*, **280**, 1238–1244.

Peckover, S. (2002a). Focusing upon children and men in situations of domestic violence: an analysis of the gendered nature of British health visiting. *Health & Social Care in the Community*, **10**, 254–261.

Peckover, S. (2002b). Supporting and policing mothers: an analysis of the disciplinary practices of health visiting. *Journal of Advanced Nursing*, **38**, 369–377.

Peckover, S. (2013). From 'public health' to 'safeguarding children': British health visiting in policy, practice and research. *Children & Society*, **27**, 116–126.

Pickles, A., Le Couteur, A., Leadbitter, K., et al. (2016). Parent-mediated social communication therapy for young children with autism (PACT): long-term follow-up of a randomised controlled trial. *The Lancet*, **388**, 2501–2509.

Pritchard, J.E. (2005). Strengthening women's health visiting work with women. *Journal of Advanced Nursing*, **51**, 236–244.

Pritchett, R., Minnis, H., Puckering, C., Rajendran, G., and Wilson, P. (2012). Can behaviour during immunisation be used to identify attachment patterns? A feasibility study. *International Journal of Nursing Studies*, **50**, 386–391.

Puckering, C., Allely, C., Doolin, O., et al. (2014). Association between parent-infant interactions in infancy and disruptive behaviour disorders at age seven: a nested, case-control ALSPAC study. *BMC Pediatrics*, **14**, 223.

Royal College of General Practitioners and the National Society for the Prevention of Cruelty to Children (2014). Safeguarding Children and Young People: The RCGP/NSPCC Safeguarding Children Toolkit for General Practice. [online] Available at: http://www.rcgp.org.uk/clinical-and-research/toolkits/the-rcgp-nspcc-safeguarding-children-toolkit-for-general-practice.aspx.

Scottish Executive Health Department. (2005). *Health for all Children 4: Guidance to implementation in Scotland 2005*. Edinburgh, HMSO. Available at: http://www.scotland.gov.uk/Publications/2005/04/15161325/13269.

Shepherd, M.L. (2011). Behind the scales: child and family health nurses taking care of women's emotional wellbeing. *Contemporary Nurse*, **37**, 137–148.

Sim, F., O'Dowd, J., Thompson, L., et al. (2013). Language and social/emotional problems identified at a universal developmental assessment at 30 months. *BMC Pediatrics*, **13**, 206.

Thompson, L., McConnachie, A., and **Wilson, P.** (2012). A universal 30-month child health assessment focussed on social and emotional development. *Journal of Nursing Education and Practice*, **13**, 13–22.

Whittaker, K. and **Cowley, S.** (2012). An effective programme is not enough: a review of factors associated with poor attendance and engagement with parenting support programmes. *Children & Society*, **26**, 138–149.

Wilson, C., Hogg, R., Henderson, M., and **Wilson, P.** (2013). Patterns of primary care service use by families with young children. *Family Practice*, **30**, 679–694.

Wilson, C., Thompson, L., McConnachie, A., and **Wilson, P.** (2012). Matching parenting support needs to service provision in a universal 13-month child health surveillance visit. *Child: Care, Health & Development*, **38**, 665–674.

Wilson, P. and **Mullin, A.** (2010). Child neglect: what has it to do with general practice? *British Journal of General Practice*, **60**, 5–6.

Wilson, P., Barbour, R., Furnivall, J., et al. (2008a). The work of health visitors and school nurses with children with emotional, behavioural and psychological problems: findings from a Scottish Needs Assessment. *Journal of Advanced Nursing*, **61**, 445–455.

Wilson, P., Barbour, R., Graham, C., Currie, M., Puckering, C., and **Minnis, H.** (2008b). Health visitors' assessments of parent-child relationships: a focus group study. *International Journal of Nursing Studies*, **45**, 1137–1147.

Wilson, P., McQuaige, F., Thompson, L., and **McConnachie, A.** (2013). Language delay is not predictable from available risk factors. *The ScientificWorld Journal*, **2013**, Art. ID 947018.

Wilson, P., Minnis, H., Puckering, C., and **Gillberg, C.** (2009). Should we aspire to screen preschool children for conduct disorder? *Archives of Disease in Childhood*, **94**, 812–816.

Wilson, P., Thompson, L., McConnachie, A., et al. (2010). Parent-child relationships: are health visitors' judgements reliable? *Community Practitioner*, **83**, 22–25.

Winnicott, D.W. (1973). *The Child, the Family, and the Outside World*. London: Penguin.

Wood, R. and **Wilson, P.** (2012). General practitioner provision of preventive child health care: analysis of routine consultation data. *BMC Family Practice*, **13**, 73.

Wright, C.M., Jeffrey, S.K., Ross, M.K., Wallis, L., and **Wood, R.** (2009). Targeting health visitor care: lessons from Starting Well. *Archives of Disease in Childhood*, **94**, 23–27.

Zeanah, C.H., Smyke, A.T., and **Dumitrescu, A.** (2002). Attachment disturbances in young children. II: Indiscriminate behavior and instiutional care. *Journal of the American Academy of Child & Adolescent Psychiatry*, **41**, 983–989.

Section 5

Children with additional needs and children in special circumstances

Chapter 24

Supporting children with developmental disorders and disabilities

Alan Emond and James Law

Summary

This chapter:

- summarizes the importance of early identification of developmental disorders and reviews the evidence for early intervention

- explains how assessment by a multidisciplinary child development team should lead to the provision of family-friendly services coordinated by a lead professional

- discusses how children require packages of care, provided through Education, Health and Care Plans/Child Plans to optimize learning. To meet families' needs for information, family support, and respite, coordinated packages need to be commissioned from health and social care, education, and the voluntary sector.

The value of early identification

Early identification of children with an atypical or disordered pattern of development, or with significant impairments likely to result in disability, is important to:

- provide a diagnosis if possible, or a clear formulation of the child's strengths and difficulties, for the family

- investigate the cause—especially genetic abnormalities, which may affect future pregnancies

- initiate therapeutic interventions from a multidisciplinary child development team

- prevent secondary problems for the child (e.g. behaviour issues arising out of frustration)

- provide information about services and benefits to parents and carers

- coordinate service planning with early years services to facilitate access to nursery and preschool education.

If a developmental concern is identified in primary care, whether following a developmental review as part of a child health programme, or opportunistically from responding to a parent's concerns, it is important that the family can be promptly referred for assessment. Practitioners working with preschool children need to know to whom and where to refer: it helps if there is an agreed referral pathway with recommended timescales for the child to be seen at different stages. A good example is the National Autism Plan (National Autistic Society, 2003), which has standards for the initial general multidisciplinary developmental assessment, and a specialist multiagency assessment. The standard for the timescale is that the assessment should be completed and feedback given to the family within 17 weeks from referral to the multiagency assessment team.

Children born preterm are at particular risk of developmental delay and often show atypical developmental patterns. The National Institute for Health and Care Excellence (NICE) guideline NG72 (2017a) is a useful resource on the follow-up of preterm infants once they leave neonatal services, with recommended good practice on the early identification of developmental difficulties.

Initial assessment

A 'single point of entry' for referrals to a child development service can make it easier and simpler for different professionals (general practitioners, health visitors, and school nurses) to refer for assessment, and also allows effective 'triage' of referrals and allocation to appropriate members of the child development service (paediatricians, physiotherapists, occupational therapists, and speech and language therapists) for initial assessment. A single point of entry system also facilitates audit, and assists in resource allocation.

A child development service includes specialist services for assessment and management of children with disabilities including physical, learning, hearing, vision, speech, and language problems. There are different models of providing this: some services are based in child development centres, while others are community based and work out of children's centres, clinics, and on home visits. Whatever the structure of the service, communication between team members and with parents and referrers is always the key challenge. There should be a single information base to support such a team, whose work will be made most efficient within a unified management structure.

Assessment of a child must be undertaken in partnership with parents, and result in a written report and sharing information with parents and professionals. The assessment should lead to an action plan which is agreed with parents and a process for coordinating treatment. One professional in the child development service should take on the role of lead professional in order to provide a single point of contact and coordination for the family's care package. (In Scotland, the concept of the lead professional has been broadened to include universal services, with the recommended lead professional for preschool children being the health visitor, and for school-aged children, the school nurse.)

Parent support groups are an essential component of the service. A selection of useful charities and support groups is included at the end of this chapter. There should be special support for ethnic and cultural minorities, and the use of link workers can help put explanations of a child's difficulties in the family's cultural context.

Family-friendly services

Family-centred services are those where there is a genuine partnership between parents and service providers, so that parents are involved in every aspect of services for their child. Services which are accessible and offer a partnership approach where parents are involved in decision-making result in improved parent satisfaction, decreased parental stress, and improvement in child outcomes. Some underlying principles of family-friendly services are illustrated in Box 24.1

Box 24.1 Key features of family-friendly services

- Each family should have the opportunity to decide the level of involvement they wish in decision-making for their child.
- Parents should have ultimate responsibility for the care of their children.
- Each family member should be treated with respect (as individuals).
- The needs of all family members should be considered.
- The involvement of all family members should be encouraged.

Adapted from Rosenbaum, P *et al.*, Family-Centred Service: A Conceptual Framework and Research Review, *Physical and Occupational Therapy in Pediatrics*, Volume 18, Issue 1, p. 6, Copyright © 1998. Reprinted with permission from Taylor and Francis Ltd, http://www.tandfonline.com.

The factor having the strongest association with parental satisfaction is information exchange, followed by respectful and supportive care, and partnership/enabling (King et al., 1999). Parents value receiving their services from the same location, and from a multidisciplinary team that they know. For parents whose children have complex developmental disabilities, it is particularly important for their services to be coordinated and available from fewer locations. A useful tool for assessing the degree to which services are family friendly is the Measures of Processes of Care (MOPC). This validated 20-item self-report scale captures parents' perceptions of the health services they and their children are receiving. Originally developed in Canada, it has been adapted and shown to be a useful tool in UK settings (McConachie and Logan, 2003).

To be family friendly, services need to be flexible to provide individualized care, that is, children and families should receive flexible provision according to their requirements. Effective intervention for young children with disabilities also requires that joint working is coordinated between all the practitioners involved and the family. Families should be fully involved through the lead professional in creating management plans for their child, monitoring the effects of interventions, and attending regular reviews (see Box 24.2).

The lead professional role addresses the two most important aspects of family-friendly services: the provision of information and the coordination of services. It does

Box 24.2 Role of lead professional

◆ Act as the main point of contact for the child and family: to provide information, engage them in making choices, and help them navigate their way through the system.

◆ Coordinate the actions agreed as the outcome of the assessment: to ensure the delivery of integrated services to children and families according to a written care plan.

◆ Organize reviews involving the family and practitioners: to ensure action plans are implemented and to identify any unmet or additional needs for the child.

Source: data from Children's Workforce Development Council (CWDC), *Coordinating and delivering integrated service for children and young people. The Team Around the Child (TAC) and the lead professional. A guide for practitioners.* CWDC, Leeds, UK, Copyright © Children's Workforce Development Council 2009.

not include some of the wider roles of the 'key worker' concept, for example, provision of emotional support, identifying and addressing needs of all family members, speaking on behalf of the family when dealing with services, and provision of support in a crisis. To achieve these wider benefits, dedicated key workers are required, with adequate training and systems in place for support and supervision, and these usually need joint funding from health and social care.

A further extension to family-centred care is the Team Around the Child (TAC), an approach that facilitates best practice in joint working for families of children with the most complex needs. The TAC approach enables the child's key practitioners and parent/s to collaborate with each other as equal partners to achieve 'collective competence' as a team (Limbrick, 2007). This model can be time-consuming, and can only realistically be achieved for a few children with very complex needs, but in the long run, care packages are implemented more effectively and outcomes can be improved.

Relationships of child development teams with the family's primary care team, and also with hospital and tertiary specialist services, are important and should be actively managed to achieve efficiency and good communication. Joint clinics (e.g. with paediatric neurology or orthopaedics) can improve communication and planning, and reduce the number of appointments. Families with a disabled child want easy access to a wide range of therapeutic and support services without multiple assessments.

Joint agency working

When planning packages of care, it is important to look at the needs of the family as a whole as well as those of the child as an individual. This is best done by health, social services, and education departments in collaboration. To support children with disabilities and their families, health services, social care, and education services need to work cooperatively and, ideally, with shared budgets.

Wherever practicable, professionals from different agencies or disciplines should undertake joint assessments in order to minimize the number of assessments of the child and family, and to improve joint working. The Children and Families Act 2014 in England and Wales introduced the concept of Education, Health, and Care (EHC) plans as a new way of promoting joint agency working with families of children with special educational needs and disabilities (SEND). The SEND code of practice (Department for Education, 2001; Association of School and College Leaders, 2015), revised in 2015, requires health services in England to work with local authorities to provide a coordinated service for children with special educational needs, and clarifies the role of health practitioners, early years workers, and special educational needs coordinators (SENCOs). Where it is decided to provide special educational needs support, the practitioners and the SENCO should agree, in consultation with the parent, the outcomes they are seeking, the interventions, and the support to be put in place. This EHC plan has to be reviewed annually. Children in receipt of an EHC plan can be entitled to personal budgets.

The implementation of the EHC plans is proceeding at different rates across England. The aim was to transfer all children with a statement of special needs, or in receipt of early years support action plus or school action plus, onto an EHC plan by 2018. The early experience has been that only the more disabled children are receiving EHC plans, fewer than previously had statements of special needs.

Training in the use of the EHC plans and the role of health practitioners in the SEND process is provided by the National Children's Bureau (Council for Disabled Children, 2017).

Guidance from the Department of Health (2016) on the commissioning of packages of care for children with complex health needs is provided in the *National Framework for Children and Young People's Continuing Care.*

To enable planning from the earliest stage, clinical commissioning groups are required by the Children and Families Act 2014 to notify local authorities of children who they believe have special educational needs or who will go on to develop special educational needs.

In Scotland, The Children and Young People (Scotland) Act 2014 (Scottish government, 2014) ensures a single planning framework—a Child's Plan—will be available for children who require extra support that is not generally available to address a child's or young person's needs and improve their well-being. The Child's Plan is part of the Getting it Right for Every Child (GIRFEC) approach to promote, support, and safeguard the well-being of children and young people (Gov.scot, 2017). Good practice is described in 'Supporting Children's Learning Code of Practice' (Gov.scot, 2010).

In Wales, departments across the Welsh Government are working together to develop an early years framework (Gov.wales, 2016) to support a consistent national approach to the assessment, tracking, and monitoring of children's developmental progress, from birth to age 7.

Respite

Respite care is short-term substitute care for children with significant disabilities, and is provided by someone other than parents or the usual carers of the child. It should form part of a support package based on the particular needs of individual children and their families. Assessment of need and provision of respite is usually the responsibility of social services. However, organizing respite services for children with complex healthcare needs will require health and social services to cooperate. Regular support can be paid for by direct payments from personal budgets, short respite breaks can be funded by social services disability teams, and some local authorities run a Family Link scheme, whereby families develop a relationship with a family with a child with special needs, and offer short-term respite for an hour or two or even overnight. Information for local authorities on how to provide short break care to disabled children is provided online (Gov.uk, 2011).

Care packages

Efficient processes should be in place for obtaining agreement about and funding for unusual or expensive packages of care, placements, or equipment. Guidance is given in the *National Framework for Children and Young People's Continuing Care*, (Department of Health, 2016) which describes the process of agreeing individual continuing care packages for children whose needs cannot be met by existing specialist services. The Framework is not prescriptive about what should be provided, but sets out the principles, timelines, and stages of assessing and arranging a package of care. An Assessment Tool Kit aids identification of continuing care needs, a Decision Support Tool aims to help local decision-making, and an exemplar care pathway is based on the Association for Children's Palliative Care core care pathway for children and young people with life-threatening or life-limiting conditions and their families (Togetherforshortlives, 2013).

Moving

It is important that there is prompt transfer of information and care when a child moves or professionals involved change. This is particularly important for children who are 'looked after' or are part of a travelling family. Efficient transfer of community child health records (immunization details, special educational needs, and medical history), primary care records, and specialist services information is needed, as well as referral to appropriate specialists. Personal Child Health Records and copies of professional letters and reports assist rapid information transfer and encourage full involvement of parents in their child's care (see Chapter 29).

Sharing of information

Parents value the providing of information about their child's condition as a crucial feature of family-friendly services. Health professionals also need to share information about an individual child to allow other services to fulfil their duties and to facilitate smooth inter-agency working, for example, for those with special educational needs, 'looked after' children, child protection investigations, and children with complex needs. Parents should receive copies of all reports and correspondence. Parents' permission (and where appropriate the child's assent) should be obtained for all interventions, but this is not essential if the child is thought to be at risk of significant harm. The child's welfare is paramount.

Rarely, a parent's concerns about a child's development are not confirmed by the specialist assessment. To avoid over-investigation, and to prevent emotional abuse and neglect of children, clinicians need to follow guidelines on fabricated and induced illnesses (NICE, 2009).

Evidence-based early interventions in children with developmental disorders

It is outside the scope of this review to systematically review and critically appraise all the evidence supporting early interventions in children with developmental conditions. In recent years, both NICE and the Scottish Intercollegiate Guidelines Network (SIGN) have published evidence-based guidelines on identification and management of many developmental conditions. For detailed information on what works and recommended good practice, commissioners of the child health programme and practitioners are referred to the guidance and assets available on the websites: http://www.nice.org.uk and http://www.sign.ac.uk. SIGN guideline recommendations are now available in an app, for use on mobile devices and tablets.

Learning difficulty/disability

A learning disability has an onset in early childhood, and is defined as a low intellectual ability (usually an IQ below 70 (less than two standard deviation units below the mean)), with significant impairment of social or adaptive functioning. Learning difficulties are a common feature of many developmental disorders (e.g. autistic spectrum conditions (ASC)) and genetic conditions (e.g. Down syndrome). Children presenting in the preschool period with atypical development and with delayed cognitive attainments need to be assessed by a multidisciplinary child development team, and supportive interventions at home and at nursery made available.

Many young children with significant learning impairments present with challenging behaviour which is regarded as age inappropriate. NICE guideline NG11 (2015) on intellectual disability with challenging behaviour recommends preschool classroom-based interventions for children aged 3–5 years with emerging behaviour that challenges.

Autism spectrum conditions

NICE (2011) clinical guideline CG128 on autism in children and young people recommends that services for children with autism should be provided through local, specialist, community-based, multidisciplinary teams. A range of interventions are available to minimize the impact of the core difficulties in young children with ASC (Kendall et al., 2013). Communication can be helped by providing visual supports as pictures or symbols which are meaningful to the child, for example, the Picture Exchange Communication System (PECS) (Pyramid Educational Consultants, 2017), a widely used UK-based functional communication system that develops communication and social skills in preschool children with autism. To help with the social communication difficulties in young children with ASC, NICE recommends play-based strategies (adjusted to the child's developmental level) with parents, carers, and teachers to increase joint attention, engagement, and reciprocal communication.

Parent-mediated inventions in ASC were subject to a Cochrane review (Oono et al., 2013) which identified six small studies of parent interventions with child assessment outcome measures. A random effects meta-analysis suggested an overall effect of intervention compared with control in terms of reducing autism symptom severity.

The evidence base for effectiveness of interventions for challenging behaviour and sleep disturbance in young children with ASC is weak, and although NICE makes sensible recommendations for helping parents manage children with these difficulties, most are based on clinical experience and expert group opinion (Kendall et al., 2013).

Attention deficit hyperactivity disorder

Although the core symptoms of attention deficit hyperactivity disorder (ADHD) are often apparent from an early age, to support a diagnosis, the symptoms of inattention, overactivity, and impulsiveness must be age inappropriate, persistent, and pervasive. NICE guideline NG72 (2017a) recommends that if a young child's behavioural problems are having an adverse impact on their development or family life, parents should be offered a parent training/education programme in the first instance. These are reviewed in Chapter 10. If the problems persist, referral to a secondary care clinician (child and adolescent mental health services or paediatrics) with expertise in diagnosis should be made.

Diagnosis of ADHD in the early years must be based on a detailed clinical history with reporting of symptoms by different carers, made by experienced clinicians with a good understanding of the wide ranges of normal child development, reinforced by good observations of the child's behaviour in different settings (home and nursery). Co-occurring conditions, such as autistic spectrum difficulties, need to be considered, and the mental health of the parents carefully assessed. Following the diagnosis of ADHD in a child of preschool age, the child's nursery should be contacted to explain the diagnosis and severity of impairment, and the care plan, and to highlight any special educational needs identified (Kendall et al., 2008).

All young children with ADHD should avoid caffeine-containing drinks. Removal of food colourings may be helpful in ADHD patients with food sensitivities. If there appears to be a link between specific foods and ADHD symptoms, then parents should be asked to keep a diary of food and drinks taken and ADHD behaviour. If the diary supports a relationship between specific foods and behaviour, then referral to a dietician is recommended. There is some weak evidence that free fatty acid supplementation (omega 3 and/or 6) may have small beneficial effects on ADHD symptoms (Sonuga-Barke et al., 2013), but these treatments are not supported by NICE.

Most ADHD guidelines do not recommend the use of medication before the age of 6 years (Taylor et al., 2004; Kendall et al., 2008). The prescription and monitoring of pharmacological medication for ADHD should be under the supervision of trained specialists, although shared care for repeat prescriptions can be cost-effective and convenient for parents.

Motor disabilities

Cerebral palsy (CP) is a heterogeneous condition, and age at diagnosis and referral to specialist child development teams varies widely. All children with delayed motor milestones (e.g. not sitting by 8 months, not walking by 18 months—corrected for gestational age), or infants showing early asymmetry of hand function before 1 year corrected, should be referred to a child development service for further assessment.

Early interventions in infants at high risk of CP (e.g. extreme preterms, those recovering from birth asphyxia) show more benefit on cognitive skills than motor development. In general, the effect of developmental programmes on motor development is small and does not persist beyond infancy. A comprehensive review (Hadders-Algra, 2014) concluded that virtually no evidence is available on the effect of early intervention in infants developing CP, as the studies available are underpowered or suffered from overlap in the contents of intervention in study and control groups. In children with established CP, an individual goal-direct approach appears most beneficial. NICE clinical guideline CG85 (2012) provides clear advice on management of spasticity, and NICE guideline NG62 (2017b) contains evidence-based advice on managing common problems in CP such as feeding, drooling, constipation, and sleeping.

Once a diagnosis of CP is made, families should be encouraged from an early age to use assistive devices such as adaptive seating to promote upright sitting, computer tablets to encourage communication, and power mobility to promote exploration of the environment. The assistive devices may promote the child's social and cognitive development, and more evidence on the effect of the assistive devices is needed.

Developmental coordination disorder (DCD), also known as dyspraxia, is a condition affecting physical coordination that causes a child to perform less well than expected in daily activities for his or her age, and impacts on educational attainment. Although usually not diagnosed until after the age of 5 years, children with DCD often show delayed early motor milestones and are late in demonstrating hand preference. Immature skills in activities of daily living (such as feeding and dressing) or delay in fine motor skills (such as writing and drawing) are often the reason for referral. Because of the overlap between DCD and other developmental traits such as social communication difficulties, children suspected of the condition should be referred to a paediatrician for a holistic developmental assessment and to an occupational therapist for evaluation of motor skills. Children can be helped by adaptive cutlery and pens, and benefit from an understanding by family and teachers that they need more time and encouragement to complete motor tasks. Evidence for the sustained benefit of early intervention to improve motor coordination is weak, but children and families value interventions to improve participation. Morgan and Long (2012) reported that parents wanted interventions that enabled their child to participate regularly in his or her chosen motor activities within the community and which created social participation opportunities. Children also valued their ability to engage in self-care and play activities. Interventions in early years settings for children based on play include 'animal fun' (Piek et al., 2015).

Developmental speech and language disorders

It is estimated that approximately 5–8% of children may have speech and/or language impairment (Boyle et al., 1996; Tomblin et al., 1997), of which a significant proportion will have primary speech and/or language disorders. Prevalence estimates for boys are higher than for girls, 8% and 6% respectively (Nelson et al., 2006). Most recent UK prevalence estimates come from a screening of 7267 4–5-year-old children in Surrey, indicating a population prevalence estimate of language disorder of 9.9%. The prevalence of language disorder of unknown origin was estimated to be 7.6%, while the prevalence of language impairment associated with intellectual disability and/or existing medical diagnosis was 2.3% (Norbury et al., 2016).

In the UK, approximately 85,000–90,000 children aged 2–6 years old are referred to speech and language therapists each year (Broomfield and Dodd, 2004), and 18–31% of children aged 19–21 months from a disadvantaged community have been found to have language delay that warrants referral for specialist assessment (Pickstone, 2003). This figure would normally be of the order of 10–16%.

There have been a number of systematic reviews of the evidence underpinning interventions for these children through randomized control trials and quasi-experimental studies (Law et al., 1998, 2003, 2017). The broad picture is that children with low language skills are commonly identified in the second or third year of life. Initially, interventions tend to focus around promoting the interaction between parent and child: for example, raising the parent's awareness of communication skills and what can be done to promote them, or increasing the amount of interaction and turn taking (Roberts and Kaiser, 2011). Interventions commonly emphasize the development of vocabulary skills (Marulis and Neuman, 2010) and then, depending on the profile of need, may focus on phonological awareness and pre-reading skills, on narrative (story telling) skills, and in the case of children with speech difficulties, on the development of expressive phonology and motor control over the speech apparatus (Dodd, 2013). For some children, the principal difficulties are associated with underdeveloped grammatical and morphological skills, relative to age-matched peers (Ebbels, 2013). Increasingly, children's needs are met within the context of the classroom.

Systematic reviews suggest interventions may be effective for a number of areas of speech and language, including expressive, phonology, and pragmatic language. The picture remains less clear for interventions targeting a child's receptive language or verbal comprehension. Intervention has been shown to be effective, in the short term at least, from preschool and throughout the school years; however, a majority of studies focus on intervention in the early years. A child's socio-economic status may impact the effectiveness of intervention (greater impact for higher socio-economic status children). This leads us to question whether despite their effectiveness, are interventions enough to sufficiently 'close the gap' between high and low achievers? A striking finding from systematic reviews is the substantial impact of indirect approaches on children's language skills. This creates a case for widening the range of practitioners able to identify difficulties and administer intervention, considering the contribution of parents and primary care workers such as health visitors and nursery staff, or teachers.

Developmental speech and language disorders are commonly associated with high levels of co-morbidity whether in terms of related sensory, developmental, or educational difficulties. Clinicians in child development teams may be asked to assess children with ADHD or ASC and speech and language difficulties may be a feature of the child's profile. Thus it is important to be aware of the need to ensure that the child's communication skills are assessed less in absolute terms (very few children do not speak at all) but relative to their peers. If children are under the care of a multidisciplinary child development team, their histories will have been well documented and they should have been comprehensively observed, so the assessment may be relatively straightforward. However, in practice, many children with developmental speech and language disorders are not referred to such teams and the primary source of specialist support will be the speech and language therapist. The key to meeting the needs of these children is a combination of parental report and careful observation of the child's communicative behaviours in the context of sound knowledge of what to expect of children at different developmental stages. How parents perceive the needs of their child is central to the management of the child's needs (Roulstone et al., 2015).

Learning links

- e-Learning for Healthcare course—'HCP 06: Development and Behaviour': https://portal.e-lfh.org.uk
- SEND training at Council for Disabled Children: https://councilfordisabledchildren.org.uk.

Support helplines for parents

- Contact a Family helpline:
  - Email: helpline@cafamily.org.uk
  - Telephone: 0808 808 3555.
- Independent Parental Special Education Advice (IPSEA) advice line: telephone: 0800 018 4016.

Useful websites

- The ADHD Foundation: http://www.adhdfoundation.org.uk/
- AFASIC: https://www.afasic.org.uk/
- Child Autism UK: http://www.childautism.org.uk/
- DCD: http://dyspraxiafoundation.org.uk/
- Down's Syndrome Society: http://www.downs-syndrome.org.uk/
- ICAN: http://www.ican.org.uk/

- Mencap: https://www.mencap.org.uk/
- Movement Matters: http://www.movementmattersuk.org/
- National Autistic Society: www.nas.org.uk/
- Scope: https://www.scope.org.uk/
- The Communication Trust: https://www.thecommunicationtrust.org.uk/
- UKAP—the UK ADHD partnership: www.ukadhd.com/.

Recommendations

- All professionals working with preschool children need to have a good understanding of child development, and be able to distinguish atypical patterns of development from developmental delay. (*Evidence: strong.*)
- Children causing parents and professionals concern about their developmental progress should be referred for assessment by a multidisciplinary child development service, as many developmental traits and disorders overlap, and have associated co-morbid conditions. (*Evidence: strong.*)
- Close involvement with parents is needed through a nominated lead professional, paying attention to their expectations and actively involving them in decision-making. (*Good practice.*)
- Services to support children with disabilities should be family centred, and commissioners should ensure that providers regularly evaluate parent satisfaction with the service. (*Evidence: moderate.*)
- Where possible, interventions can be delivered directly through parents, once they have been provided with training by specialist practitioners. (*Evidence: moderate.*)
- It is important that those working directly with young children with developmental disabilities in health, education, and social services sectors work closely together to ensure that children are provided with the best opportunities. (*Evidence: strong.*)
- Children with additional needs should be supported by a multi-agency plan (EHC plan/child's plan). (*Evidence: strong.*)

References

Association of School and College Leaders (2015). Summary of Special Education Needs (SEN) Code of Practice. [online] Available at: https://www.ascl.org.uk/download. E808B657-D080-4DE5-A3445A3F5751A309.html [Accessed 25 Sep. 2017].

Boyle, J., Gillham, B., and **Smith, N.** (1996). Screening for early language delay in the 18–36-month age-range: the predictive validity of tests of production and implications for practice. *Child Language Teaching and Therapy,* **12**, 113–127.

Broomfield, J. and Dodd, B. (2004). Children with speech and language disability: caseload characteristics. *International Journal of Language and Communication Disorders*, **39**, 303–324.

Council for Disabled Children (2017). Homepage. [online] Available at: https://councilfordisabledchildren.org.uk/ [Accessed 25 Sep. 2017].

Department for Education. (2001). Special Educational Needs Code of Practice. DfES/581/2001 [online]. Available from https://www.gov.uk/government/uploads/system/uploads/attachment_data/file/273877/special_educational_needs_code_of_practice.pdf [Accessed 20 Sep. 2016].

Department of Health (2016). *National Framework for Children and Young People's Continuing Care*. Gateway reference 13509. London: Department of Health.

Dodd, B. (2013). *Differential Diagnosis and Treatment of Children with Speech Disorder*. London: Whurr Publishers.

Ebbels, S. (2013). Effectiveness of intervention for grammar in school-aged children with primary language impairments: a review of the evidence. *Child Language Teaching and Therapy*, **30**, 7–40.

Gov.scot (2010). Supporting children's learning code of practice (revised edition). [online] Available at: http://www.gov.scot/Publications/2011/04/04090720/0 [Accessed 25 Sep. 2017].

Gov.scot (2017). Getting it right for every child (GIRFEC). [online] Available at: http://www.gov.scot/Topics/People/Young-People/gettingitright [Accessed 25 Sep. 2017].

Gov.uk (2011). Short break care: how local authorities should provide it. [online] Available at: https://www.gov.uk/government/publications/short-breaks-for-carers-of-disabled-children [Accessed 25 Sep. 2017].

Gov.wales (2016). Healthy Child Wales Programme. [online] Available at: http://gov.wales/topics/health/publications/health/reports/healthy-child/?lang=en [Accessed 25 Sep. 2017].

Hadders-Algra, M. (2014). Early diagnosis and early intervention in cerebral palsy. *Frontiers in Neurology*, **5**, 185.

Kendall, T., Megnin-Viggars, O., Gould, N., Taylor, C., Burt, L.C., and Baird, G. (2013). Management of autism in children and young people: summary of NICE and SIGN guidance. *BMJ*, **347**, f4865.

Kendall, T., Taylor, E., Perez, A., and Taylor, C. (2008). Guidelines: diagnosis and management of attention-deficit/hyperactivity disorder in children, young people, and adults: summary of NICE guidance. *BMJ*, **337**, 751–753.

King, G., King, S., Rosenbaum, P., and Goffin, R. (1999). Family-centred caregiving and well-being of parents of children with disabilities: linking process with outcome. *Journal of Pediatric Psychology*, **24**, 41–53.

Law, J., Boyle, J., Harris, F., Harkness, A., and Nye, C. (1998). Screening for speech and language delay: a systematic review of the literature. Executive Summary. *Health Technology Assessment*, **2**, 9.

Law, J., Garrett, Z., and Nye, C. (2003). Speech and language therapy interventions for children with primary speech and language delay or disorder. *Cochrane Database of Systematic Reviews*, **3**, CD004110.

Law, J., Charlton, J., Dockrell, J., Gascoigne, M., McKean, C., and Theakston, A. (2017). *Early Language Development: Needs, Provision and Intervention for Preschool Children from Socio-Economically Disadvantage Backgrounds*. London: Education Endowment Foundation.

Limbrick, P. (Ed.) (2017). *Family-Centred Support for Children with Disabilities and Special Needs: A Collection of Essays*. Herefordshire: Interconnections.

Marulis, L.M. and Neuman, B. (2010). The effects of vocabulary intervention on young children's word learning: a meta-analysis. *Review of Educational Research*, **80**, 300–335.

McConachie, H. and Logan, S. (2003). Validation of the measure of processes of care for use when there is no Child Development Centre. *Child: Care, Health and Development*, **29**, 35–45.

Morgan, R. and Long, T. (2012). The effectiveness of occupational therapy intervention for children with developmental coordination disorder: review of the qualitative literature. *British Journal of Occupational Therapy*, **75**, 10–18.

National Autistic Society (2003). *National Autism Plan for Children*. London: National Autistic Society.

National Institute for Health and Care Excellence (NICE) (2009). Child maltreatment: when to suspect maltreatment in under 18s. Clinical guideline [CG89] (Last updated Oct. 2017). [online] Available at: https://www.nice.org.uk/guidance/cg89.

National Institute for Health and Care Excellence (NICE) (2011). Autism spectrum disorder in under 19s: recognition, referral and diagnosis. Clinical guideline [CG128] (Last updated Dec. 2017). [online] Available at: https://www.nice.org.uk/guidance/cg128.

National Institute for Health and Care Excellence (NICE) (2012). Spasticity in under 19s: management. Clinical guideline [CG145] (Last updated Nov. 2016). [online] Available at: https://www.nice.org.uk/guidance/cg145.

National Institute for Health and Care Excellence (NICE) (2015). Challenging behaviour and learning disabilities: prevention and interventions for people with learning disabilities whose behaviour challenges. Guideline [NG11]. [online] Available at: https://www.nice.org.uk/guidance/ng11.

National Institute for Health and Care Excellence (NICE) (2017a). Developmental follow-up of children and young people born preterm. Guideline [NG72]. [online] Available at: https://www.nice.org.uk/guidance/ng72.

National Institute for Health and Care Excellence (NICE) (2017b). Cerebral palsy in under 25s: assessment and management. Guideline [NG62]. [online] Available at: https://www.nice.org.uk/guidance/ng62.

Nelson, H.D., Nygren, P., Walker, M., and Panoscha, R. (2006). Screening for speech and language delay in preschool children: systematic evidence review for the US Preventive Services Task Force. *Pediatrics*, **117**, e298–e319.

Norbury, C.F., Gooch, D., Wray, C., et al. (2016). The impact of nonverbal ability on prevalence and clinical presentation of language disorder: evidence from a population study. *Journal of Child Psychology and Psychiatry*, **57**, 1247–1257.

Oono, I.P., Honey, E.J., and McConachie, H. (2013). Parent-mediated early intervention for young children with autism spectrum disorders (ASD). *Cochrane Database of Systematic Reviews*, **4**, CD009774.

Pickstone, C. (2003). A pilot study of paraprofessional screening of child language in community settings. *Child Language Teaching and Therapy*, **19**, 49–65.

Piek, J.P., Kane, R., Rigoli, D., et al. (2015). Does the Animal Fun program improve social-emotional and behavioural outcomes in children aged 4-6 years? *Human Movement Science*, **43**, 155–163.

Pyramid Educational Consultants (2017). Picture Exchange Communication System (PECS)˚. [online] Available at: http://www.pecs.com [Accessed 25 Sep. 2017].

Roberts, M. and Kaiser, A. (2011). The effectiveness of parent-implemented language interventions: a meta-analysis. *American Journal of Speech-Language Pathology*, **20**, 180–199.

Roulstone, S.E., Marshall, J.E., Powell, G.G., et al. (2015). *Evidence-Based Intervention for Preschool Children with Primary Speech and Language Impairments: Child Talk—An Exploratory Mixed-Methods Study.* Southampton: NIHR Journals Library. Available at: https://www.ncbi.nlm.nih.gov/books/NBK311174/.

Scottish government (2014). The Children & Young People (Scotland) Act. [online] CYPCS. Available at: https://www.cypcs.org.uk/policy/children-young-people-scotland-act [Accessed 25 Sep. 2017].

Sonuga-Barke, E.J.S., Brandeis, D., Cortese, S., et al. (2013). **European ADHD Guidelines Group.** Nonpharmacological interventions for ADHD: systematic review and meta-analyses of randomized controlled trials of dietary and psychological treatments. *American Journal of Psychiatry*, **170**, 275–289.

Taylor, E., Döpfner, M., Sergeant, J., et al. (2004). European clinical guidelines for hyperkinetic disorder: first upgrade. *European Child and Adolescent Psychiatry*, **13**(Suppl 1), I7–I30.

Togetherforshortlives (2013). Core Care Pathway. [online] Available at: https://www. togetherforshortlives.org.uk/resource/core-care-pathway/ [Accessed 25 Sep. 2017].

Tomblin, J.B., Smith, E., and Zhang, X.Y. (1997). Epidemiology of specific language impairment: prenatal and perinatal risk factors. *Journal of Communication Disorders*, **30**, 325–344.

Chapter 25

Safeguarding

Alison M. Kemp

Summary

This chapter:

- discusses the epidemiology and definitions of child abuse and neglect

- addresses the roles and responsibilities of healthcare practitioners in safeguarding children, with a focus on child protection and the prevention of child maltreatment

- summarizes the legal framework for child protection in the UK

- provides signposting to resources for practitioners, managers, and commissioners.

The chapter should be read in conjunction with guidance from the National Institute for Health and Care Excellence (NICE), 'Child maltreatment: when to suspect maltreatment in under 18s' (NICE, 2009). For a more in-depth understanding of child protection, the reader is referred to the Royal College of Paediatrics and Child Health (RCPCH) online resource on child protection evidence (RCPCH, 2016).

Introduction and definitions

'Whilst local authorities play a lead role, safeguarding children and protecting them from harm is everyone's responsibility. Everyone who comes into contact with children and families has a role to play.' (Gov.uk, 2015)

Box 25.1 outlines the definitions of child abuse and neglect taken from the UK Government guidance 'Working Together to Safeguard Children' (Gov.uk, 2015). While distinct categories are defined, there is considerable overlap between the nature and types of abuse that individual children may experience.

While domestic abuse (DA) is not included within these definitions, the NSPCC recognize that 'Domestic abuse can seriously harm children and young people. Witnessing domestic abuse is child abuse, and teenagers can suffer domestic abuse in their relationships'. DA is an incident or series of incidents of abusive behaviour used by one person to control and dominate another. Most DA is experienced by women and is generally perpetrated by a partner or ex-partner and ranges from verbal abuse, intimidation, and isolation, to serious physical and sexual assault, and homicide.

Box 25.1 Definitions of child abuse and neglect

Physical abuse: may involve hitting, shaking, throwing, poisoning, burning or scalding, drowning, suffocating, or otherwise causing physical harm to a child. Physical harm may also be caused when a parent or carer fabricates the symptoms of, or deliberately induces, illness in a child.

Sexual abuse: forcing or enticing a child or young person to take part in sexual activities, not necessarily involving a high level of violence, whether or not the child is aware of what is happening. The activities may involve physical contact, including assault by penetration (e.g. rape or oral sex) or non-penetrative acts such as masturbation, kissing, rubbing, and touching outside of clothing. They may also include non-contact activities, such as involving children in looking at, or in the production of, sexual images, watching sexual activities, encouraging children to behave in sexually inappropriate ways, or grooming a child in preparation for abuse (including via the internet). Sexual abuse is not solely perpetrated by adult males. Women can also commit acts of sexual abuse, as can other children.

Emotional abuse: the persistent emotional maltreatment of a child such as to cause severe and persistent adverse effects on the child's emotional development. It may involve conveying to a child that they are worthless or unloved, inadequate, or valued only insofar as they meet the needs of another person. It may include not giving the child opportunities to express their views, deliberately silencing them, or 'making fun' of what they say or how they communicate. It may feature age or developmentally inappropriate expectations being imposed on children. These may include interactions that are beyond a child's developmental capability, as well as overprotection and limitation of exploration and learning, or preventing the child participating in normal social interaction. It may involve seeing or hearing the ill treatment of another. It may involve serious bullying (including cyber bullying), causing children frequently to feel frightened or in danger, or the exploitation or corruption of children. Some level of emotional abuse is involved in all types of maltreatment of a child, though it may occur alone.

Neglect: the persistent failure to meet a child's basic physical and/or psychological needs, likely to result in the serious impairment of the child's health or development. Neglect may occur during pregnancy as a result of maternal substance abuse. Once a child is born, neglect may involve a parent or carer failing to:

♦ provide adequate food, clothing, and shelter (including exclusion from home or abandonment)

♦ protect a child from physical and emotional harm or danger

♦ ensure adequate supervision (including the use of inadequate caregivers)

♦ ensure access to appropriate medical care or treatment.

It may also include neglect of, or unresponsiveness to, a child's basic emotional needs (emotional neglect).

Adapted from HM Government, *Working together to safeguard children: A guide to interagency working to safeguard and promote the welfare of children*, © Crown copyright 2017, under the Open Government Licence v3.0, available from https://www.gov.uk/government/uploads/system/uploads/attachment_data/file/592101/Working_Together_to_Safeguard_Children_20170213.pdf.

One of the most recent and burgeoning forms of child abuse happens online. The NSPCC use the following working definition for online abuse—the use of technology to manipulate, exploit, coerce or intimidate a child to (but not limited to): engage in sexual activity; produce sexual material/content; force children to look at or watch sexual activities; encourage a child to behave in a sexually inappropriate way or groom a child in preparation for sexual abuse (either online or off line). It can involve directing others, or coordinating the abuse of children online. As with other forms of sexual abuse, online abuse can be misunderstood by the child and others as being consensual, occurring without the child's immediate recognition or understanding of abusive or exploitative conduct. The fear of what might happen if they do not comply can also be a significant influencing factor.

While a number of these issues may involve adolescents, children are accessing the internet at an increasingly young age. Practitioners who are primarily involved with pre-school children have the opportunity to work within the family home and may become aware of issues in older members of sibling groups.

Child maltreatment is a rapidly changing field and practitioners must be aware of issues such as child trafficking, modern slavery, female genital mutilation, online grooming and abuse, 'organizational' abuse, and emotional abuse presenting as 'spiritual' abuse. In addition, there are the safeguarding needs of vulnerable children who may have disabilities. The *Safeguarding Disabled Children* (Murray and Osbourne, 2009) practice guidance recognizes that disabled children have additional needs caused by barriers, impairments, and heightened vulnerability and sets out possible indicators of abuse and neglect. Families who fail to engage with healthcare workers, children who are looked after, refugees and asylum seekers, and the issues of forced marriage and 'honour-based' violence must also be considered.

Child safeguarding legislation

Between 1989 and 2015, a series of Children's Acts have provided a framework of child safeguarding legislation for England (gov.uk, 2015) and Wales (gov.wales, 2006); The Children (Northern Ireland) Order 1995 (NSPCC, 2017a) and the Children (Scotland) Act 1995 and 2014 (2014) share the same principles. Statutory guidance (National Guidance for Child Protection in Scotland, 2014) sets out the framework to promote the welfare of children and to protect them from harm. Child protection is devolved; each nation has its own guidance on interagency working aiming to protect children from maltreatment, preventing impairment of children's health or development, ensuring that children are growing up in circumstances in which care is safe and effective; enabling children to have optimum life chances and to enter adulthood successfully. Safeguarding is the underpinning philosophy of all child health programmes. For definitions, see Box 25.2.

The legislation brings all local government functions of children's welfare and education under the statutory authority of local directors of children's services. They determine the jurisdiction of and the approach to decision-making about children's welfare by the courts, and establish the responsibilities of public agencies (e.g. NHS) to deliver safeguarding services for children and young people under 18 years of age.

Box 25.2 Safeguarding terminology and definitions

Children in need: a child who is unlikely to achieve or maintain a reasonable level of health or development, or whose health and development is likely to be significantly or further impaired, without the provision of services; or a child who is disabled.

In Scotland, The Children and Young People (Scotland) Act 2014 is about improving the well-being of children and young people in Scotland. The Act is wide ranging and includes key parts of the 'Getting it Right for Every Child' approach, commonly known as GIRFEC (Gov.scot, 2017). GIRFEC is the national approach to improving outcomes and supporting the well-being of children and young people by offering the right help at the right time from the right people. It includes guidance on corporate parenting and looked after children.

Child in need status has ceased to exist in Wales following the Social Services and Well-being (Wales) Act (2014) that came into force in 2016. Children in need has been replaced by a duty on the local authority to assess a child who appears to need care and support in addition to, or instead of, the care and support provided by their family

Child protection is part of safeguarding and denotes the protection of children who have suffered from or are likely to suffer significant harm, defined as 'ill treatment or the impairment of health or development' determined by comparing the child's health and development with what could reasonably be expected from a similar child' and reaching a threshold that justifies compulsory intervention in family life in the best interests of children, and gives local authorities a duty to make enquiries to decide whether they should take action to safeguard or promote the welfare of a child who is suffering or likely to suffer significant harm.

Source: data from HM Government, *Working together to safeguard children: A guide to inter-agency working to safeguard and promote the welfare of children*, © Crown copyright 2017, available from https://www.gov.uk/government/uploads/system/uploads/attachment_data/file/592101/Working_Together_to_Safeguard_Children_20170213.pdf. Contains public sector information licensed under the Open Government Licence v3.0.

Within the UK, the safeguarding principals are reinforced further within the United Nations Convention on the Rights of the Child (Unicef UK, 2017) ratified in the UK in 1991. Article 19 states that all children have a right to be protected from 'all forms of physical or mental violence, injury or abuse, neglect or negligent treatment, maltreatment or exploitation including sexual abuse, while in the care of parent(s), legal guardian(s) or any other person who has care of the child'.

Duty to report maltreatment

While, with the exception of female genital mutilation, reporting suspicion of maltreatment is not mandated in the UK, all health professionals have a duty to report any suspicion of maltreatment to the local authority children's social care to ensure early recognition and intervention to protect children. Although there is no legal requirement to report in England and Wales, there are specific guidelines and procedures in place for people who work with children. Scotland's national guidance for child protection refers to 'collective responsibilities' to protect children. In Northern Ireland, it is an offence not to report an arrestable offence, including those against children, to the police.

The size of the problem

It is impossible to know the full extent of maltreatment in children in the UK. Estimates are based upon low-quality evidence, provided from the cases that are identified or from surveys of the life experiences of young people. In short, the problem is considerable. National government statistics (NSPCC, 2017b) estimate that 57,345 children were subject to a child protection plan or on a child protection register in 2015. This amounted to 49,690 in England, 2751 in Scotland, 2935 in Wales, and 1969 in Northern Ireland. These figures have increased over the past 5 years with surges in online child abuse.

The World Health Organization (WHO) 'European Report on Preventing Maltreatment' (2013) combined a number of international community surveys and gave the following estimated prevalence of maltreatment in childhood: physical abuse, 22.9%; emotional abuse, 29.1%; physical neglect, 16.3%; emotional neglect, 18.4%; and sexual abuse, 13.4% in girls and 5.7% in boys. The NSPCC (2016) provides an analysis of the statistics related to child maltreatment across the UK. The key findings are set out in Table 25.1

Roles and responsibilities of health professionals

'Working Together to Safeguard Children' in England (Gov.uk, 2015) and Wales recognizes that 'Health professionals are in a strong position to identify welfare needs or safeguarding concerns regarding individual children and, where appropriate, provide support'. Northern Ireland (Department of Health, 2017) has a similar document. The Scottish Government has produced specific guidance for health professionals, NHS services, and health boards (National Guidance for Child Protection in Scotland, 2014). The child protection role extends to all of those who work directly with children and families and there are clear standards for safeguarding within all healthcare organizations (see Boxes 25.3 and 25.4). Within health boards, these standards are led and maintained at a senior level.

Safeguarding training: all healthcare professionals who work with children must have the appropriate competences to recognize child maltreatment and its consequences and to take effective action as appropriate to their role. It is the duty of employers to ensure that those working for them have the appropriate levels of training (see Box 25.4).

In 2014, the third edition of the inter-collegiate document 'Safeguarding children and young people: roles and competencies for healthcare staff' (RCPCH, 2014) was published. The document lists the six levels of competencies expected of staff working in the NHS. It lists clearly which level each type of healthcare

Table 25.1 The increasing burden of child maltreatment in the UK

Police-recorded child sexual offences (2010/2011–2014/2015)	Increased significantly across all four nations in the UK, from a 48% increase in Wales to 80% rise in England
Police-recorded offences of cruelty and neglect (2010/2011–2014/2015)	Increased, in every nation apart from Scotland—up 60% in Northern Ireland, up 48% in Wales, and up 46% in England.
Number of children subject to a child protection plan or on a child protection register (2010/2011–2014/2015)	Increased by 24% across the UK
Number of children becoming looked after due to neglect or abuse (2010/2011–2014/2015)	Increased by 11% in Wales and 17% in England. In Scotland, numbers have stabilized since 2012, with a decrease of 83 (<1%) in 2016 from 2015
Self-reported abuse and neglect and family violence	18.6% of 11–17-year-olds and 25.3% of 18–24-year-olds surveyed describe a lifetime exposure to abuse or neglect. 19.8% and 27.8% respectively described lifetime exposure to family violence
Online offences against children	Since 2010/2011, there has been a 134% increase in recorded offences of this kind in England, a 184% increase in Wales, a 292% increase in Northern Ireland, and a 168% increase in Scotland ChildLine counselling about sexting has increased by 15% since 2014
Child trafficking	The National Crime Agency estimated 732 children were trafficked in 2014, an increase of 22% on the previous year. 38% were from Asia, 28% from Europe, and 27% from Africa
Mortality	In 2014/2015, there were 75 child homicides and in 2014, 42 deaths from assault or undetermined cause across the UK. These figures have declined steadily over the past 30 years

Source: data from Bentley H et al., *How safe are our children? The most compressive overview of child protection in the UK 2016*, NSPCC, London, UK, Copyright © 2016 NSPCC, available from https://www.nspcc.org.uk/globalassets/documents/research-reports/how-safe-children-2016-report.pdf.

professional needs and sets out a clear syllabus of core competencies, skills, knowledge, attitudes, and values that are required at each level together with criteria for assessment. General practitioners, health visitors, and paediatricians are all expected to have level 3 training and competencies. Training can be provided in a flexible manner, encompassing different learning styles and opportunities and should be updated on a 3-yearly basis. Online training packages are signposted in the 'Learning links' box at the end of this chapter.

Box 25.3 Roles in safeguarding for healthcare professionals within their job description

- To recognize children in need of support and/or safeguarding, and parents who may need extra help in bringing up their children.
- To contribute to enquiries about a child and family.
- To assess the needs of children and contribute to an assessment of the capacity of parents to meet their children's needs.
- To plan and provide support to vulnerable children and families.
- To participate in child protection conferences.
- To plan support for children at risk of significant harm.
- To provide therapeutic help to abused children and parents under stress (e.g. mental illness).
- To play a part, through the child protection plan, in safeguarding children from significant harm; and contributing to case reviews.
- To provide reports and police statements if requested.
- To present evidence in court as a professional witness to fact within family and/ or criminal courts if required.

Adapted from HM Government, *Working together to safeguard children: A guide to inter-agency working to safeguard and promote the welfare of children*, © Crown copyright 2017, under the Open Government Licence v3.0, available from https://www.gov.uk/government/uploads/system/uploads/attachment_data/file/592101/Working_Together_to_Safeguard_Children_20170213.pdf.

Box 25.4 Level of safeguarding training expected of different tiers of healthcare professionals

- Level 1: all staff including non-clinical managers and staff working in healthcare settings.
- Level 2: minimum level required for non-clinical and clinical staff who have some degree of contact with children and young people and/or parents/carers.
- Level 3: clinical staff working with children, young people, and their parents/carers and who could potentially contribute to assessing, planning, intervening, and evaluating the needs of a child or young person and parenting capacity where there are safeguarding/child protection concerns.
- Level 4: named professionals (in Scotland—paediatrician with a special interest in child protection).
- Level 5: designated professionals (in Scotland—lead paediatrician for child protection).

Adapted with permission from *Safeguarding Children and Young People: Roles and Competences for Health Care Staff, Intercollegiate Document, Third edition*, Copyright © March 2014. Published by the Royal College of Paediatrics and Child Health 2014 on behalf of the contributing organisations (see pdf) available from https://www.rcpch.ac.uk/resources/safeguarding-children-young-people-roles-competences-healthcare-staff. This document is being revised and an update is planned for 2019.

Recognizing child maltreatment

The consequences of maltreatment are profound and often have lifelong effects. Studies published in the US (Felitti et al., 1998) were the first to identify a series of adverse childhood experiences (ACEs) that include maltreatment and the magnitude of their consequences in later life (Anda et al., 2006). See Box 25.5.

Surveys from Europe, Australia, New Zealand, and the US, and more recently within the UK (Bellis et al., 2014b), all confirm that the larger the numbers of ACEs that an individual experiences, the greater the increase in their risks of adverse future health and well-being outcomes.

Representative population surveys in England (Bellis et al., 2014a) and Wales (Public Health Wales, 2015) confirmed that an estimated 46–47% of adults surveyed had experienced at least one ACE before the age of 18 years and 8.3% in England and 14% in Wales had experienced four or more ACEs. There is growing evidence that these experiences early in childhood are associated with later health-harming behaviours (drug and alcohol abuse, risky sexual behaviour), victimization, violence, poor educational outcomes, crime (Dregan and Gulliford, 2012), future physical illness (cancers, diabetes), and mental health problems in adulthood (Felitti et al., 1998). A systematic review of health consequences of ACEs that included 42 studies (Kalmakis and Chandler, 2015) adds scientific weight to these findings, but does raise caution when generalizing results that are predominantly based upon self-report. Most published literature addresses the consequences in adulthood and does not explore the evolution of the consequences of ACEs throughout childhood or factors that promote resilience.

Exposure to ACEs can impair brain development and development of the nervous and hormonal systems (Danese and McEwen, 2012). This results in vulnerability to ill health in children who maintain a chronic level of stress and high state of anxiety, alertness, and fear of further emotional of physical trauma. Post-traumatic stress disorder has been reported as a consequence of abuse in up to 25% of children who have

Box 25.5 Adverse childhood experiences

◆ All forms of child abuse and neglect (physical, sexual, and emotional abuse, physical and emotional neglect).

◆ Inter-personal violence.

◆ Household alcohol or drug abuse.

◆ Household mental illness.

◆ Criminality and incarceration in the household.

◆ Parental separation or divorce.

Source: data from Robert F Anda *et al.*, 'The enduring effects of abuse and related adverse experiences in childhood. A convergence of evidence from neurobiology and epidemiology,' *European Archives of Psychiatry and Clinical Neuroscience*, Volume 256, Issue 3, pp. 174–186, Copyright © 2006 Steinkopff-Verlag. https://doi.org/10.1007/s00406-005-0624-4.

been abused (Widom et al., 2007). Consequent adverse health-seeking behaviours together with learnt experiences in those who have suffered from ACEs increase the risk of repeating the cycle of abuse in the future generation.

These findings from research confirm the profound lifelong consequences of maltreatment in childhood, and emphasize the importance of early recognition and intervention to prevent ACEs and the long-term adverse effects on health and well-being. Comparative analyses of children who have not experienced ACEs reassure us that 'Stable and protective childhoods are critical factors in the development of resilience to health-harming behaviors' (Bellis et al., 2014a).

Prevention of child maltreatment

The three approaches to prevention of maltreatment require participation from healthcare professionals. Primary prevention relies upon an understanding of the risk factors and triggers for maltreatment and universal prevention programmes, directed at the general population with the aim of preventing maltreatment before it occurs. Secondary prevention requires early recognition of children at risk of maltreatment and early child protection intervention with the family. Tertiary prevention reduces harmful impacts when child maltreatment has occurred.

The WHO 'European Report on Preventing Maltreatment' (2013) sets out an evidence-informed public health approach to the reduction of child maltreatment. The report states clearly that while child protection has long been recognized as a social care and legal responsibility: 'Health systems have a key role not only in providing high-quality services for children who experience violence, but also in detecting and supporting families at risk. The health sector is also best placed to advocate for preventive approaches within an evaluative framework'.

Understanding the risk factors for maltreatment

The WHO report summarizes findings from systematic reviews (Whitaker et al., 2008; Stith et al., 2009) and population studies, informing an understanding of which risk factors are associated with maltreatment and which are preventable, and identifies protective factors. Risk factors are identified according to those that relate to parents, carers, and perpetrators and those that relate to the child, or family interactions. The more risk factors that are present for a child, the greater the risk of maltreatment. Maltreatment is rarely a one-off event and risk factors contribute to persistently abusive environments.

Parental factors

Young or single parents, social isolation, unemployment (Paavilainen et al., 2001), and parents of low socio-economic status or low educational attainment (Sidebotham et al., 2006) have an association with maltreatment. These risks are likely to be related to inexperience, low financial resources, poor cognitive skills, poor social support, and the increased stress levels that ensue (Budd et al., 2000). All can impair optimal parenting (Woodward et al., 2007). Ethnicity and immigrant status have only been shown to be a risk factor in studies based in the US. High socio-economic status has a small protective effect (Stith et al., 2009). These risk factors inform targeted parent preventative interventions (e.g. Family Nurse Partnership, Flying Start, and Triple P).

Individual risk factors in parents

Alcohol and drug abuse (Dube et al., 2001; Bellis et al., 2006) can have lifelong profound effects on the child if taken in pregnancy (e.g. fetal alcohol disorder). Postnatally, they affect a parent's capacity to cope and care, cognitive abilities, and cause disinhibition. If a parent has suffered child abuse as a child, there is an association with perpetration of physical and sexual abuse as a parent. The proposed mechanism by which maltreatment is proliferated across generations is complicated and likely to be related to the association between ACEs and adult health risks, behaviours, and violence. However, not all victims of child abuse go on to abuse their own children.

Maternal mental health issues (e.g. depression, anxiety, and other psychiatric conditions) are recognized ACEs and are strongly associated with maltreatment (Sidebotham et al., 2006), especially fatal cases, and are consistent findings in serious case reviews (Brandon et al., 2012). The associated inconsistent mood swings, indifference, irritability, paranoia, and delusions can all impair the quality of parenting.

Studies of caregivers who have abused their children have identified that they show 'deficits in emotional recognition, and show less warmth, compassion and concern for others and greater anxiety and discomfort from other people's negative experiences' (de Paul et al., 2008). These characteristics make it difficult for parents to recognize and respond to a child's emotional needs appropriately (Asla et al., 2011); they may have unrealistic expectations of behaviour which are often not age appropriate, and emotional responses to children can be inconsistent. These factors can impair the child's emotional development and lead to attachment problems. In a similar manner, parental stress causes anger or hostility that can adversely affect child care and parent–child relationships.

Child factors

Low birthweight, prematurity, and neonatal complications are associated with maltreatment (Sidebotham et al., 2006). These risk factors are often related to perinatal stress and may affect the parents' ability to attach with their child. Children with disabilities are three times more likely to suffer physical or sexual violence and four times more likely to suffer emotional abuse or neglect than non-disabled children (Jones et al., 2012). Disability results in additional stress and extended dependency on parents. The parental stress that ensues, the impaired communication skills enabling children to disclose abuse, and the increased prevalence of institutional care all contribute to increased risks of maltreatment.

Parent–child relationships and family factors

Children of parents who believe in corporal punishment are at a high risk of physical abuse (Akmatov, 2011). Dysfunctional families, those with poor family cohesion (e.g. following divorce), insecure attachment, and intimate partner violence have an association with maltreatment. A UK study of serious child maltreatment identified an association with domestic violence in two-thirds of cases. Negative attitudes towards children and those perceived to be a problem increase the risk of maltreatment, particularly emotional neglect (Stith et al., 2009).

Protective factors

The evidence base behind protective factors is poorly developed. Protective factors include social support, supportive family environment, strong social networks, strong parent–child relationship with secure attachment, and stable parental relationships, and all can modify the likelihood of maltreatment for children living with multiple risk factors. These in turn build parental confidence, self-esteem, and resilience. All characterize good parenting skills, which in turn contribute to the positive emotional development of children. Social support and parental employment provide parents with supportive networks with peers and wider members of society. Social support for teenage mothers has been shown to reduce the risk of maltreatment (Li et al., 2011).

Prevention of maltreatment: what works?

With the profound long-term effects of maltreatment, one could argue that primary prevention has the potential to be more cost-effective than secondary or tertiary prevention. Yet the financial, policy, and legal investment is heavily weighted towards the recognition of the risks of maltreatment and secondary or tertiary interventions. In 2009, Mikton and Butchart published a systematic review of 26 reviews exploring the effect of child maltreatment interventions. The WHO 'European Report on Preventing Maltreatment' (2013) also evaluated the evidence. The findings from these two publications support the following.

Early childhood home interventions

Early childhood home interventions are often targeted at high-risk groups and have been shown to be effective at reducing family risk factors for maltreatment (Mikton and Butchart, 2009). There are limited data on whether they reduced maltreatment events. Great weight has been given to the beneficial effects of the Nurse-Family Partnership reducing child abuse in a 15-year follow-up in the United States (Olds et al., 1997). However, a more recent evaluation of the short-term benefits of the same programme (Family-Nurse Partnership) in England was less persuasive (Robling et al., 2016) (see Chapter 32) The Early Start programme in New Zealand has been well evaluated and shown to reduce child maltreatment (Fergusson et al., 2005).

Parent education programmes

Parent education programmes delivered to groups showed a positive benefit and reduced risk factors for maltreatment; these are reviewed in Chapter 9.

Child sexual abuse prevention programmes

Child sexual abuse prevention programmes are usually based in schools and teach pupils self-protection, how to recognize inappropriate and harmful situations, how to say no, etc. Mikton et al. (2009) concluded that these programmes were effective at promoting knowledge and protective factors but there was limited evidence presented about reduction of sexual abuse. Some studies reported negative factors related to children becoming fearful of touch and anxious about sexual abuse.

Preventing abusive head trauma

Hospital-based interventions with parents of newborn children that included a pledge not to shake the baby have been associated with a 47% reduction in abusive head trauma. The most recent evaluation of this programme in a 'before and after study' suggests that it 'was not associated with a reduction in AHT [paediatric abusive head trauma] hospitalization rates but was associated with improved self-reported parental knowledge that was retained for 7 months' (Dias et al., 2017). The programme has been revised and adopted in parts of the UK, and evaluations are awaited. Other interventions include programmes aimed to manage the baby—these have been shown to increase knowledge about crying and some of the factors that may influence abusive head trauma (Barr et al., 2009).

Corporal punishment

A legal ban on corporal punishment in Sweden failed to reduce the number of deaths or assaults on children; however, it did influence and improve the social attitude towards physical punishment (Durrant et al., 2017).

While there is some evidence to support some community-based interventions more research is required to develop and evaluate interventions that are fit for purpose.

Secondary and tertiary prevention

The key to secondary prevention is to recognize children at risk of maltreatment in order to implement effective interventions early. For the healthcare professional, this relies upon an understanding of the risk factors already discussed and being able to prioritize, target, or access effective interventions and resources for such families. Prevention programmes may be targeted at neighbourhoods that have a high incidence of these risk factors and include local parenting programmes, school-based parenting teaching, parent support groups, more intensive home visiting, and respite for families of children with special needs.

Recognizing maltreatment

In 2009, NICE published evidence and consensus-based guidance around the recognition of child maltreatment. The guidance set out referral pathways for health professionals on the course of action to be taken when they 'consider' or 'suspect' maltreatment. Child health surveillance, and regular and opportunistic points of contact with any healthcare professional provide a framework where safeguarding issues should be considered at each contact.

The health professional may *consider* maltreatment as one possible explanation for the alerting feature or where maltreatment is included in the differential diagnosis. On the other hand, the health professional may *suspect* maltreatment where they have a serious level of concern but not confirmation of maltreatment. All healthcare practitioners should be aware of and act upon the NICE guidance (2009) which stresses the importance of:

♦ listening carefully to the child and parents

♦ recording the history, symptoms, physical signs, and investigation findings carefully and accurately

♦ assessing the child's appearance, demeanour, and interaction with their parent/carer.

A careful evaluation of any explanations for injury is necessary and can raise suspicions of maltreatment where the explanation of a physical injury is absent, implausible, inadequate or inconsistent with the child/young person's age development, medical condition, and normal activities; between parents or carers; between accounts over time; or based upon cultural practices

If the practitioner is *considering* maltreatment, it is advised that they alert and discuss the matter with their line manager and explore the situation more widely, gathering other collateral information and arranging to review the child. When there is a greater level of *suspicion*, then a referral to children's social care is recommended following local child protection procedures.

The guidance provides a comprehensive list of physical features, clinical presentations, behaviours, and parent–child interactions to alert healthcare professions to possible child maltreatment.

This guidance was reviewed in 2014 and it was deemed that there was little new evidence to justify an update.

Evidence-based resources

The Cardiff Child Protection Systematic Review Group has produced a series of systematic reviews (CORE- info) that identify and critically appraise the evidence behind the recognition and investigation of child physical abuse and neglect. This programme of research has been taken over by the RCPCH who are updating the reviews on a regular basis and providing results on their website (RCPCH, 2016).

Together with the NSPCC, the Core-info group have produced a series of leaflets (RCPCH, 2017) derived from the scientific evidence base that highlight the essential features to look out for across various injury types: bruising, burns, fractures, oral injury, head injury, and neglect at different ages. These are useful aide-memoires and teaching resources.

Child Protection Companion: while frontline practitioners are unlikely to be involved in the clinical investigation of children with suspected maltreatment, the investigation strategies and procedures are set out in the second edition of the RCPCH (2013) publication which can be accessed from the RCPCH electronic platform. The document is evidence based where possible and includes many wider child maltreatment related issues. The volume is available on Pediatric Care Online and is updated as new information becomes available.

The Royal College of General Practice (RCGP) toolkit is a series of practical workbooks for GPs and the primary healthcare team to recognize when a child, under the age of 18, may be at risk of abuse. The toolkit (RCGP, 2017) is available for download in PDF format. This second edition provides an update of the evidence-based review and focuses on evidence for the physical signs of child sexual abuse in girls and boys.

Acting upon child maltreatment concerns

If a healthcare professional suspects child maltreatment, they should refer the child to the children's social care team (Gov.uk, 2015). Many areas have established a Multi-Agency Safeguarding Hub (MASH) as a single point of entry for safeguarding referrals where the police, local authorities, and other agencies are co-located and can effectively share information to mitigate the risk of anyone slipping through the safeguarding net.

The level of immediate risk to the child will be assessed and the social care team will decide whether the case meets the statutory threshold to be considered by local authority children's social care for assessment or suggest other sources of more suitable support. This information should be fed back to the healthcare professional.

If there is an immediate risk to the child and other children in the household, an emergency protection order, exclusion order, or child assessment order may be undertaken. The police have the power to remove a child to a place of safety for up to 72 hours without a court order if necessary. Once the immediate safety of the child has been addressed, a strategy discussion between children's social care, the police, and health and other relevant agencies should take place to share information and decide whether a child protection enquiry is needed. If the child is thought to be at risk of significant harm, a case conference will be held where all the relevant agencies and the family share information, identify risks, and outline whether any action should be taken to safeguard and promote the welfare of the child.

If it is deemed necessary to protect the child and siblings, the child will become the subject of a child protection plan (or its equivalent according to devolved child protection procedures). This is a detailed interagency plan setting out what must be done to protect a child from further harm, to promote the child's health and development, and ways to support the family to promote the child's welfare. The child protection plan should clarify the responsibilities of professionals, parents, and agencies and the actions to be taken by whom and when, with reviews to monitor progress. Healthcare professionals can be key participants within a child protection plan and may be requested to undertake further healthcare assessment, monitoring, and medical intervention as required. Health visitors and family nurses have a key role in supporting families of young children who are subject to a child protection plan and supporting those with wider safeguarding needs as participants in child in need reviews, core groups, network meetings, and looked after children reviews.

Learning links

- E-Learning for health have developed an intercollegiate e-learning package: https://www.e-lfh.org.uk/programmes/safeguarding-children/
- The NSPCC have a good online introductory safeguarding course: https://www.nspcc.org.uk/learning
- The RCPCH offers a number of training products in safeguarding children and young people: http://www.rcpch.ac.uk/e-learning.

Recommendations

- Ensure healthcare professionals familiarize themselves with the guidance relevant to child protection issues, national legal frameworks, and statutory requirements of child protection. (*Evidence: strong.*)
- Provide training in safeguarding for healthcare professionals to achieve the competencies that are appropriate to their clinical discipline and level of involvement and contact with children. (*Evidence: moderate.*)
- Practitioners should be competent in working with families to identify children at risk of maltreatment and prevent ACEs. (*Evidence: moderate.*)
- Provider organizations should provide time and training opportunities for all employees working with children to gain the required safeguarding competencies, and ensure there is adequate time and supervision within job plans to enable safeguarding to be undertaken to a high standard across the NHS. (*Evidence: moderate.*)

Acknowledgements

This chapter contains public sector information licensed under the Open Government Licence v3.0.

References

Akmatov, M.K. (2011). Child abuse in 28 developing and transitional countries – results from the multiple indicator cluster surveys. *International Journal of Epidemiology*, **40**, 219–227.

Anda, R.F., Felitti, V.J., and Bremner, J.D. (2006). The enduring effects of abuse and related adverse experiences in childhood. A convergence of evidence from neurobiology and epidemiology. *European Archives of Psychiatry and Clinical Neuroscience*, **256**, 174–186.

Asla, N., de Paul, J., and Perez-Albeniz, A. (2011). Emotion recognition in fathers and mothers at high-risk for child physical abuse. *Child Abuse & Neglect*, **35**, 712–721.

Barr, R.G., Barr, M., Fujiwara, T., et al. (2009). Do educational materials change knowledge and behaviour about crying and shaken baby syndrome? A randomized controlled trial. *CMAJ: Canadian Medical Association Journal*, **180**, 727–733.

Bellis, M.A., Hughes, S., and Hughes, K. (2006). *Child Maltreatment and Alcohol.* Geneva: World Health Organization.

Bellis, M.A., Hughes, K., Leckenby, N., Perkins, C., and Lowey, H. (2014a). National household survey of adverse childhood experiences and their relationship with resilience to health-harming behaviors in England. *BMC Medicine*, **12**, 72.

Bellis, M.A., Lowey, H., Leckenby, N., Hughes, K., and Harrison, D. (2014b). Adverse childhood experiences: retrospective study to determine their impact on adult health behaviours and health outcomes in a UK population. *Journal of Public Health*, **36**, 81–91.

Brandon, M., Sidebotham, P., Bailey, S., and Megson, M. (2012). *New Learning from Serious Case Reviews: A Two Year Report for 2009–2011.* London, Department for Education.

Budd, K.S., Heilman, N.E., and Kane, D. (2000). Psychosocial correlates of child abuse potential in multiply disadvantaged adolescent mothers. *Child Abuse & Neglect*, **24**, 611–625.

Children (Scotland) Act 1995 and 2014 (2014). [online] Available at: http://www.legislation. gov.uk/asp/2014/8/pdfs/asp_20140008_en.pdf [Accessed 2 Oct. 2017].

Danese, A. and McEwen, B. (2012). Adverse childhood experiences, allostasis, allostatic load, and age-related disease. *Physiology and Behavior*, **106**, 29–39.

Department of Health (2017). Co-operating to Safeguard Children and Young People in Northern Ireland. [online] Available at: https://www.health-ni.gov.uk/publications/co-operating-safeguard-children-and-young-people-northern-ireland [Accessed 2 Oct. 2017].

de Paul, J., Pérez-Albéniz, A., Guibert, M., Asla, N., and Ormaechea, A. (2008). Dispositional empathy in neglectful mothers and mothers at high risk for child physical abuse. *Journal of Interpersonal Violence*, **23**, 670–684.

Dias, M.S., Rottmund, C.M., Cappos, K.M., et al. (2017). Association of a postnatal parent education program for abusive head trauma with subsequent pediatric abusive head trauma hospitalization rates. *JAMA Pediatrics*, **71**, 223–229.

Dregan, A. and Gulliford, M.C. (2012). Foster care, residential care and public care placement patterns are associated with adult life trajectories; population-based cohort study. *Social Psychiatry and Psychiatric Epidemiology*, **47**, 1517–1526.

Dube, S.R., Anda, R.F., Felitti, V.J., et al. (2001). Growing up with parental alcohol abuse: exposure to childhood abuse, neglect and household dysfunction. *Child Abuse & Neglect*, **25**, 1627–1640.

Durrant, J.E., Fallon, B., Lefebvre, R., et al. (2017). Defining reasonable force: does it advance child protection? *Child Abuse & Neglect*, **71**, 32–43.

Felitti, V.J., Anda, R.F., Nordenberg, D., et al. (1998). Relationship of childhood abuse and household dysfunction to many of the leading causes of death in adults: the Adverse Childhood Experiences (ACE) Study. *American Journal of Preventive Medicine*, **14**, 245–258.

Gov.scot (2017). What is GIRFEC? [online] Available at: http://www.gov.scot/Topics/People/Young-People/gettingitright/what-is-girfec [Accessed 2 Oct. 2017].

Gov.uk (2015). Working together to safeguard children. [online] Available at: https://www.gov.uk/government/publications/working-together-to-safeguard-children--2 [Accessed 2 Oct. 2017].

Gov.wales (2006). Safeguarding Children – Working Together Under the Children Act 2004. [online] Available at: http://gov.wales/topics/health/publications/socialcare/circular/nafwc1207/?lang=en [Accessed 2 Oct. 2017].

Fergusson, D.M., Grant, H., Horwood, L.J., and Ridder, E.M. (2005). Randomized trial of the Early Start program of home visitation. *Pediatrics*, **116**, e803–e809.

Jones, L., Bellis, M.A., Wood, S., et al. (2012). Prevalence and risk of violence against children with disabilities: a systematic review and meta- analysis of observational studies. *The Lancet*, **380**, 899–907.

Kalmakis, K.A. and Chandler, G.E. (2015). Health consequences of adverse childhood experiences: a systematic review. *Journal of the American Association of Nurse Practitioners*, **27**, 457–465.

Li, F., Godinet, M.T., and Arnsberger, P. (2011). Protective factors among families with children at risk of maltreatment: follow up to early school years. *Children and Youth Services review*, **33**, 139–148.

Mikton, C. and Butchart, A. (2009). Child maltreatment prevention: a systematic review of reviews. *Bulletin of the World Health Organization*, **87**, 353–361.

Murray, M. and Osborne, C. (2009). *Safeguarding Disabled Children: Practice Guidance*. London: Department for Children, Schools and Families.

National Guidance for Child Protection in Scotland (2014). [online] Available at: http://www.cne-siar.gov.uk/childProtectionCommittee/documents/Guidelines2014.pdf [Accessed 10 Sep. 2017].

National Institute for Health and Care Excellence (NICE) (2009). Child maltreatment: when to suspect maltreatment in under 18s. Clinical guideline [CG89]. (Last updated Oct. 2017). [online] Available at: https://www.nice.org.uk/guidance/cg89.

NSPCC (2016). How safe are our children? [online] NSPCC. Available at: https://www.nspcc.org.uk/globalassets/documents/research-reports/how-safe-children-2016-report.pdf [Accessed 2 Oct. 2017].

NSPCC (2017a). Legislation, policy and guidance. [online] Available at: https://www.nspcc.org.uk/preventing-abuse/child-protection-system/northern-ireland/legislation-policy-guidance/ [Accessed 2 Oct. 2017].

NSPCC (2017b). Child protection plan and register statistics: UK 2012–2016. [online] NSPCC. Available at: https://www.nspcc.org.uk/globalassets/documents/statistics-and-information/child-protection-register-statistics-united-kingdom.pdf [Accessed 2 Oct. 2017].

Olds, D.L., Eckenrode, J., Henderson, C.R., et al. (1997). Long-term effects of home visitation on maternal life course and child abuse and neglect: fifteen-year follow-up of a randomized trial. *JAMA*, **278**, 637–643.

Paavilainen, E., Astedt-Kurki, P., Paunonen-Ilmonen, M., and Laippala, P. (2001). Risk factors of child maltreatment within the family: towards a knowledgeable base of family nursing. *International Journal of Nursing Studies*, **38**, 297–303.

Public Health Wales (2015). [online] Adverse childhood experiences and their impact on health-harming behaviours in the Welsh adult population. [online] Available at: http://www.cph.org.uk/wp-content/uploads/2016/01/ACE-Report-FINAL-E.pdf [Accessed 2 Oct. 2017].

Robling, M., Bekkers, M.J., Bell, K., et al. (2016). Effectiveness of a nurse-led intensive home-visitation programme for first-time teenage mothers (Building Blocks): a pragmatic randomised controlled trial. *The Lancet*, **387**, 146–155.

Royal College of General Practitioners (RCGP) (2014). Safeguarding Children Toolkit for General Practice. [online] Available at: http://www.rcgp.org.uk/clinical-and-research/toolkits/the-rcgp-nspcc-safeguarding-children-toolkit-for-general-practice.aspx [Accessed 2 Oct. 2017].

Royal College of Paediatrics and Child Health (RCPCH) (2014). *Safeguarding Children and Young People: Roles and Competences for Health Care Staff*. London: RCPCH. Available at: https://www.rcpch.ac.uk/resources/safeguarding-children-young-people-roles-competences-healthcare-staff [Accessed 2 Oct. 2017].

Royal College of Paediatrics and Child Health (RCPCH) (2016). Child Protection Evidence. [online] Available at: https://www.rcpch.ac.uk/key-topics/child-protection/evidence-reviews [Accessed 2 Oct. 2017].

Royal College of Paediatrics and Child Health (RCPCH) (2017). About the Child Protection Companion. [online] Available at: https://www.rcpch.ac.uk/improving-child-health/child-protection/about-child-protection-companion/about-child-protection-comp [Accessed 2 Oct. 2017].

Sidebotham, P., Heron, J., ALSPAC Study Team (2006). Child maltreatment in the "children of the nineties": a cohort study of risk factors. *Child Abuse & Neglect*, **30**, 497–522.

Social Services and Well-being (Wales) Act (2014). Available at: https://socialcare.wales/hub/sswbact [Accessed 10 Sep. 2017].

Stith, S.M., Liu, T.L., Davies, C., et al. (2009). Risk factors in child maltreatment: a meta-analytic review of the literature. *Aggression and Violent Behavior*, **14**, 13–29.

Unicef UK (2017). UN Convention on the Rights of the Child (UNCRC). [online] Available at: https://www.unicef.org.uk/what-we-do/un-convention-child-rights/ [Accessed 2 Oct. 2017].

Widom, C.S., Dumont, K.A., Czaja, S.J. (2007). A prospective investigation of major depressive disorder and comorbidity in abused and neglected children grown up. *Archives of General Psychiatry*, **64**, 49–56.

Whitaker, D.J., Le, B., Karl Hanson, R., et al. (2008). Risk factors for the perpetration of child sexual abuse: a review and meta-analysis. *Child Abuse & Neglect*, **32**, 529–548.

Woodward, L.J., Fergusson, D.M., Chesney, A., and Horwood, L.J. (2007). Punitive parenting practices of contemporary young parents. *New Zealand Medical Journal*, **120**, U2866.

World Health Organization (2013). European report on preventing child maltreatment. [online] Available at: http://www.euro.who.int/__data/assets/pdf_file/0019/217018/European-Report-on-Preventing-Child-Maltreatment.pdf [Accessed 2 Oct. 2017].

Chapter 26

Gypsy/Traveller, migrant, and refugee children

Louise Condon and Julie Mytton

Summary

This chapter:

- reviews the health needs of children living in special circumstances due to migration or refugee status, or being of Gypsy, Roma, or Traveller ethnicity

- discusses the reasons why children from these groups require focused health promotion, and the factors that influence their ability to access preventive services

- describes interventions to improve their physical and mental health through the child health programmes.

Introduction

There is a lack of data about the health status and needs of all Travellers and migrants. A significant barrier is that routinely collected data may record ethnic group, but not migration variables such as country of birth, length of residence, or immigration status (Jayaweera, 2014). Similarly, there is a lack of data on the health status of Travellers and their children due to the 2011 census categories not being routinely used in health records.

Who are Gypsies/Travellers?

This group includes English, Welsh, and Scottish Gypsies, Irish Travellers, New Age Travellers, Boat People, and Show People (van Cleemput, 2010). Gypsies and Irish Travellers were included as an ethnic group for the first time in the 2011 Census, and 58,000 people (0.1% of the usual resident population of England and Wales) identified themselves as being a 'Gypsy or Irish Traveller'. Numbers responding were limited by factors such as low literacy among respondents.

Gypsies and Irish Travellers are more likely to be aged under 20 years, and almost half of census respondents had dependent children (Office for National Statistics, 2014). Numbers with no qualifications were almost three times higher than for England and

Wales as a whole, and fewer people were economically active. Only a quarter of Gypsy/ Travellers lived in a caravan or other mobile/temporary structure, with the rest living in 'bricks and mortar'. In Scotland's census, 0.1% of the population self-identified as Gypsy/Travellers, and 0.6% in Ireland.

An estimated 10–12 million Roma people (also known as Gypsies, Travellers, Manouches, Ashkali, Sinti, and Boyash) live across Europe, and are the largest ethnic minority in the European Union (EU). They are at risk of discrimination and unequal access to employment, education and health (European Commission, 2017).

Who are migrants?

A migrant is a person born abroad who intends to stay in the country of settlement for at least 1 year (United Nations Statistical Commission, 1998). Migration to the UK has increased since the accession of new member states to the EU in the 2000s. In 2015, approximately 13% of the UK population were foreign born (Migration Observatory, 2017). Currently about a third of UK migrants were born in other EU member states with a fifth from South Asia (India, Pakistan, Bangladesh, and Sri Lanka) (Rutter, 2015).

Most migrants come to the UK to work, with smaller numbers arriving to study or as family migrants. Migrants differ from UK-born workers in being more highly educated, less likely to be unemployed, and younger (Rienzo, 2017). Migrants often live in precarious social and financial circumstances due to low pay, paired with high housing and living costs (Pemberton et al., 2014). Children of migrants are a growing sector of the population, with over a quarter (27.5%) of live births in 2015 being to mothers born outside the UK (Office for National Statistics, 2016).

Who are refugees and asylum seekers?

A refugee has left their homeland due to a fear of persecution for reasons of race, religion, nationality, or membership of a particular social group or political opinion, and has received a positive decision from the authorities on their asylum claim. To become an asylum applicant and be legally recognized as a refugee in Britain, migrants need to be on UK territory. Consequently, many migrants fleeing from war and persecution resort to 'illegal' means to get to Europe, increasing the risk of injury and death.

In 2016, refugees comprised 0.24% of the UK population, with 10% of applications from unaccompanied asylum-seeking children (UASCs) (Refugee Council, 2017a). A UASC is aged under 18 years, not in the care of a responsible adult, and has applied for asylum in their own right. In 2016, only 8% of UASC were less than 14 years old; most child asylum seekers are under 5 years old, and arrive with their parents.

The health of Gypsy, Roma, and Traveller children

Gypsy/Travellers in the UK have poorer health and a higher risk of mortality than other socio-economically matched groups. Levels of anxiety and depression are higher than other ethnic groups as are rates of stillbirth and premature death of offspring (Parry et al., 2007). Despite high health needs, there is a low uptake of health services

(Peters et al., 2009). Reluctance by some general practitioner practices to register transient Travellers reduces access to healthcare (van Cleemput, 2010).

Preventive healthcare is underused by Gypsy/Travellers, (Parry et al., 2007) which has been attributed to low health expectations, fear about potential diagnoses, and structural constraints such as a lack of caravan sites and stopping places (van Cleemput et al., 2007). Variable uptake of childhood immunization contributes to outbreaks of measles and whooping cough (Dar et al., 2013). Gypsy/Travellers are less likely to visit a dentist, or practice nurse, to contact NHS Direct, or to be registered with a general practitioner (Peters et al., 2009). They are more likely to smoke, have below-average consumption of fruit and vegetables, and are less likely to breastfeed (Pinkney, 2012). In Roma communities, low mental well-being, high levels of stress, and unhealthy lifestyles (high rates of smoking and alcohol use, suboptimal intake of fruit and vegetables) (Warwick-Booth et al., 2017) impact the health of babies and children. While breastfeeding is practised commonly prior to migration, duration of breastfeeding can decline once resident in the UK (Dar et al., 2012).

There is a higher prevalence of communicable and non-communicable disease and risk of malnutrition among Roma children (Janevic et al., 2010), with greater prevalence of low birthweight, lower vaccination coverage, and environmental risks (Cook et al., 2013). Mothers lack access to maternity care and can experience discriminatory treatment (Watson and Downe, 2017).

The health of the children of migrants

Health outcomes vary according to migration histories and experience but current evidence suggests poorer health outcomes for all non-UK born individuals (Jayaweera and Quigley, 2010). While the health of migrants is frequently good at the time of migration, health status can subsequently decline (Rechel et al., 2013). The Millennium Cohort Study showed that for every additional 5 years spent in the UK, the likelihood of mothers smoking during pregnancy increased by 31% and they were 5% less likely to breastfeed for at least 4 months (Hawkins et al., 2008). These behaviour changes have been attributed to acculturation (incomers adopting the prevalent health behaviours of the host population) but are increasingly linked to structural factors, such as housing, and other wider determinants of health (Condon and McClean, 2017). Migrant children, especially non-Europeans, are at higher risk for overweight and obesity than other European children (Labree et al., 2011).

The health of refugee and asylum seeker children

An asylum seeker entering the UK must immediately make an asylum application or they may be denied welfare support and accommodation (Asylum Aid, 2017). Many refugees are now dispersed to areas which lack specialist services and where health service staff have little warning of their arrival. Almost all asylum seekers are not allowed to work, are not entitled to council housing, and live on state support which can be as little as £5 per day (Refugee Council, 2017b), and many asylum seeker families cannot pay for basics such as clothing or nappies (Children's Society, 2012).

Those refused asylum are not entitled to financial support and can become homeless (Refugee Council, 2017b). Where there is no recourse to public funds, local authorities have a duty to provide support for a child in need (Home Office, 2016); such provision is likely to be very limited.

Although refugee women are at higher risk of adverse outcomes in pregnancy and birth, maternity care in the NHS is chargeable for most women who do not have indefinite leave to remain in the UK. Maternity care must be offered regardless of a woman's ability to pay, but in practice, many pregnant women are deterred from accessing care, and late booking and missed appointments are common (Feldman, 2016). Frequent moves and lack of interpretation and translation also create barriers to accessing healthcare care (Renton et al., 2016). Although some refugees migrate from countries with high rates of HIV, formula milk is not universally provided to HIV-positive refugee mothers (National Aids Trust, 2017).

Refugee children are vulnerable to mental health problems such as anxiety and depression, sleep disorders, self-harm, and post-traumatic stress disorder (Children's Society, 2012). The UK government has the power to detain people seeking refuge, and in the 12 months prior to March 2017, 51 children were locked up in immigrant detention, despite a promise in 2010 to end this practice (Refugee Council, 2017c). Tuberculosis is prevalent in some migrant populations (Feldman, 2013; Public Health England, 2016) but there is lower uptake of immunizations and screening in non-UK born populations. Dental problems are common among asylum seekers, which affects sleeping, eating, and speech (Renton et al., 2016).

Effectiveness of interventions to improve health through the delivery of a child health programme

A literature review of studies undertaken in the UK to improve the health of Traveller, migrant, and refugee children's health through prevention, screening, surveillance, and health promotion identified very limited evidence. Where found, it related specifically to interventions to promote mother–child bonding or positive parenting, highlighting a focus on individual factors rather than the wider determinants of health. The principles of good practice identified and the recommendations made as a result of the review may apply to children from other vulnerable groups, such as homeless families.

Gypsies, Travellers, and Roma

No UK-based studies of evaluated interventions to improve access or uptake of preventive healthcare, screening or health promotion for Gypsy/Travellers or Roma parents and children were identified. The National Institute for Health and Care Excellence (NICE) has produced guidance for local authorities on best practice in providing services for communities who do not normally access health and social care services (NICE, 2014). NICE recommend understanding the characteristics and needs of the local community, and using that information to develop, commission, and deliver local services that meet those needs. Success is more likely if these activities are undertaken in partnership with the community and led by local health champions.

Services, such as specialist health visiting, are valued by Gypsy/Traveller communities (Jackson et al., 2017). The Institute for Health Visiting Good Practice Guidance recommends that understanding culture and values is essential for building trusting relationships and key areas for health promotion include immunization and injury prevention (see 'Learning links' at the end of this chapter).

Refugees and asylum seekers

One case study and one participatory action research study evaluated culturally sensitive community-based services to support the mental health of women from specific countries or ethnic groups: Afghanistan (Hughes, 2014) and West Africa (O'Shaunessey et al., 2012). Both studies identified the strengths and resources from the mothers' cultural and religious backgrounds which, within a safe setting and supported by a trusted link worker, were built upon to enable mothers to address the needs of their children. The study designs mean it is not possible to determine that an intervention will have a specific clinically relevant effect, but these two studies have indicated an area for further research. (Quality of evidence—needs further research; strength of evidence—moderate).

Migrants

One quasi-experimental intervention study to improve mother–infant bonding in Chinese migrant mothers living in social isolation in Northern Ireland was identified (Yuan and Freeman, 2011). Mothers were non-randomly allocated to a social support programme delivered in the guise of an infant oral health education programme, or a no-treatment comparison group. Using questionnaires at baseline and follow up to 12 months, mothers in the intervention arm had better bonding scores than those in the comparison arm. Oral health outcomes were not assessed. (Quality of evidence: moderate; strength of evidence; low (single study)). The Institute for Health Visiting Good Practice Guidance recommends engaging families in health promotion through discussion of usual health behaviours in their country of origin, encouraging continuation of healthy behaviours, and sign posting to services and information (see 'Learning links' at the end of this chapter).

Facilitators and barriers to accessing the child health programme

A literature review of studies exploring the barriers and facilitators to health promotion services provides insights into the factors influencing access.

Gypsies, Roma, and Travellers

Qualitative studies exploring facilitators and barriers to parents and children accessing preventive health services in the UK were identified for infant feeding (Condon and Salmon, 2015), preschool children's health (Dion, 2008), and immunization uptake (Jackson et al., 2017). Barriers to accessing Healthy Child Programme topics that were reported across more than one study included (i) a sense of fatalism and disempowerment, (ii) low literacy not being recognized by health practitioners, (iii) poor understanding of spoken and written English among Roma families, (iv) a cultural tradition of living in the present and not arranging appointments in the future, and (v) the fact that managing poor housing conditions, low income, and discrimination are likely to take priority over actions to improve health or prevent ill health. Factors that facilitate access to preventive healthcare across more than one study included (i) health professionals who understand cultural sensitivities (e.g. breastfeeding in public or giving the HPV vaccine before children are sexually active); (ii) valuing health information delivered orally, especially through trusted and familiar health professionals; and (iii) younger generations being more likely to read, write, and be internet literate; additionally, as they travel less they are more likely to have a location where they return to and can receive post. (Quality of evidence: high; strength of evidence: high.)

Refugees and asylum seekers

Four qualitative studies explored facilitators and barriers to parents and children accessing preventive health services in the UK for infant feeding (Hufton and Raven, 2016), safeguarding (Burchill, 2011), and maternity care (Bridle, 2012; Lepherd and Haith-Cooper, 2016). Barriers reported across more than one study included (i) lack of knowledge of the health system, including entitlement to services and where access is free; (ii) not being registered with a general practitioner or difficulty registering; (iii) not speaking or reading English; (iv) a fear of deportation arising from engagement with health services; and (v) disruption to the delivery of health services due to dispersal. Factors facilitating access to health promotion reported across more than one study included (i) awareness by staff of religious/cultural traditions and practices (e.g. female genital mutilation); (ii) having trusted health professionals; and (iii) the use of non-written information to deliver healthcare messages (e.g. orally, or through pictures or DVDs). (Quality of evidence: moderate; strength of evidence: high.)

Migrants

Five qualitative and one mixed methods study explored facilitators and barriers to parents and children accessing preventive health services in the UK for preschool children's general health (Abbott and Riga, 2007), maternity care (Balaam et al., 2013; Phillimore, 2016), infant feeding (Choudhry and Wallace, 2012), and supporting children with disabilities (Croot et al., 2012). These included a range of ethnic groups: Bangladeshi (Abbott and Riga, 2007), South Asian (Choudhry and Wallace, 2012), Pakistani (Croot et al., 2012), EU migrants (Balaam et al., 2013; Richards et al., 2014), and one study explored any migrant to the UK in the last 5 years (Philimore, 2016). Barriers to accessing Healthy Child Programme services reported in more than one study included (i) limited English combined with lack of interpreting, advocacy, or translating services, risks of miscommunication, and mistrust of health practitioners; (ii) not understanding what services are available or how to use them; (iii) not being registered with a general practitioner; (iv) economic reasons for not being able to engage with health services (such as inability to afford travel costs or childcare for siblings); (v) a sense of fatalism or disempowerment; and (vi) prioritizing religious/

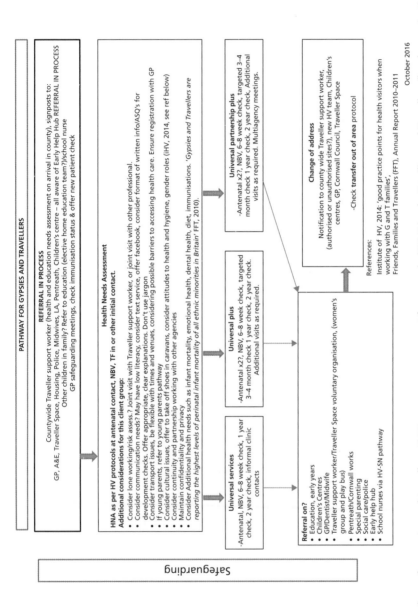

PATHWAY FOR GYPSIES AND TRAVELLERS

Safeguarding

REFERRAL IN PROCESS

Countywide Traveller support worker (health and education needs assessment on arrival in county), signposts to:
GP, A&E, Traveller Space, Housing, Police, Midwives, LA, Pentreath, Children's centre – all aware of Early Help Hub REFERRAL IN PROCESS
Other children in family? Refer to education (elective home education team?)/school nurse
GP safeguarding meetings, check immunisation status & offer new patient check

Health Needs Assessment

HNA as per HV protocols at antenatal contact, NBV, TF in or other initial contact.
Additional considerations for this client group:
- Consider lone working/risk assess.? Joint visit with Traveller support worker, or joint visit with other professional.
- Consider communication needs? May have low literacy, consider text service, offer facebook, consider format of written info/ASQ's for development checks. Offer appropriate, clear explanations. Don't use jargon
- Consider transport issues, be flexible with times and venues, considering possible barriers to accessing health care. Ensure registration with GP
- If young parents, refer to young parents pathway
- Consider cultural issues, offer to take off shoes in caravans, consider attitudes to health and hygiene, gender roles (iHV, 2014, see ref below)
- Consider continuity and partnership working with other agencies
- Maintain confidentiality and privacy
- Consider Additional health needs such as infant mortality, emotional health, dental health, diet, immunisations. *'Gypsies and Travellers are reporting the highest levels of perinatal infant mortality of all ethnic minorities in Britain'* FFT, 2010).

Universal services
-Antenatal, NBV, 6–8 week check, 1 year check, 2 year check, informal clinic contacts

Referral on?
- Education, early years
- Children's Centres
- GP/Dentist/Midwife
- Traveller support worker/Traveller Space voluntary organisation, (women's group and play bus)
- Pentreath/Cornwall works
- Special parenting
- Social care/police
- Early help hub
- School nurses via HV-SN pathway

Universal plus
-Antenatal x27, NBV, 6–8 week check, targeted 3–4 month check 1 year check, 2 year check. Additional visits as required.

Universal partnership plus
-Antenatal x27, NBV, 6–8 week check, targeted 3–4 month check 1 year check, 2 year check, Additional visits as required. Multiagency meetings.

Change of address
Notification to county wide Traveller support worker, (authorised or unauthorised sites?), new HV team, Children's centres, GP, Cornwall Council), Traveller Space

-Check **transfer out of area** protocol

References:
Institute of HV, 2014: 'good practice points for health visitors when working with G and T families',
Friends, Families and Travellers (FFT), Annual Report 2010–2011

October 2016

Fig. 26.1 Pathway for gypsies and travellers. CAF, common assessment framework; FFT, Friends, Families and Travellers (local organization); HV, health visitor; LA, local authority; NBV, new birth visit; SN, school nurse; TAC, team around the child; TF in, transfer in visit.

Reproduced with permission from the Cornwall Partnership NHS Foundation Trust. Source: data from Beach H et al., *Good Practice Points for Health Visitors, Working with Traveller and Gypsy families*, Institute of Health Visiting, Copyright © Institute of Health Visiting 2014, available from https://search3.openobjects.com/mediamanager/herts/enterprise/files/02_mg_traveller_families.pdf.

cultural traditions (such as fasting) over individual health needs. Factors that facilitated service use included (i) practitioner sensitivity to cultural traditions and to the community's understanding of specific health conditions; (ii) having good advocacy, interpreting, and translation services available; (iii) developing trusted relationships with community members, often by continuity of care; and (iv) the ability to deliver individualized information. (Quality of evidence: moderate to high; strength of evidence: moderate.)

Good practice in child health promotion

Many local areas develop their own resources to ensure that the children of Travellers, migrants, and refugees have access to child health programmes. Figure 26.1 is a flowchart devised by the Health Visitor Champion for Gypsy, Traveller, and Migrant families in Redruth, Cornwall. In addition to a usually resident population of Gypsy/Travellers, many others visit Cornwall over the summer. This flowchart provides guidance for health visiting and school nursing teams on delivering health promotion.

Learning links

- Institute for Health Visiting: http://ihv.org.uk/wp-content/uploads/2016/11/GPP_Migrant_Familes_V1_2.pdf
- Institute for Health Visiting: http://ihv.org.uk/wp-content/uploads/2015/09/02-MG_Traveller-Families.pdf.

Recommendations

- All health professionals and support staff working on CHPs should be given cultural competence training including an understanding of how cultural beliefs inform health behaviours, and how these evolve with subsequent generations. (*Evidence: strong.*)
- Practitioners should have access to effective means of communication with families, through link workers, interpreting services, or advocates. Dependence on family members for translation is *not* good practice. (*Evidence: strong.*)
- Health promotion advice and information should be available in non-written forms, such as video clips. (*Good practice.*)
- All families should be asked for their ethnic group and whether they have migrated when they present to NHS services. Health records should include service users' migrant, Traveller, refugee, or asylum seeker status for monitoring purposes and to aid optimal access to child health promotion services. (*Good practice.*)

References

Abbott, S. and **Riga, M.** (2007). Delivering services to the Bangladeshi community: the views of healthcare professionals in East London. *Public Health*, **121**, 935–941.

Asylum Aid (2017). The Asylum Process Made Simple. [online] Available at: http://www.asylumaid.org.uk/the-asylum-process-made-simple/ [Accessed 11 July 2017].

Balaam, M.-C., Akerjordet, K., Lyberg, A., et al. (2013). A qualitative review of migrant women's perceptions of their needs and experiences related to pregnancy and childbirth. *Journal of Advanced Nursing*, **69**, 1919–1930.

Bridle, L. (2012). Asylum seekers and refugees accessing maternity care – literature review and discussion. *MIDIRS Midwifery Digest*, **22**, 7–12.

Burchill, J. (2011). Safeguarding vulnerable families: work with refugees and asylum seekers. *Community Practitioner*, **84**, 23–26.

Choudhry, K. and Wallace, L. (2012). 'Breast is not always best': South Asian women's experiences of infant feeding in the UK within an acculturation framework. *Maternal and Child Nutrition*, **8**, 72–87.

Condon, L. and McClean, S. (2017). Maintaining pre-school children's health and wellbeing in the UK: a qualitative study of the views of migrant parents. *Journal of Public Health*, **39**, 455–463.

Condon, L. and Salmon, D. (2015). 'You likes your way, we got our own way': Gypsy/Travellers' views on infant feeding and health professional support. *Health Expectations*, **18**, 784–795.

Cook, B., Wayne, G., Valentine, A., Lessios, A., and Yeh, E. (2013). Revisiting the evidence on health and health care disparities among the Roma: a systematic review 2003–2012. *International Journal of Public Health*, **58**, 885–911.

Croot, E., Grant, G., Mathers, N., and Cooper, C. (2012). Coping strategies used by Pakistani parents living in the United Kingdom and caring for a severely disabled child. *Disability and Rehabilitation*, **34**, 1540–1549.

Dar, N., Egan, J., Edgar, F., and Harkins, C. (2012). What shapes future infant feeding choices? The views of young people from three cultural backgrounds. [online] Available at: http://www.gcph.co.uk/assets/0000/3623/Infant_feeding_choices_cultural_FINAL_2012.pdf [Accessed 11 July 2017].

Dar, O., Gobin, M., Hogarth, S., Lane, C., and Ramsay, M. (2013). Mapping the Gypsy Traveller community in England: what we know about their health service provision and childhood immunization uptake. *Journal of Public Health*, **35**, 404–412.

Dion, X. (2008). Gypsies and Travellers: cultural influences on health. *Community Practitioner*, **81**, 31–34.

European Commission (2017). EU and Roma. [online] Available at: http://ec.europa.eu/justice/discrimination/roma/index_en.htm [Accessed 11 July 2017].

Feldman, R. (2013). *When Maternity Doesn't Matter. Dispersing Pregnant Women Seeking Asylum. A Joint Report of the Refugee Council and Maternity Action*. London: Maternity Action.

Feldman, R. (2016). Maternity care for undocumented migrant women: the impact of charging for care. *British Journal of Midwifery*, **24**, 52–59.

Hawkins, S., Lamb, K., Cole, T., and Law, C. (2008). Influence of moving to the UK on maternal health behaviours: prospective cohort study. *British Medical Journal*, **336**, 1052.

Home Office (2016). Public funds. [online] Available at: https://www.gov.uk/government/publications/public-funds [Accessed 14 July 2017].

Hufton, E. and **Raven, J.** (2016). Exploring the infant feeding practise of immigrant women in the North West of England: a case study of asylum seekers and refugees in Liverpool and Manchester. *Maternal and Child Nutrition*, **12**, 299–313.

Hughes, G. (2014). Finding a voice through 'The Tree of Life': A strength-based approach to mental health for refugee children and families in schools. *Clinical Child Psychology and Psychiatry*, **19**, 139–153.

Jackson, C., **Bedford, H., Cheater, F**, et al. (2017). Needles, jabs and jags: a qualitative exploration of barriers and facilitators to child and adult immunisation among Gypsies, Travellers and Roma. *BMC Public Health*, **17**, 254.

Janevic, T., **Petrovic, O., Bjelic, I.**, and **Kubera, A.** (2010). Risk factors for childhood malnutrition in Roma settlements in Serbia. *BMC Public Health*, **10**, 509.

Jayaweera H. (2014). Health of migrants in the UK: what do we know? [online] Available at: http://www.migrationobservatory.ox.ac.uk/resources/briefings/health-of-migrants-in-the-uk-what-do-we-know/ [Accessed 11 July 2017].

Jayaweera, H. and **Quigley, M.** (2010). Health status, health behaviour and healthcare use among migrants in the UK: evidence from mothers in the Millennium Cohort Study. *Social Science & Medicine*, **71**, 1002–1010.

Labree, L., **Van De Mheen, H., Rutten, F.**, and **Foets, M.** (2011). Differences in overweight and obesity among children from migrant and native origin: a systematic review of the European literature. *Obesity Reviews*, **12**, e535–e547.

Lepherd, E. and **Haith-Cooper, M.** (2016). Pregnant and seeking asylum: exploring women's experiences 'from booking to baby'. *British Journal of Midwifery*, **24**, 130–136.

Migration Observatory (2017) . Migrants in the UK: an overview. [online] University of Oxford. Available at: http://www.migrationobservatory.ox.ac.uk/resources/briefings/migrants-in-the-uk-an-overview/ [Accessed 11 July 2017].

National Aids Trust (2017). Policy briefing: access to formula milk for mothers living with HIV in the UK. [online] Available at: http://www.nat.org.uk/sites/default/files/publications/Access%20to%20Formula%20Milk%20Briefing%20FINAL.pdf [Accessed 11 July 2017].

National Institute for Health and Care Excellence (NICE) (2014). Improving access to health and social care services for people who do not routinely use them. Local Government Briefing [LGB14]. [online] Available at: https://www.nice.org.uk/advice/lgb14/chapter/Introduction [Accessed 2 July 2017].

Office for National Statistics (2014). *What Does the 2011 Census Tell us about the Characteristics of Gypsy or Irish Travellers in England and Wales?* London: Office for National Statistics. Available at: https://www.ons.gov.uk/peoplepopulationandcommunity/culturalidentity/ethnicity/articles/whatdoesthe2011censustellusaboutthecharacteristicsofgypsyoririshtravellersinenglandandwales/2014-01-21 [Accessed 11 July 2017].

Office for National Statistics. Statistical bulletin: Parents' country of birth, England and Wales, 2016. [online] Available at: https://www.ons.gov.uk/peoplepopulationandcommunity/birthsdeathsandmarriages/livebirths/bulletins/parentscountryofbirthenglandandwales/2015#main-points [Accessed 11 July 2017].

O'Shaughnessy, R., **Nelki, J., Chiumento, A., Hassan, A.**, and **Rahman, A.** (2012). Sweet mother: evaluation of a pilot mental health service for asylum-seeking mothers and babies. *Journal of Public Mental Health*, **11**(4), 214–228. doi:http://dx.doi.org/10.1108/17465721211289392.

Parry, G., Van Cleemput, P., Peters, J., Walters, S., Thomas, K., and Cooper, C. (2007). Health status of Gypsy/Travellers in England. *Journal of Epidemiology and Community Health*, **61**, 198–204.

Pemberton, S., Phillimore, J., and Robinson, D. (2014). Causes and experiences of poverty among economic migrants in the UK. [online] Available at: http://www.birmingham.ac.uk/Documents/college-social-sciences/social-policy/iris/2014/working-paper-series/IRiS-WP-4-2014.pdf [Accessed 11 July 2017].

Peters, J., Parry, G.D., Van Cleemput, P., Moore, J., Cooper, C.L. and Walters, S.J. (2009). Health and use of health services: a comparison between Gypsy/Travellers and other ethnic groups. *Ethnicity & Health*, **14**, 359–377.

Philimore, J. (2016). Migrant maternity in an era of superdiversity: new migrants' access to and experience of antenatal care in the West Midlands, UK, 2016. *Social Science and Medicine*, **148**, 152–159.

Pinkney, K. (2012). The practice and attitudes of Gypsy and Traveller women towards early infant feeding. *Community Practitioner*, **85**, 26–29.

Public Health England (2016). Tuberculosis in England. [online] Available at: https://www.gov.uk/government/uploads/system/uploads/attachment_data/file/581238/TB_Annual_Report_2016_GTW2309_errata_v1.2.pdf [Accessed 13 July 2017].

Rechel, B., Mladovsky, P., Ingleby, D., Mackenbach, J., and McKee, M. (2013). Migration and health in an increasingly diverse Europe. *The Lancet*, **381**, 1235–1245.

Refugee Council (2017a). Children in the asylum system. [online] Available at: https://www.refugeecouncil.org.uk/assets/0004/0485/Children_in_the_Asylum_System_May_2017.pdf [Accessed 11 July 2017].

Refugee Council (2017b). The truth about refugees and asylum. [online] Available at: https://www.refugeecouncil.org.uk/assets/0004/0315/Ref_C_TILII_APRIL_2017_FINAL [Accessed 11 July 2017].

Refugee Council (2017c). Top 20 facts about refugees and asylum seekers. [online] Available at: https://www.refugeecouncil.org.uk/latest/news/4935_top_20_facts_about_refugees_and_asylum_seekers [Accessed 11 July 2017].

Renton, Z., Hamblin, E., and Clements, K. (2016). *Delivering the Healthy Child Programme for Young Refugee and Migrant Children*. London: National Children's Bureau. Available at: https://www.ncb.org.uk/sites/default/files/field/attachment/delivering_hcp_for_young_refugee_and_migrant_children.pdf [Accessed 11 July 2017].

Richards, J., Kilner, M., Brierley, S., and Stroud, L. (2014). Maternal and infant health of Eastern Europeans in Bradford, UK: a qualitative study. *Community Practitioner*, **87**, 33–36.

Rienzo, C. (2017). Migration Observatory briefing: Characteristics and outcomes of Migrants in the UK Labour Market. [online] Available at: http://www.migrationobservatory.ox.ac.uk/briefings/characteristics-and-outcomes-migrants-uk-labour-market [Accessed 11 July 2017].

Rutter, J. (2015). *Moving Up and Getting On: Migration, Integration and Social Cohesion in the UK*. London: Policy Press.

The Children's Society (2012). Into the unknown: children's journeys through the asylum process. [online] Available at: https://www.childrenssociety.org.uk/sites/default/files/tcs/into-the-unknown--childrens-journeys-through-the-asylum-process--the-childrens-society.pdf [Accessed 13 July 2017].

United Nations Statistical Commission (1998). Statistical Standards and Studies - No. 49. [online] Available at: http://www.unece.org/fileadmin/DAM/stats/documents/statistical_standards_&_studies/49.e.pdf [Accessed 11 July 2017].

Van Cleemput, P. (2010). Social exclusion of Gypsy/Travellers: health impact. *Journal of Research in Nursing*, **15**, 315–327.

Van Cleemput, P., Parry, G., Thomas, K., Peters, J., and Cooper, C. (2007). Health-related beliefs and experiences of Gypsy/Travellers: a qualitative study. *Journal of Epidemiology & Community Health*, **61**, 205–210.

Warwick-Booth, L., Trigwell, J., Kinsella, K., Jeffreys, K., Sankar, D., and Dolezalova, M. (2017). Health within the Leeds Migrant Roma Community; an exploration of health status and needs within one UK Area. *Health*, **9**, 669–684.

Watson, H. and Downe, S. (2017). Discrimination against childbearing Romani women in maternity care in Europe: a mixed-methods systematic review. *Reproductive Health*, **14**, 1.

Yuan, S. and Freeman, R. (2011). Can social support in the guise of an oral health education intervention promote mother–infant bonding in Chinese immigrant mothers and their infants? *Health Education Journal*, **70**, 57–66.

Chapter 27

Looked after and adopted children

Douglas Simkiss

Summary

This chapter:

◆ introduces the legal and human rights framework for fostered and adopted children in the UK

◆ describes what looked after children tell us is important

◆ outlines the evidence for looked after children having health promotion, attachment, mental, and physical health needs

◆ makes some recommendations on the most effective interventions.

Introduction

Looked after children are children who have been accommodated by a local authority. It is a relatively common event. On any particular day, around 1 in 200 children are looked after, in a year, approaching 1 in 100 children will have been in care; and birth cohort studies show that around 1 in 30 adults spent some time as a looked after child (Department for Education, 2016; Viner and Taylor, 2005). The most common reason for children becoming looked after is maltreatment (Department for Education, 2016).

The United Nations Convention on the Rights of the Child (United Nations General Assembly, 1989) and the Children Act 1989 state that children should live in their birth family if at all possible, and many looked after children do return to their parents; a few are placed back home under a care order and so remain looked after. Others will go to live with extended family members and these placements may be formalized through a Special Guardianship Order. Some children remain as looked after children living in foster care or, rarely for children aged 7 or less, in children's homes. For some young children, when the parents and extended family are unable to care for them, a plan for adoption is made and children are legally part of a new family with the granting of an adoption order; this is the only situation when parental responsibility is withdrawn from a birth parent.

This chapter will explain why these children are so vulnerable and the current evidence for effective interventions. In many areas, the evidence is based on observational studies (which are moderate quality), or clinical series and opinions.

Looked after children's views

As part of the National Institute for Health and Care Excellence (NICE) guidance on looked after children (NICE, 2010), a qualitative review of the 'experiences, views and preferences of looked after children and young people and their families and carers about the care system' was published (Jones et al., 2011). This is a good place to start to understand the impact of becoming and remaining a looked after child and what children want from being looked after. The review used evidence from 50 studies and identified 17 themes. The most relevant themes for health professionals working with these children are as follows.

Love

Looked after children reported that (i) love and affection is desired but is often lacking in their lives; (ii) love, or the lack of it, has a significant impact on their emotional well-being, in particular their self-esteem; (iii) for some looked after children, training and payment for foster carers undermines the sense that they are wanted or loved; and (iv) an unmet need for love and affection is perceived by some looked after children to have a profound and lasting impact on their future outcomes.

A sense of belonging

Looked after children reported that (i) a sense of belonging is desirable, yet often lacking in their lives; (ii) their sense of identity is compromised by a lack of sense of belonging; (iii) frequent moves and lack of permanence are a characteristic of being looked after that undermines any sense of belonging and therefore has a negative emotional impact for them; (iv) a potential barrier to achieving the desired state of belonging is the conflict that arises for looked after children of being part of two families simultaneously, their birth family and their carer's family; and (v) achieving a sense of belonging and identity is compromised further when they are placed with carers from different ethnic and cultural backgrounds.

Having someone to talk to

Looked after children reported that (i) opportunities to talk to someone about their concerns were often not available, but they appreciated when they were; and (ii) they were often mistrustful of talking to professionals as they could not be sure what they said would be kept confidential.

Professionals

Looked after children raised the following concerns: (i) the issue of continuity in their relationships with professionals; (ii) the negative impact of a lack of continuity; (iii) a desire to form a personal relationship with professionals; (iv) to have professionals who listen, who are accessible; and (v) who can be relied upon to be there for them and have the ability to get things done.

Health promotion needs

Immunization rates for looked after children are rising (87%) but are consistently lower than the general population (94%) (Department for Education, 2013). The reasons for this poor uptake of a fundamental health promotion intervention are to do with neglect and residential mobility before and during care, and the more complicated process for ensuring consent has been given for immunization. Attention to detail is required to compile a complete immunization record for some looked after children. The intervention of providing immunization information to social workers was not, by itself, effective in increasing immunizations for looked after children in one area (Ashton-Key and Jorge, 2003). An immunization look-up tool (Health notes, 2013) and the Public Health England (2017) advice sheet on vaccination of individuals of uncertain or incomplete immunization status are good tools to guide further immunization.

Dental decay is a common form of neglect (Harris et al., 2009) and so looked after children are at high risk and regular dental checks are part of the reporting framework for looked after children (Department for Education, 2013). The Faculty of Dentistry in the Royal College of Surgeons recommends children start to see a dentist 6-monthly from when their teeth first erupt (see Chapter 13).

The residential mobility of looked after children increases the risk that components of the child health programme may not have been done or, if done, results requiring action are not addressed. Examples include abnormal antenatal results for hepatitis B, HIV or syphilis serology requiring treatment, abnormal neonatal Guthrie results, and incomplete newborn hearing screen results not being followed up. For older children entering care, neglect may mean that previous child health programme contacts and activities have not been done and there should be a careful review of the information to facilitate access to appropriate health promotion and screening activities that have been missed.

Attachment

The emotional experiences of the first 2 years of life have a major impact on long-term emotional well-being and NICE has published guidance on promoting secure attachment in children and young people who are adopted from care, in care or at high risk of going into care (NICE, 2015). Children whose caregivers respond sensitively to their needs at times of distress and fear in infancy and early childhood develop secure attachments. They have better outcomes than non-securely attached children in social and emotional development, educational achievement, and mental health.

Attachment patterns and difficulties in children and young people are largely determined by the nature of the caregiving they receive. Repeated changes of primary caregiver, or neglectful and maltreating behaviour from primary caregivers who persistently disregard the child's attachment needs, are the main contributors to attachment difficulties.

Early attachment relations are thought to be crucial for later social relationships and for the development of capacities for emotional and stress regulation, and self-control. Children and young people who have had insecure attachments are more likely to struggle in these areas and to have emotional and behavioural difficulties. This is a key issue for looked after children as their experiences of child abuse and neglect lead to more insecure and disorganized patterns of attachment than in the general population and these attachment difficulties may evolve into coercive, controlling, or compulsive caregiving patterns in children of preschool age or older.

The NICE guideline on promoting secure attachment recommends that health and social care provider organizations should train key workers in:

♦ 'recognising and assessing attachment difficulties and parenting quality, including parental sensitivity

♦ recognising and assessing multiple socioeconomic factors (for example, low income, single or young parents) that together are associated with an increased risk of attachment difficulties

♦ recognising and assessing other difficulties, including coexisting mental health problems and the consequences of maltreatment, including trauma

♦ knowing when and how to refer for evidence-based interventions for attachment difficulties' (NICE, 2015)[‡].

It also recommends that health and social care professionals should offer a child or young person who may have attachment difficulties, and their parents or carers, a comprehensive assessment before any intervention.

For preschool-age children with attachment difficulties, the NICE guidance recommends that health and social care professionals should offer a video feedback programme to foster carers, special guardians, and adoptive parents (NICE, 2015).

There is good evidence to support the use of video feedback programmes, which should be delivered in the parental home by a trained health or social care worker experienced in working with children and young people and

♦ 'consist of 10 sessions (each lasting at least 60 minutes) over 3–4 months

♦ include filming the parents interacting with their child for 10–20 minutes every session

♦ include the health or social care worker watching the video with the parents to:

  ♦ highlight parental sensitivity, responsiveness and communication

- highlight parental strengths
  - acknowledge positive changes in the behaviour of the parents and child'
    (NICE, 2015)[†].

If there is little improvement to parental sensitivity or the child's attachment after ten sessions of a video feedback programme for foster carers, special guardians, and adoptive parents of preschool-age children, NICE guidance advises to arrange a multiagency review before going ahead with more sessions or other interventions. If foster carers, special guardians, or adoptive parents do not want to take part in a video feedback programme, offer parental sensitivity and behaviour training, though this has less evidence to support it as an intervention.

Mental health

The most comprehensive review of the mental health of looked after children was published in 2003 (Meltzer et al., 2003; Ford et al., 2007). An update of this work is underway by the Office for National Statistics, but is not due to report until 2018 (House of Commons Education Committee, 2016) so currently our best data are from more than a decade ago. This large epidemiological study gathered data from more than a thousand children in care, used the Strengths and Difficulties Questionnaire (SDQ) completed by two adults and was able to compare the data with children living at home who had been studied using the same methodology. Looked after children have high rates of mental illness at entry into care and the rate falls only slowly over time in care. Figure 27.1 shows data on the prevalence of mental disorders compared to the general population by type.

A recent review of the quality of evidence for what works in preventing and treating poor mental health in looked after children was published in 2014 by the Rees Centre at the University of Oxford and the NSPCC (Luke et al., 2014). This report sets out the current evidence base for prevention and treatment interventions for looked after children and is summarized below.

The effectiveness of assessments of mental health and well-being for looked after children

The SDQ provides a good estimate of the prevalence of mental health conditions, allowing the identification of children with psychiatric diagnoses based on the Development and Well-Being Assessment (DAWBA).

Caregivers' and teachers' responses on the SDQ are more useful than self-reports and their use as a screening tool during routine health assessments for looked after children increases the detection rate of socio-emotional difficulties. A score of 14 is

---

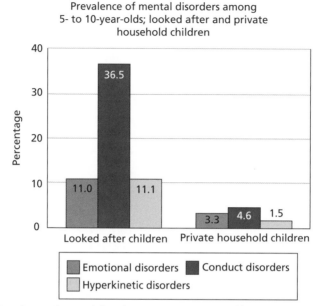

Fig. 27.1 Prevalence of mental disorders among 5–10-year-olds.

Reproduced under the Open Government License v.3.0 from Meltzer H et al., *The mental health of young people looked after by local authorities in England*, Office of National Statistics, London, UK, © Crown Copyright 2003, available from http://webarchive.nationalarchives.gov.uk/20121006174025/ http://www.dh.gov.uk/prod_consum_dh/groups/dh_digitalassets/@dh/@en/documents/digitalasset/dh_ 4060689.pdf.

considered the threshold for further intervention, although each individual score should be considered, including for lower overall scores.

The SDQ, Child Behaviour Checklist (CBCL), Children's Global Assessment Scale (CGAS), and DAWBA can help clinicians determine children's clinical needs, though the SDQ, CBCL, and CGAS may be more useful as broad measures of well-being than for assessing specific conditions. The DAWBA's use of different types of questions and added focus on patterns, duration, and impact of symptoms may explain why it is most effectively used by clinicians, especially with complex cases where clinical judgements are needed. The reliability of assessments depends on who is completing the instrument, in what context, and the skills of the person interpreting them.

The effectiveness of specific interventions

The quality of the research makes it difficult to say a particular intervention or factor has been shown to be clinically effective, leaving a set of common principles that require more rigorous testing. These are, firstly, that structured programmes focusing directly on the child are more effective when they have core components with some flexibility to meet individual needs, and a 'joined-up' approach from services with follow-up support. Secondly, approaches to behavioural issues that focus on the carer (and thereby indirectly on the child) are more effective when they are underpinned by a combination of attachment theory and social learning theory that informs relationship building, focusing on caregiver sensitivity and attunement, positive reinforcement, behavioural consequences, and limit-setting. Thirdly, approaches to behavioural and emotional issues are more likely to be effective when they include some focus on developing relationships and understanding, targeting both the caregiver's understanding of the causes of children's behaviour and the young person's understanding of their own emotions and identity. Fourthly, consistent approaches that reflect fidelity to the programme are associated with better outcomes, and, finally, high levels of commitment from both carers and young people enhance the efficacy of the interventions.

Looked after children have complex histories and needs, and it is unlikely that a single intervention or one that focuses only on the child will address all of these needs. However, few interventions take the mixed approach needed to target both the child and their environment including their carer, school, and social worker, even though there are indications that for some children this might be the most effective strategy. Of the interventions reviewed by Luke et al. (2014), the most promising was Fostering Changes, which shows improvements in carer-rated behaviours, including in one randomized controlled trial, but did not have long-term follow-up.

Recommendations for interventions

The review of the interventions targeted at preventing problems and enhancing the mental health and well-being of looked after children undertaken by Luke et al. (2014) suggests that policymakers and care providers need to consider the conditions under which interventions are effective and the longer-term sustainability of the reported effects. The key messages from the review were that effective intervention programmes can be based on social learning as well as improving attachment. Interventions should be flexible to individual needs and involve a 'joined-up' approach from services. Support for children and carers needs to be consistent, and follow-up should continue after the end of the intervention. Foster carer training needs to ensure that carers are supported to be able to generalize the experience gained from working with one child and apply it to their work with other children (Luke et al., 2014).

Physical health

There is some evidence that looked after children have common physical health issues that are not identified before they enter care; these include undescended testes, strabismus, chronic secretory otitis media, head lice and scabies, as well as incomplete immunization (Hill and Watkin, 2003; Simkiss, 2012). There are also more complex health needs that occur more frequently in this group of children. These include exposure to drugs and alcohol *in utero* with neonatal abstinence syndrome or fetal alcohol spectrum disorders, and an increased risk of vertical transmission of infections and disability, including learning disability (Simkiss, 2012).

These health needs are well recognized and the governments of the four countries of the UK have created health assessment processes to identify and address all health issues. The detail of the process and legislative framework differs in each country and is set out in detail in the intercollegiate role framework developed by the Royal College of Nursing, Royal College of General Practitioners, and Royal College of Paediatrics and Child Health (RCPCH, 2015). However, the essence is the same; a comprehensive health assessment when entering care and regular ongoing health assessments. The review health assessments should ensure that actions from the previous healthcare plan are complete and should have a health promotion focus (Department for Education and Department of Health, 2015; Royal College of Paediatrics and Child Health, 2015). The issue of continuity of professional relationship raised by looked after children (NICE, 2010; Jones et al., 2011) is important to consider as local systems are created.

Developmental and educational needs

There is good evidence that the experience of neglect has an impact on developmental progress as well as emotional and behavioural consequences. While many looked after children make good developmental progress in care, ongoing developmental concerns are common. There are good national data on educational attainment for looked after children, their high prevalence of special educational needs, and Education, Health, and Care plans compared to other children (Figures 27.2 and 27.3).

These educational needs are also more prevalent in adopted children than children who have never been in care. The NICE guidance on attachment identified interventions schools can employ to promote secure attachment and have a positive impact on developmental progress and educational attainment (NICE, 2015, 2016).

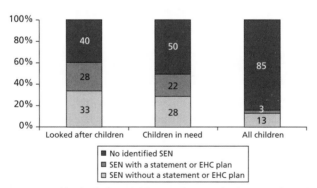

Fig. 27.2 Percentage of looked after children with special educational needs (SEN). EHC, Education, Health, and Care.

Reproduced under the Open Government Licence v3.0 from Department of Education, *Outcomes for children looked after by local authorities in England, 31 March 2015*, © Crown Copyright 2016, available from https://www.gov.uk/government/statistics/outcomes-for-children-looked-after-by-las-31-march-2015. Includes data from CLA-NPD, CIN-NPD, school census.

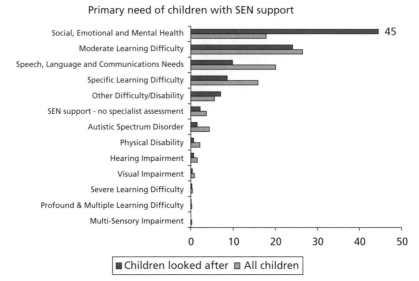

Fig. 27.3 Type of special educational need (SEN) and disability in looked after children.

Reproduced under the Open Government Licence v3.0 from Department of Education, *Outcomes for children looked after by local authorities in England, 31 March 2015*, © Crown Copyright 2016, available from https://www.gov.uk/government/statistics/outcomes-for-children-looked-after-by-las-31-march-2015. Includes data from CLA-NPD, school census.

Conclusion

Looked after children are a vulnerable group with significant health promotion needs. They are at risk of attachment difficulties and unidentified physical and mental health needs. They often have developmental and educational concerns. Effective professional relationships can be therapeutic and there are interventions to promote health and well-being for looked after children.

Learning links

◆ Module 4 ('Safeguarding') by e-Learning for Healthcare provides learning sessions on vulnerable children including looked after children: http://www.e-lfh.org.uk/programmes/healthy-child-programme/more-information/.

Recommendations

◆ When children enter care, a review should be undertaken of their receipt of recommended screening and preventative services, their uptake of immunizations, and any unmet needs identified. (*Evidence: strong.*)

- Foster carers, special guardians, and adoptive parents should be offered a video feedback programme for working with preschool-age children with attachment difficulties. (*Evidence: strong.*)
- Practitioners should focus on school readiness for looked after children. (*Evidence: strong.*)
- Provider organizations should prioritize the health needs and the service provided to looked after children placed out of area (*Evidence: moderate.*)
- Adopted children with significant and ongoing health needs require specialist support. (*Evidence: moderate.*)

References

Ashton-Key, M. and **Jorge, E.** (2003). Does providing social services with information and advice on immunisation status of 'looked after children' improve uptake? *Archives of Disease in Childhood,* **88,** 299–301.

Children Act 1989. London: The Stationery Office. Available at: http://www.legislation.gov.uk/ukpga/1989/41/contents [Accessed 25 Sep. 2017].

Department for Education (2013). *Outcomes for Children Looked After by Local Authorities in England, year ending 31 March 2013.* London: Department for Education.

Department for Education (2016). *Children Looked After in England (Including Adoption) Year Ending 31 March 2016.* SFR 41/2016. London: Department for Education.

Department for Education and Department of Health (2015). Promoting the health and well-being of looked-after children: statutory guidance on the planning, commissioning and delivery of health services for looked-after children. [online] Available at: https://www.gov.uk/government/publications/promoting-the-health-and-wellbeing-of-looked-after-children--2.

Ford, T., Vostanis, P., Meltzer, H., and **Goodman, R.** (2007). Psychiatric disorder among British children looked after by local authorities; comparison with children living in private households. *British Journal of Psychiatry,* **190,** 319–325.

Harris, J.C., Elcock, C., Sidebotham, P.D., and **Welbury, R.R.** (2009). Safeguarding children in dentistry: 2. Do paediatric dentists neglect child dental neglect? *British Dental Journal,* **206,** 465–470.

Health notes (2013). Is this looked after child fully immunised? A comparison of records and the development of an immunisation look-up tool. *Adoption & Fostering,* **37,** 212–219.

Hill, C.M. and **Watkins, J.** (2003). Statutory health assessments for looked after children: what do they achieve? *Child: Care, Health & Development,* **29,** 3–13.

House of Commons Education Committee (2016). *Mental Health and Well-Being of Looked-After Children.* House of Commons HC 481. London: The Stationery Office.

Jones, R., Everson-Hock, E.S., Papaioannou, D., et al. (2011). Factors associated with outcomes for looked-after children and young people: a correlates review of the literature. *Child: Care, Health and Development,* **37,** 613–622.

Luke, N., Sinclair, I., Woolgar, M., and **Sebba, J.** (2014). *What Works in Preventing and Treating Poor Mental Health in Looked After Children?* Impact and Evidence Series. London: NSPCC/Rees Centre.

Meltzer, H., Gatward, R., Corbin, T., Goodman, R., and Ford, T. (2003). *The Mental Health of Young People Looked After by Local Authorities in England*. London: The Stationery Office.

National Institute for Health and Care Excellence (NICE) (2010). Promoting the quality of life of looked-after children and young people. Quality standard [QS31]. [online] Available at: https://www.nice.org.uk/guidance/qs31

National Institute for Health and Care Excellence (NICE) (2015). Children's attachment: attachment in children and young people who are adopted from care, in care or at high risk of going into care. NICE guideline [NG26]. [online] Available at: https://www. nice.org.uk/guidance/ng26

National Institute for Health and Care Excellence (NICE) (2016). Children's attachment. Quality standard [QS133]. [online] Available at: https://www.nice.org.uk/guidance/qs133

Public Health England (2017). Vaccination of individuals with uncertain or incomplete immunisation status. [online] Available at: www.gov.uk/government/publications/ vaccination-of-individuals-with-uncertain-or-incomplete-immunisation-status.

Royal College of Paediatrics and Child Health (RCPCH) (2015). Looked after children: Knowledge, skills and competences of healthcare staff. Intercollegiate Role Framework. [online] Available at: http://www.rcpch.ac.uk/system/files/protected/page/ Looked%20After%20Children%202015_0.pdf.

Simkiss, D. (2012). Outcomes for looked after children and young people. *Paediatrics and Child Health*, **22**, 388–392.

United Nations General Assembly (1989). *Convention on the Rights of the Child, 20 November 1989*. New York: United Nations. Available at: http://www.ohchr.org/Documents/ ProfessionalInterest/crc.pdf [Accessed 26 Nov. 2016].

Viner, R.M. and Taylor B. (2005). Adult health and social outcomes of children who have been in public care: population-based study. *Pediatrics*, **115**, 894–899.

Section 6

Components of a healthy child programme

Chapter 28

Recommended universal components by age across the UK

Alison Burton

Summary

This chapter:

- provides an overview of current policy on the provision of a universal child health programme across the four nations of the UK
- describes the common shared themes and principles, and summarizes the four individual programmes and their policy context.

Overview

The core child health programme (CHP) starts in the antenatal period and consists of the following key elements: screening, child health surveillance, health protection, and health promotion. The four UK universal CHPs are similar and share common objectives. They are based on the proposition that a progressive or proportionate universal approach provides a foundation for predicting risk and preventing problems from developing and for early identification of need, and timely, targeted interventions reducing the need for more complex intensive and costly interventions at a later stage. A universal programme provides an opportunity for the health visitor to visit every child at home and undertake a holistic assessment of child and family needs encompassing, physical, and psychosocial assessment of the family and home environment.

There is some variation between countries in the number and intensity of core contacts, where those contacts may take place, and who should undertake them. Currently England has the fewest number of core contacts and Scotland has the most contacts and highest-intensity programme with eight home visits by the health visitor scheduled in the first year.

Content

The core content covered by the CHP consists of promoting attachment, supporting transition to parenthood and couples relationships, and care of the infant—including breastfeeding, health and well-being, sleeping, safety, child development, growth monitoring, immunization, oral health promotion, infant mental health, and social and emotional well-being.

Family health includes perinatal mental health, parental health, domestic violence, smoking, drugs, alcohol, healthy eating, physical activity, inter-parental relationships, parenting, contraception, and sexual health. Delivery of the CHP also considers other factors which can impact on health and well-being, parenting and family function, such as wider determinants of health—housing, financial issues, and employment (Table 28.1).

Table 28.1 Core schedule across all UK countries

Core offer to all babies in UK	Age	Screening	Immunization	Health visitor (HV) contacts
Pregnancy	From 10 weeks	Antenatal screening programmes	Pertussis and influenza vaccination	Up to 1 HV contact (Wales—first baby only)
Birth to 2 years	72 hours	Newborn infant physical examination		
	5 (8) days	Newborn bloodspot screen		
	10–14 (21) days			New birth visit
	By 8 weeks	Infant physical examination	1st primary immunization	HV contact
	By 4 weeks	Newborn hearing screen		
	12 weeks		2nd primary immunization	
	16 weeks		3rd primary immunization	
	By 1 year			At least 1 HV contact
	12–13 months		Booster immunizations and menC vaccine and measles, mumps and rubella vaccine	
2–5years	2–2.5 years			HV contact
	By 4 years		Preschool immunization	

Source: data from Public Health England, *Guidance to support the commissioning of the healthy child programme 0 to 19: health visiting and school nursing services (commissioning guide 2)*, PHE Publication Gateway Reference 2017762, © Crown Copyright 2018, available from https://www.gov.uk/government/uploads/system/uploads/attachment_data/file/686930/best_start_in_life_and_beyond_commissioning_guidance_2.pdf. Contains public sector information licensed under the Open Government Licence v3.0.

Table 28.2 Schedule of universal core offer in England

England	Age	Core offer	
Pregnancy	28 weeks	Antenatal contact	
0–3 years	10–21 days	HV new birth visit	
	6–8 weeks	HV-led contact	
	1 year	HV-led contact	
	2–2.5 years	HV-led contact	Ages and Stages Questionnaire (ASQ) developmental review Integrated review with early years setting

HV, health visitor.

Source: data from Public Health England, *Guidance to support the commissioning of the healthy child programme 0 to 19: health visiting and school nursing services (commissioning guide 2)*, PHE Publication Gateway Reference 2017762, © Crown Copyright 2018, available from https://www.gov.uk/government/uploads/system/uploads/attachment_data/file/686930/best_start_in_life_and_beyond_commissioning_guidance_2.pdf. Contains public sector information licensed under the Open Government Licence v3.0.

Summary of the national programmes in the four UK countries

England

Policy context

The current universal offer for infants and young children in England is the 'Healthy Child Programme: Pregnancy and the First 5 Years of Life' published in 2009. In 2010, the coalition government announced its commitment to expand the number of health visitors in England by 50% or 4200 health visitors by March 2015 (Gov.uk, 2011). Alongside the expansion programme a new 4–5–6 service model was published outlining four levels of service, five universal contacts, and six high-impact areas, key public health outcomes where health visiting can significantly improve outcomes for babies and young children (Figure 28.1). The high-impact areas were refreshed in 2016 and expanded to include six high-impact areas for school nursing (Gov.uk, 2014).

The aims of the programme are increased access, improved outcomes for children, increased service user satisfaction, and a reduction in health inequalities. An 'Early Years Profile' to monitor outcomes and measure progress has been developed and is available as an interactive tool to enable local areas to view their data and benchmark against national and statistical neighbour rates (Public Health England, 2016).

The Health and Social Care Act 2012 transferred the responsibility for public health from the NHS to local government. Local authorities became responsible for commissioning the majority of public health services for the population with the exception of

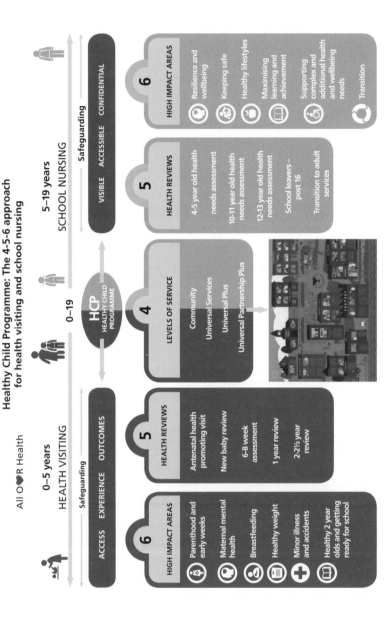

Fig. 28.1 The 4–5–6 service model.

Box 28.1 The mandated reviews of the Healthy Child Programme in England

◆ Antenatal health promoting visit from 28 weeks.

◆ New baby review between 10 and 21 days.

◆ 6–8-week assessment.

◆ 1-year assessment.

◆ 2- to 2½-year review.

Reproduced under the Open Government Licence v3.0 from Public Health England, *Review of mandation for the universal health visiting service*, PHE Publications Gateway Number 2016409, © Crown Copyright 2016, available from https://www.gov.uk/government/uploads/system/uploads/attachment_data/file/592893/Review_of_mandation_universal_health_visiting_service.pdf.

---

immunization and screening services which transferred to NHS England and Public Health services for 0–5-year-olds were also transferred to NHS England for 2 years to deliver the Health Visitor Implementation Plan and the expansion of Family Nurse Partnerships.

The final part of the public health transfer (i.e. the 0–5s public health services) was completed on 1 October 2016. To ensure a safe transfer, maintain service delivery, and promote stability post transfer, regulations were put in place to require local authorities to commission the delivery of specific universal elements of the Healthy Child Programme. The five 'mandated' reviews are outlined in Box 28.1.

In 2015, Public Health England issued further guidance (Gov.uk, 2016) to support local government in commissioning seamless services from birth to age 19 years: including a visualization of the 4–5–6 model of delivery (Gov.uk, 2016). A further review of the Healthy Child Programme is expected in 2019.

The universal reviews are the foundations for a progressive universal approach of prevention, early identification and intervention, and integrated delivery of early support and help for all children based on child and family needs (Table 28.2).

Scotland

Policy context

The Scottish Government is investing resources into the early years. Current policy is aimed at strengthening the universal offer for all families with very young children. For example, during the current parliament the Scottish Government has pledged to:

◆ provide every newborn with a 'baby box' of essential items

◆ expand the number of health visitors

- extend the Family Nurse Partnership to support every new teenage mother
- provide 30 hours childcare a week for all 3- and 4-year-olds and vulnerable 2-year-olds
- from Spring 2016 ensure that all pregnant women are given free vitamins.

In October 2015, the Scottish Government published a Universal Health Visiting Pathway along with a set of tools and resources supporting delivery. The toolkit includes resources and assessment tools including a Minimum Child Health Surveillance Data Set, assessment tools appropriate to the child's age, health promotion resources, continuing professional development/e-learning, and evidence resources for practitioners (Gov.scot, 2015). The pathway integrates the work of health visitors with children's services to create a joined-up whole system, with a consistent approach across all agencies. Getting it Right for Every Child (GIRFEC) (http://www.gov.scot/Topics/People/Young-People/gettingitright) is the national approach in Scotland to improving outcomes and supporting the well-being of children and young people. A key outcome of the GIRFEC is for all children to have a named professional; the health visitor is the named professional for all children from birth to age 5 years.

The universal pathway consists of 11 home visits, eight of which take place in the first year (Table 28.3). Contact starts in the antenatal period with an antenatal letter

Table 28.3 Schedule of universal core offer in Scotland

Scotland	Age	Core offer	
Pregnancy	Pre-birth	Antenatal letter	
	Antenatal contact 32–34/40	Home visit	
0–2 years	11–14 days	New baby home visit	
	3–5 weeks	Two home visits	
	6–8 weeks	Home visit	
	3 months	Home visit	
	4 months	Home visit	
	6 months	Home visit	Review GIRFEC assessment
	8 months	Home visit	
	13–15 months	Home visit	Developmental and well-being review
3–5 years	27–30 months	Home visit	Developmental and well-being review
	4–5 years	Home visit	Developmental and well-being review

Source: data from Scottish Government, *Getting It Right For Every Child (GIRFEC)*, © Crown Copyright 2018, available from http://www.gov.scot/Topics/People/Young-People/gettingitright. Contains public sector information licensed under the Open Government Licence v3.0.

followed by a home visit at 32–34 weeks. There are a further eight home visits by the age of 8 months; an assessment, using the GIRFEC framework and Health Plan Indicator where additional family needs are identified, is undertaken for every family with a formal review at age 6 months. Three formal developmental reviews are undertaken at 13–15 months, 27–30 months, and 4–5 years followed by a handover from the health visitor to the incoming named person who is usually an education professional. Full roll-out of the new programme is being led through the Scottish health boards and is expected to take around 2 years with the aim that universal coverage is achieved by 2018.

Wales

Policy context

Following a review of current provision of early years services, the Welsh Government and NHS Wales published the Healthy Child Wales Programme (HCWP) in September 2016 (Gov.wales, 2016). The programme was launched by the Minister for Public Health and Social Services at the all Wales Health Visitor conference on 1 October 2016. The programme sets out a schedule of planned contacts children and their families can expect from their health boards—from maternity service handover to the first years of schooling (0–7 years). The HCWP includes a consistent range of evidence-based preventive and early intervention measures, and advice and guidance to support parenting and healthy lifestyle choices. The universal contacts cover three areas of intervention; screening, immunization, and monitoring and supporting child development.

Responsibility for implementing the HCWP rests with the health boards. While the Welsh Government recognizes that not all areas will be starting from the same place in terms of current delivery, it is expected that the universal core offer will be fully implemented by October 2018.

There are various tools currently used to support health visitors in making a professional assessment of family resilience. To further improve this area of work, the University of South Wales and Welsh health visitors have worked in partnership to develop a fully validated all Wales Health Visiting Family Resilience Assessment Instrument Tool (FRAIT). The aims of the FRAIT are to identify protective factors within families as well as to identify additional need alongside potential safeguarding concerns. FRAIT will be used at key stages throughout a child's first 5 years of life and, if appropriate, a plan will be agreed with families encompassing interventions and reviews to evaluate progress.

Building on the FRAIT initiative, an all Wales Health Visiting Acuity Tool is in development, which will enable each health board to more accurately determine local workforce requirements through the application of a standardized tool.

A full review of the HCWP will be conducted 3 years after its introduction to ensure it takes into account the emerging evidence base Table 28.4 is a summary of the universal contacts set out in the HCWP.

Table 28.4 Schedule of universal core offer in Wales

Wales	Age	Core offer	
Pregnancy	10–40 weeks	Routine antenatal care	
	28 weeks	Targeted HV visit	1st baby Learning difficulties Safeguarding Emotional/mental health Fetal health condition Multiple pregnancy
0–2 years	14 days	New birth home visit	Maternal mental health assessment Family resilience assessment
	6–8 weeks	GP contact	Physical examination
	8 weeks	HV clinic contact	Growth assessment
	12 weeks	HV clinic contact	Growth assessment
	16 weeks	HV clinic contact	Growth assessment
	6 months	HV clinic contact	Weaning and baby safety advice, family resilience assessment
	15 months	HV home visit contact	Assessment of growth and development Family resilience assessment
2–5 years	27 months	HV home visit contact	Assessment of growth and development Family resilience assessment
	3.5 years	HV home visit contact	Assessment of growth and development Family resilience assessment
	4/5 years	Handover from HV to school nurse	
School	4–7 years	School nurse service	Vision and growth screening Hearing impairment screening Child Measurement programme

GP, general practitioner; HV, health visitor.

Source: data from Welsh Government, *Healthy Child Wales Programme*, © Crown Copyright 2016, available from http://gov.wales/topics/health/publications/health/reports/healthy-child/?lang=en. Contains public sector information licensed under the Open Government Licence v3.0.

Northern Ireland

Policy context

'Healthy Child, Healthy Future: A Framework for the Universal Child Health Promotion Programme in Northern Ireland' was published in May 2010 to be commissioned as one programme covering all stages of childhood (Department of Health,

2010). It provides guidance on the schedule, delivery mechanisms, and content of the CHP 0–19 years. The programme is a universal service requiring a number of set contacts to identify health needs, provide screening and surveillance, and where necessary early intervention and specialist interventions according to need, consisting of two core elements: health improvement and health protection. It is underpinned by seven principles:

1. 'A whole child approach
2. A major emphasis on parenting support and positive parenting
3. The application of new information about neurological development and child development
4. The inclusion of changing public health priorities
5. An increased focus on vulnerable families, underpinned by a model of progressive universalism
6. An emphasis on integrated services
7. The use of new technologies and scientific developments' (Department of Health, 2010).

Table 28.5 Schedule of universal core offer in Northern Ireland

Northern Ireland	Age	Core offer	
Pregnancy	12–40 weeks	Routine antenatal care delivered by midwives	
	28 weeks	Health visitor home visit	May be earlier if indicated
0–2 years	Birth–10 days	Postnatal care	
	10–14 days	Health visitor home visit	
	6–8 weeks	Health visitor home visit	
	14–16 weeks	Health visitor contact	Home or other as appropriate
	6–9 months	Health visitor-led contact	Home or other as appropriate
	1 year	Health visitor home visit	
	2–2.5 years	Health visitor home visit	
3–5 years	3 years	Health visitor-led contact	Early years and group settings
	4–4.5 years	Health visitor-led contact	Record review Clinic or telephone as appropriate prior to handover to school nursing service

Source: data from Department of Health, Understanding the Needs of Children in Northern Ireland (UNCNI), *Thresholds of Need Model*, © Crown Copyright 2010, available from https://www.health-ni.gov.uk/publications/thresholds-need-model. Contains public sector information licensed under the Open Government Licence v3.0.

The programme is delivered on four levels based on the Understanding the Needs of Children in Northern Ireland (UNOCINI) 'thresholds of need' model (Department of Health, Social Services and Public Safety, 2008)

◆ '*Level 1: base population*. Children 0–18 years, including children and families who may require occasional advice, support and/or information.

◆ *Level 2: children with additional needs*. Vulnerable children who may be at risk if social exclusion.

◆ *Level 3: children in need*. Children with complex needs that may be chronic and enduring.

◆ *Level 4: children with complex and/or acute needs*. Children in need of rehabilitation; children with critical and/or high-risk needs; children in need of safeguarding (inc. LAC [looked after children]); children with complex and enduring needs' (UNOCINI, 2010).

The thresholds promote the use of a common format, language, and understanding of needs among key agencies and professionals working in Northern Ireland with the aim of supporting integration and joined-up delivery of services (Table 28.5).

Learning links

◆ e-Learning for Health—'Healthy Child programme': https://www.e-lfh.org.uk/programmes/healthy-child-programme/

◆ e-Learning for Health—'Ages and Stages': https://www.e-lfh.org.uk/programmes/ages-and-stages-questionnaires/.

Recommendations

◆ Commission an evidence-based CHP in each devolved nation and ensure that adequate resources are provided to deliver a quality service to the whole population based on the principle of proportionate universalism. (*Evidence: strong.*)

◆ Evaluation of coverage and measures of outcomes should be built into each CHP. (*Evidence: strong.*)

◆ Ensure clarity about the competencies required from practitioners to deliver the programme. (*Evidence: strong.*)

Acknowledgement

This chapter contains public sector information licensed under the Open Government Licence v3.0.

References

Department of Health (2010). Healthy Child, Healthy Future: A Framework for the Universal Child Health Promotion Programme in Northern Ireland. [online] Available at: https://www.health-ni.gov.uk/sites/default/files/publications/dhssps/healthychildhealthyfuture.pdf [Accessed 2 Oct. 2017].

Department of Health, Social Services and Public Safety (2008). Understanding the Needs of Children in Northern Ireland. [online] Available at: https://www.health-ni.gov.uk/sites/default/files/publications/dhssps/unocini-guidance.pdf [Accessed 25 Sep. 2017].

Gov.scot (2015). Universal Health Visiting Pathway in Scotland - Pre Birth to Pre School. [online] Available at: http://www.gov.scot/Publications/2015/10/9697 [Accessed 25 Sep. 2017].

Gov.uk (2011). Health visitor implementation plan 2011 to 2015. [online] Available at: https://www.gov.uk/government/publications/health-visitor-implementation-plan-2011-to-2015 [Accessed 25 Sep. 2017].

Gov.uk (2014). Supporting public health: children, young people and families. [online] Available at: https://www.gov.uk/government/publications/commissioning-of-public-health-services-for-children [Accessed 25 Sep. 2017].

Gov.uk (2016). Healthy child programme 0 to 19: health visitor and school nurse commissioning. [online] Available at: https://www.gov.uk/government/publications/healthy-child-programme-0-to-19-health-visitor-and-school-nurse-commissioning [Accessed 29 Sep. 2017].

Gov.wales (2016). Healthy Child Wales Programme. [online] Available at: http://gov.wales/topics/health/publications/health/reports/healthy-child/?lang=en [Accessed 2 Oct. 2017].

Public Health England (2016). Public Health Profiles. [online] Available at: https://fingertips.phe.org.uk/profile-group/child-health/profile/child-health-early-years [Accessed 25 Sep. 2017].

UNOCINI (2010). Understanding the Needs of Children in Northern Ireland: Thresholds of Need Model. [online] Available at: https://www.health-ni.gov.uk/publications/thresholds-need-model [Accessed 29 Sep. 2017].

Chapter 29

Personal child health record

Helen Bedford

Summary

This chapter

+ describes the Personal Child Health Record (PCHR) used in all four UK countries, reflecting the content of the local child health programme

+ discusses why use of the PCHR is suboptimal in some population groups and by some groups of health professionals

+ reviews the potential benefits and pitfalls of the development of digital ePCHRs.

Background to development of the current Personal Child Health Record

Parents have individually been holding records of their child's growth and development for over 100 years. However, the first 'Parent-Held Record' to be used on a population basis was developed by Professor David Morley in 1959 for use in Nigeria. A simple health and weight chart, it was known as the 'Road-to-Health Chart' (Cuthbertson and Morley, 1962). Mothers valued the chart and kept it safely; it improved their participation in their child's growth and development as well as enabling sharing of information between professionals (Morley, 1973). Use of the chart had positive health outcomes for children (Cuthbertson and Morley, 1962). The Road-to-Health Chart was adapted and adopted by the World Health Organization and UNICEF and versions are still used in low-income countries.

In England, Personal Child Health Records (PCHRs) were developed and used locally in the 1980s, notably in Oxfordshire (Saffin and Macfarlane, 1988). In 1990, a British Paediatric Association (now Royal College of Paediatrics and Child Health (RCPCH)) multidisciplinary working group led by Dr Aidan Macfarlane recommended the development of a national PCHR. It included some details about the appearance and content but allowed flexibility for districts and boards to modify it according to local needs (British Paediatric Association, 1990).

This record was adopted widely in England but in time, the adaptations districts made for local use, which often included adding locally produced information and health promotion material, resulted in a plethora of versions with considerable variation in both content and appearance. Although the original prototype had a red cover, and was known as 'The Red Book', by 2003, PCHRs with blue, green, yellow, and white covers were in use in different districts. This variation in content was a potential limitation both for parents moving from district to district and for health professionals, who could not easily and quickly navigate the different records.

In 2003, as part of *Health for all children*, 4th edition (HFAC4) (Hall and Elliman, 2003), the PCHR was extensively reviewed. This review was informed by a survey of 166 trusts and health authorities (response rate 84%) about their use of and policies with respect to the record; a review of the content of records provided by surveyed districts; discussions at a 1999 national conference; and discussions of the PCHR working group set up under the auspices of HFAC4 and with other experts in the field. On the basis of these findings and using the best features from existing records, in 2004 a new core standard record was developed based on the child health programme (CHP). This included a description of the programme, pages to record details of the child's birth, results from the screening programmes, as well as immunization and child health reviews. Pages were included for parents to make notes and to record their child's developmental firsts. However, detailed health promotion material was deliberately not included in the core record for a number of reasons:

♦ The PCHR is a record of health and development. Adding detailed health promotion would make the record bulky potentially compromising parents' use.

♦ At that time, the Department of Health produced a hard copy publication, *Birth to Five*, containing detailed health promotion which was issued to all new mothers. This was produced with input by health promotion and design experts to ensure that parents had access to high-quality consistent information in an appropriate format.

Since 2004, most areas in England have used the standard core record, although many include additional pages particularly with local details; some continue to include health promotion information; and a few areas have developed their own record.

In 2009, the PCHR was extensively revised again to include the new World Health Organization growth charts (Wright et al., 2010). In developing the growth charts, parents were consulted and their input influenced the design of the charts and the explanatory text to accompany the PCHR charts was informed by their information requirements and need for explanation of the process of growth monitoring (Sachs et al., 2012). More recent developments include improved signposting to other resources and the inclusion of website addresses and QR codes.

The PCHR is updated as the CHP changes, for example, to include additional screening tests and changes to the immunization schedule. However, a limitation of a paper-based PCHR is the challenge of keeping it up to date and ensuring that parents are always issued with the most up-to-date version (to avoid wastage, districts tend to use up old stock) and the difficulty of issuing revised single pages to parents with existing records.

Ethos of the record

The PCHR provides an holistic overview of a child's health and development which is often not available in other records such as general practitioner (GP) or hospital records. The ethos of parents holding their child's record is that, by having a complete overview of the child's health and development in one place, including the parent's perspective, it allows the parent to gain a better understanding of their child's health and development; encourages partnership with health professionals; and improves communication between health professionals, ultimately leading to improved child health outcomes.

PCHRs in the UK

The four UK countries have all developed a standard record applicable for their country reflecting the CHP but there are similarities in appearance and content. In England, a multidisciplinary PCHR committee set up under the auspices of the RCPCH oversees the content and development of the record. The Department of Health in Wales, the Scottish Government, and the Public Health Agency in partnership with the Department of Health in Northern Ireland have this responsibility. In Wales and Northern Ireland, the PCHR has recently been reviewed and extensively revised to reflect their respective CHPs. In England, Wales, and Scotland, these standard core versions signpost to appropriate health promotion resources: in England (Nhs.uk, 2016) to NHS Choices, in Scotland to 'Ready Steady Baby' (Readysteadybaby.org.uk, 2017), and in Wales to 'Bump Baby and Beyond' which is available in both hard copy, distributed by midwives, and digital formats (Wales.nhs.uk, 2017), while the Northern Ireland version does contain some health promotion material.

Requests from organizations representing parents of children with specific conditions and others to include pages in the record describing signs and symptoms of specific conditions are considered in England by the RCPCH PCHR committee. However, as a general principle, information about specific conditions is best included in the relevant health promotion information resource.

PCHR inserts

Specific inserts have been developed for some groups of children with additional needs. For example, the Down Syndrome Medical Interest Group (DSMIG) developed a special PCHR insert for babies with Down syndrome; this contains information for parents and professionals about the health and well-being of babies born with Down syndrome, details of additional health checks that may be required, as well as Down syndrome growth charts (DSMIG, 2017). In Northern Ireland, an insert is being developed for babies who have been admitted to the neonatal unit.

Use by parents of the PCHR

There is strong evidence that the PCHR is generally used well at least in the first years of life but social inequalities in use exist. In a large representative study of 18,503 parents of 9-month-old children born in 2000–2002 in the four UK countries, 93% of mothers produced their child's PCHR and 85% of mothers showed effective use of their child's PCHR defined by producing their child's PCHR, consulting it, and having the baby's most recent weight recorded in the record. Last weight was recorded in 97% of PCHRs consulted. However, effective use was lower in children previously admitted to hospital, and in association with factors reflecting social disadvantage, including residence in disadvantaged communities, young maternal age, large family size, and lone parent status (Walton et al., 2006).

The limited research conducted evaluating the use of and attitudes to the PCHR suggests that parents value the record and use it mainly for monitoring their child's growth, for recording their developmental firsts, and to remind themselves of the immunization schedule (Hampshire et al., 2004). There is some evidence that its main value is not as a health promotion tool (Wright and Reynolds, 2006).

Use by health professionals of the PCHR

Several studies have reported PCHRs to be used mainly by health visitors, less well by GPs, who report finding it difficult knowing where to record information (Hampshire et al., 2004; Wright and Reynolds, 2006; Walton and Bedford, 2007), and least by hospital staff, although this could be a reflection of parents being less likely to take their PCHRs to hospital appointments (Moss, 2005). However as Aidan Macfarlane observed over 25 years ago: 'How well it [the PCHR] works does not only depend on its use by parents but even more so on its use by, and the value attached to it by, doctors and nurses both in the community and hospital. If it is valued by them, then the parents will value it too, will not lose it, and will bring it with them to all contacts with the primary and secondary care providers to share the information so as to ensure the better care of their child' (Macfarlane, 1992). This remains the case in 2018.

It is particularly important that parents are provided with an explanation and shown the content of the record and how to use it, but this does not always happen (Walton and Bedford, 2007). Parents need to be given 'permission' to use and to write in the record. Ideally, the PCHR should be issued to parents in the antenatal period, giving them time to become familiar with its content and allowing information to be recorded from birth. The mandated health visitor antenatal contact at 28 weeks in England is an ideal time to introduce the PCHR which, as a fundamental part of the CHP, can be used to inform parents about recommended screening tests, reviews, and immunization.

Future developments of the PCHR

The development of the PCHR has always been a dynamic ongoing process and the latest development is a digital PCHR (ePCHR). In 2016, NHS England published its vision for how child health information can support parents and professionals in providing the highest quality care for children (NHS England, 2016). The report commended the PCHR and highlighted the need to ensure that its ethos is taken forward and transferred to a digital platform to provide improvements in services to parents, families, carers, children, and young people. It was observed that as the PCHR is a cross- professionally agreed summary record with a core record dataset agreed nationally, the PCHR content will form the basis of the core child dataset.

If its vision is realized, use of an ePCHR would have considerable benefits, enabling timely, seamless data flow from and into GP systems and Child Health Information Systems into and from the ePCHR. Electronic links would give parents easier access to health promotion material, and use of electronic messaging for immunization appointments may have a positive impact on immunization uptake rates (Jacobson Vann et al., 2005). For a child attending the emergency department in a hospital many miles from home, the ready availability of a complete record of their health and development will be extremely valuable to ensure effective management and ongoing care with information about their hospital attendance instantly available for their home GP and HV.

However, some important issues also need to be considered as use of a digital record may have the potential to further disadvantage the already disadvantaged particularly for those with poor digital literacy skills. An ePCHR produced by an independent company, which mirrors the content of the national standard core PCHR, was piloted in two English NHS Trusts. In a small qualitative study, interviews were conducted with implementation staff (mainly IT staff) ($n = 11$), parents ($n = 12$), and health visitors ($n = 12$) to identify factors affecting participation in the ePCHR. Health visitors reported finding the technology complex, especially enrolling new parents. Concerns were expressed by health visitors and parents about the security of the health information if held by a multinational company rather than the NHS. The authors describe the digital divide as being a barrier in some areas with a lack of high- speed broadband connections in rural areas posing a significant challenge, as well as some families being unable to afford the technical equipment or internet services required to access the online tool (O'Connor, 2016). Although this was a small study, insight into these limitations will be useful in further development of the digital version. An ePCHR is currently being rolled out in some districts.

Conclusion

The PCHR is a well-established and highly valued part of the CHP. However, its use is suboptimal in some population groups and by some professionals. The development of a digital record shows promise but key issues need addressing and ongoing evaluation is important.

Learning links

- The National standard for PCHR: http://www.rcpch.ac.uk/improving-child-health/public-health/personal-child-health-record/personal-child-health-record
- eRedbook, an online version of the PCHR: https://www.eredbook.org.uk/.

Recommendations

- ◆ Advise healthcare professionals to use the PCHR (whether paper or digital) and reinforce the value of the PCHR. (*Evidence: good practice.*)
- ◆ Explain the purpose, content, and use of the PCHR at or soon after its distribution to parents. (*Evidence: good practice.*)
- ◆ Evaluate the use of PCHRs among groups who traditionally use it less well such as ethnic minorities, young parents, and the socially disadvantaged. (*Evidence: strong.*)

Acknowledgement

Text extracts from Macfarlane A. 'Personal child health records' held by parents, *Archives of disease in childhood*, Volume 67, Issue 5, pp. 571–572, Copyright © 1992 reproduced with permission from the BMJ Publishing Group.

References

British Paediatric Association (1990). *Report of the Joint Working Party on Professional and Parent Held Records Used in Child Health Surveillance*. London: British Paediatric Association.

Cuthbertson, W.F.J. and Morley, D. (1962). A health and weight chart for children from birth to five. *West African Medical Journal*, December, 237–240.

Down Syndrome Medical Interest Group (DSMIG) (2017). Personal Child Health Record (PCHR). [online] Available at: https://www.dsmig.org.uk/information-resources/personal-child-health-record-pchr/ [Accessed 26 Sep. 2017].

Hall, D. and Elliman, D. (2003). *Health for all Children* (4th edn.). Oxford: Oxford University Press.

Hampshire, A.J., Blair, M.E., Crown, N.S., et al. (2004). Variation in how mothers, health visitors and general practitioners use the personal child health record. *Child: Care, Health and Development*, **30**, 307–316.

Jacobson Vann, J.C. and Szilagyi, P. (2005). Patient reminder and recall systems to improve immunization rates. *Cochrane Database of Systematic Reviews*, **3**, CD003941.

Macfarlane, A. (1992). 'Personal child health records' held by parents. *Archives of Disease in Childhood*, **67**, 571–572.

Morley, D. (1973). The Road-to-Health card. In: *Paediatric Priorities in the Developing World*, pp. 125–147. London: Butterworths.

Moss, A.L. (2005). Is the personal child health record used in secondary care? *Child: Care, Health and Development*, **31**, 627–628.

NHS England (2016). Healthy Children: A Forward View for Child Health Information. [online] Available at: https://www.england.nhs.uk/wp-content/uploads/2016/11/healthy-children-transforming-child-health-info.pdf.

Nhs.uk (2016). Birth to five development timeline. [online] Available at: http://www.nhs.uk/Tools/Pages/birthtofive.aspx [Accessed 26 Sep. 2017].

O'Connor, S., Devlin, A.M., McGee Lennon, M., et al. (2016). Factors affecting participating in the eRedbook: a personal Child Health Record. *Nursing Informatics*, **2016**, 971–972.

Readysteadybaby.org.uk (2017). Ready Steady Baby – NHS guidance for pregnancy, labour and birth. [online] Available at: http://www.readysteadybaby.org.uk/ [Accessed 26 Sep. 2017].

Sachs, M., Sharp, L., Bedford, H., and Wright, C.M., (2012). 'Now I understand': consulting parents on chart design and parental information for the UK-WHO child growth charts. *Child: Care, Health and Development*, **38**, 435–440.

Saffin, K. and Macfarlane, A. (1988). Parent held child health and development records. *General Practice, Maternal and Child Health*, October, 288–291.

Wales.nhs.uk (2017). Bump Baby and Beyond. [online] Available at: http://www.wales.nhs.uk/documents/Pregnancy%20to%204%20Years%20Book%20FINAL%20English%20Revised%20E-Book%20Compressed.pdf [Accessed 26 Sep. 2017].

Walton, S. and Bedford, H. (2007). Parents' use and views of the national standard Personal Child Health Record: a survey in two primary care trusts. *Child: Care, Health and Development*, **33**, 744–748.

Wright, C.M. and Reynolds, L. (2006). How widely are personal child health records used and are they effective health education tools? A comparison of two records. *Child: Care, Health and Development*, **32**, 55–61.

Wright, C.M., Williams, A.F., Elliman, D., et al. (2010). Using the new UK-WHO growth charts. *BMJ*, **340**, c1140–c1140.

Chapter 30

Health and early years services

Susan Soar and Mary Malone

Summary

This chapter:

+ summarizes the evidence supporting joint working in the early years
+ discusses the rationale for the integrated health and education review at age two years
+ reviews the challenges and benefits of joint working.

Introduction

From 2010 onwards, there was rapid policy development in services for the early years of life, in which health, education, and social care provision for young children became the subject of widespread government investment and reform across the UK. Evidence from reviews of the early years foundation stage (EYFS) (Tickell, 2011), health inequalities (Marmot et al., 2010), poverty and life chances (Field, 2010), early intervention (Allen, 2011), and child protection (Munro, 2011) reinforced key messages around the importance of the early years in children's later lives, emphasizing the need for prompt and effective early intervention where children are not getting the best start in life and the need for services to work together to support families. Responding to these reviews, the UK government published a joint policy document from the Department for Education (DfE) and Department for Health (DH): 'Supporting Families in the Foundation Years' (2011). Key policy elements of the new government's offer to families included increased health visitor provision, an extended entitlement to free early education, and a policy commitment to bring together the Healthy Child Programme (HCP) review at age two to two-and-a-half years with a new EYFS progress check at age two years. This chapter sets out the current status of health and early years provision and how these policy intentions have been implemented in practice.

How is health visiting provision organized?

Child health programmes (CHPs) in the UK require input from different healthcare practitioners who all contribute to child and family health, but the health visitor has a central role in delivering the HCP. Health visitors are specialist community public health nurses who have undergone one post-qualification year of specialist education in order to promote child and family health through contacts with families at home

---

Box 30.1 The four levels of service delivery

◆ *Community*: health visitors have a broad knowledge of community needs and resources available (e.g. Children's Centres and self-help groups) and work to develop these and make sure families know about them.

◆ *Universal service*: offered to every family and ensures that each child receives elements of the Healthy Child Programme such as screening, development reviews, immunization, and parenting advice.

◆ *Universal Plus*: providing families with timely, expert advice when they need it for specific issues such as postnatal depression, and feeding or sleeping problems.

◆ *Universal Partnership Plus*: working with other agencies to provide ongoing support for families with continuing complex needs, for example, where a child has a long-term condition.

Adapted under the Open Government Licence v3.0 from Department of Health, *Health Visitor Implementation Plan 2011–15: A Call to Action*, © Crown Copyright 2011, available from https://www.gov.uk/government/uploads/system/uploads/attachment_data/file/213759/dh_124208.pdf.

---

and in child health clinics. Health visitors offer this service to all families on a caseload and this universal contact enables the health visitor to offer information, guidance, and possibly referral to other agencies as well as identifying families needing extra help (Cowley et al., 2015).

In 2011, the DH determined that health visitors should deliver four levels of service: building community capacity, universal, universal plus, and universal partnership plus. These are described in Box 30.1 (DH, 2011).

All health visitors have a commitment to safeguarding children and their work at each service level helps to do this by early identification of need, intervening for change and improvement, and referral to statutory agencies if necessary. The number of key contacts by health visitors in the different CHPs in different countries of the UK varies, and has been described in Chapter 28.

How is early years provision organized?

Healthcare and early education fall under devolved powers for the individual nations in the UK, and each has a different level of entitlement to early education and childcare (see Box 30.2).

All registered early years provision in England is governed by the EYFS, a statutory framework for curriculum and welfare requirements for children from birth to 5 years (DfE, 2017). Children may take up entitlements to free early education, or paid-for hours, within a diverse range of types of setting and provision. These are briefly summarised:

◆ *Reception and nursery class provision for children within maintained schools and academies*: normally teacher led, 959,000 places for children to access early years provision within the school sector were available in 2016 (Ofsted, 2016).

Box 30.2 Free entitlements to early education and childcare 2016–2017

England

All three- and four-year-olds are currently able to receive a universal entitlement of 570 hours of free early education per year, usually taken as 15 hours a week for 38 weeks of the year. The 2016 Childcare Act increased that entitlement to 30 hours a week for children of working parents from September 2017, subject to earnings-related criteria. Many two-year-olds are also able to access 15 hours a week of free early education, with funding targeted towards children from disadvantaged groups and families in receipt of benefits.

Scotland

The Children and Young People (Scotland) Act increased provision to 600 hours of free early education per year, for all three- and four-year-olds and vulnerable two-year-olds. This equates to 16 hours per week during term time. The Scottish Government is committed to raising the entitlement to 1140 hours per year by 2020, for all three- and four-year-old children. Models for the expansion will be trialled from September 2017.

Wales

All three- and four-year-olds are entitled to a minimum of 10 hours of free, part-time, early education in a school or funded nursery. The Welsh Government is due to pilot a scheme to extend the entitlement to 30 hours a week for children of working parents.

Northern Ireland

Parents of all three- and four-year-olds can apply to receive 12.5 hours per week of funded preschool education. These hours can only be taken as 2.5 hours per day, 5 days per week, during term time. There are no plans to extend the entitlement at present.

Source: includes public sector information licensed under the Open Government Licence v3.0.

- *Maintained nursery schools*: offer teacher-led provision and the highest proportion of provision judged good or outstanding by Ofsted, but comprise a small proportion of the sector, with 403 nursery schools providing for around 44,000 pupils nationally (Ofsted, 2016).
- *Children's centres*: originally established as part of Sure Start local programmes, these now work to 'improve outcomes for young children and their families and reduce inequalities, particularly for those families in greatest need of support' (DfE, 2013). With a remit to provide integrated early childhood services and support children's outcomes in a particular geographical area, children's centres may offer

early years provision through different providers. There were 2605 main children's centre sites with a further 731 additional sites in 2015 (All Party Parliamentary Group on Children's Centres, 2016).

♦ *Nurseries, pre-schools, and playgroups within the private, voluntary, and independent sector*: private and independent day nurseries often offer full-day provision to meet the needs of working parents while pre-schools and playgroups often offer attendance on a half-day basis. Parents can use their child's free entitlement to early education within private, voluntary, and independent settings and pay for additional hours of provision by arrangement. Reception and nursery class provision is also offered within the independent school sector.

♦ *Childminders*: offer early years provision within their own homes or occasionally on non-domestic premises and may offer the free entitlement to early education (DfE, 2017). In 2016, there were 1.28 million places available to children within the childminding, private, voluntary, and independent sectors (Ofsted, 2016).

♦ *Registered home childcarers or 'nannies'*: These are private individuals employed by families to care for children within their own home. Nannies may undertake voluntary registration on the Ofsted childcare register, enabling parents to access financial support to pay for childcare; however, they are not eligible to deliver the free entitlement to early education.

Many families also use a patchwork of unregulated provision including unregistered nannies, au pairs, babysitters, grandparents, and care provided by friends and family members. Nearly half (47%) of parents use informal childcare, with grandparents offering the most hours of care (Rutter and Evans, 2012). Both health and early years practitioners need to be aware of the wider range of individuals who may be caring for children and, where relevant, to explore with families how these other carers can contribute to a child's development and well-being.

The importance of preschool education

Longitudinal research evidence has shown the importance of high-quality early education for children's longer-term outcomes. The Effective Provision of Pre-school and School Education (EPPSE) study of over 3000 children, followed children from age three to 18 years. A key study objective was to explore the impact of pre-school on children's development, alongside family background and other factors. The study's use of a 'educational effectiveness' (or value-added) approach enabled the researchers to use statistical modelling to separate out the effects of different aspects of a child's early experiences, while the large cohort size meant that it was possible to study variation in outcomes between different groups (Sylva et al., 1999). EPPSE found that pre-school improves children's intellectual development and their social behaviour, with a group of children who remained at home doing less well at entry to school even after taking into account differences in child, family, and home learning environment characteristics (Sammons et al., 2002, 2003). An earlier start at around age 2–3 years and a longer duration of attendance in months was found to be particularly beneficial, but no particular benefit was conferred by full-time as opposed to part-time attendance

(Sammons et al., 2002, 2003). The EPPSE researchers found that the positive impact of pre-school on children's attainment in reading, writing, and mathematics was evident at age 7 (Sammons et al., 2004) and age 11 years (Sylva et al., 2008). The positive effects of pre-school were still being felt at age 17, with children who had attended a high-quality pre-school being twice as likely as those who hadn't attended pre-school to take AS-levels (Sammons et al., 2015). However, the study also found that the quality of provision was key to better child outcomes, and was associated with higher staff qualifications (particularly qualified teacher status) and effective adult–child inter-actions (Sylva et al., 2004). Attending such a pre-school was found to have a lasting effect in promoting better social/behavioural outcomes, with increased levels of self-regulation, 'prosocial' behaviour and lower 'antisocial' behaviour levels at age 11 years (Sylva et al., 2008).

The EPPSE study findings on the importance of high-quality pre-school proved hugely influential and recent years have seen significant expansion of entitlements to free early education, with 94% of 3-year-olds and 99% of 4-year-olds taking up a funded place in 2015 (Public Accounts Committee, 2016). Although entitlement to free early education should be provided without cost to parents at the point of delivery, a Parliamentary enquiry in 2016 highlighted 'unacceptable variations' in the amount of information available to parents about access to free childcare, as well as concerns that some providers offer the free entitlement only on condition that parents pay for additional hours (Public Accounts Committee, 2016).

The entitlement to free early education for three-year-olds is universal, but ac-cessing the free entitlement for 2-year-olds has been directly targeted at disadvantaged families. Criteria have included receipt of income-related benefits and entitlement prioritised for children who are looked after by the local authority, have a current statement of special educational needs and disability or an Education, Health, and Care plan, who are in receipt of Disability Living Allowance or who have left care through adoption, a child arrangements order, or a special guardianship order. While these policy initiatives have increased the number of free early-education places, up-take rates for the most disadvantaged children remain lower than anticipated. While most three- and four-year-olds take up free early education, only 90% of parents take up the offer in the most deprived areas. Take-up of free early education for two-year-olds is substantially lower, with only 58% of disadvantaged two-year-olds taking up a place (National Audit Office, 2016).

The impact of the extension of the entitlement to two-year-olds is being explored as part of the Study of Early Education and Development (SEED) research study: a new longitudinal study following over 5000 two-year-olds to school entry, then tracking children via the National Pupil Database until age seven years. This study aims to evaluate the effects of free early education on children's outcomes, the quality of provi-sion, and its value for money. The large cohort, including families across the range of disadvantage-based eligibility criteria, will enable the researchers to explore the effect of the scheme on children's outcomes across different groups. The clustering of parti-cipants in geographical areas will also enable researchers to assess the impact of the quality of local provision (Speight et al., 2015). Early reported findings from the study include the quality of childminder provision (Pia Otero and Melhuish, 2015), good practice in early education (Callanan et al., 2017), and meeting the needs of children with special educational needs and disability in the early years (Griggs and Bussard, 2017). Findings on the impact of early education up to the age of three years show that, after controlling for home environment and demographic factors, the amount of early childhood education and care received between ages two and three years was associated with positive differences in cognitive and socio-emotional outcomes, across all types of provision (Melhuish et al., 2017). The final cohort of SEED study children entered reception in September 2016, so further reporting is anticipated in the next few years.

While the impact of the extended entitlement for two-year-olds is under evaluation, the incoming Conservative government of 2015 set fresh challenges for the sector with the manifesto promise of an extension to 30 hours of early education and childcare for three- and four-year-old children of working parents. However, children's organizations have expressed concern about the focus of investment shifting towards supporting extended hours of provision for working parents, rather than investing in higher levels of qualifications and training for practitioners to support children's early learning and development (Save the Children, 2016). Alongside concerns from early years sector organisations about the funding and supply of places, it remains to be seen whether the '30 hours' policy will deliver the hoped for beneficial impacts on families.

The early intervention workforce: skillsets and competencies

The revised EYFS (2012) gives all practitioners, regardless of qualification level, specific responsibilities to guide the learning and development of children in their care, safeguard their well-being, and work with parents. The Nutbrown review (2012) identified some of the key skills and competencies necessary for working with young children, including an understanding of the social, emotional, physical, and cognitive development of children, special educational needs and disabilities, early language development, skills in observing the individual child, working effectively with families, and, not least, 'providing the warmth and love children need to develop emotionally alongside and as part of planned and spontaneous learning opportunities'. However, the qualification levels and skillsets of the early years workforce remain a matter of policy tension.

The transfer of commissioning from health to local authorities and the reduction of service provision has led to contraction of the health visitor workforce throughout England, Scotland, and Wales. This means that the relative contributions of the many different practitioners are changing and the need to align contributions of all services to promote and maintain the well-being of children and families is of paramount importance. In England, provision of the universal two-year health and development review (the two-year review) is one example of how this alignment of different professional contributions is being managed.

Reviewing health and development at age two years

The independent review of the EYFS (Tickell, 2011) recommended that early years practitioners should carry out a review of a child's progress between the age of two and three years, and share this with parents. Supported by an evidence base around the importance of the first years of life, and the rationale that parents are most receptive to support and intervention in the early years, Tickell (2011) concluded that the EYFS profile at the end of the reception year was 'too late to identify school unreadiness …' and that a review at the age of two years would give an opportunity to identify areas where children might need further support. The EYFS progress check at age two years became a statutory point of assessment within the framework, when early years practitioners must review a child's progress when they are aged between 24 and 32 months and provide parents with a short, written summary of their child's development in the three prime areas: personal, social and emotional development; communication and language; and physical development. Initially intended to be carried out as a standalone early education assessment within early years settings, the revised EYFS and accompanying supporting materials asked practitioners to encourage parents to share the written summary with their health visitor during the HCP review at two years (National Children's Bureau (NCB), 2012; DfE, 2017).

The Tickell review also highlighted the overlaps between the EYFS prime areas and the HCP review and contained a recommendation that the government 'test the feasibility of a single integrated review at age two to two-and-a-half'. The joint DfE and DH (2011) policy document 'Supporting Families in the Foundation Years' led to the establishment of the DH and DfE Joint Integrated Review Development Group, with supporting materials published by NCB (2015).

In practical terms, the Integrated Review was designed to bring together existing reviews for children at around two years of age: the EYFS progress check at two years and the CHP review at age two- to two-and-a-half years. The Integrated Review, based on the 'ecological' model of child development (Bronfenbrenner, 1979), makes use of an evidence-based validated tool, the Ages and Stages Questionnaires ASQ-3™, alongside a wider review of the child's health, learning, and development and other contextual factors, to which health visitors, early years practitioners, and parents contribute. A visual model of the review is shown in Figure 30.1.

Prior to developing the Integrated Review, researchers undertook a review of a number of potential measures of child development (Bedford et al., 2013) and reviewed the acceptability and understanding of the ASQ-3™ with parents, carers and health professionals (Kendall et al, 2014). E-learning support material developed on the basis of findings of these reviews is referenced at the end of this chapter in 'Learning links'.

The Integrated Review was piloted in a number of local authority areas and an implementation study (NCB and ICF GHK, 2014) identified two core models emerging for the review. The first was a 'separate meetings' model in which integration is achieved through information sharing of separate health and early education reviews. This model allows the input of both health and early years practitioners, but success depends on good channels of communication and strong information-sharing protocols between services. The second model was a 'joint meetings' model, in which health visitors, early years practitioners, and the family come together for a meeting in the same place. This model was felt to be most holistic in terms of allowing input from both services, but potentially more time-intensive for both health and early years practitioners (NCB and ICF GHK, 2014). A subsequent follow-up study (NCB, 2015a, 2015b) returned to two local authorities that had been involved

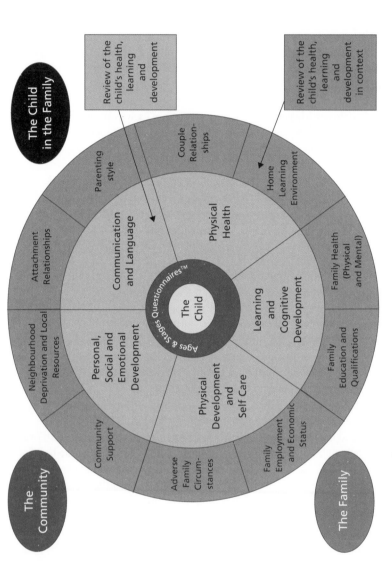

Fig. 30.1 Integrated review model.

The Integrated Review: a more detailed visual model

The Child in the Family

Review of the child's health, learning and development

Review of the child's health, learning and development in context

The Community

The Family

Parenting style

Couple Relation-ships

Attachment Relationships

Communication and Language

Physical Health

Home Learning Environment

Neighbourhood Deprivation and Local Resources

Personal, Social and Emotional Development

The Child

Ages & Stages Questionnaires™

Learning and Cognitive Development

Family Health (Physical and Mental)

Community Support

Physical Development and Self Care

Family Education and Qualifications

Adverse Family Circum-stances

Family Employment and Economic Status

in the piloting and implementation of the integrated review, to review the embedding and ongoing delivery of the review.

Findings from both the implementation study (NCB and ICF GHK, 2014) and the follow-up study (NCB, 2015a, 2015b) highlighted the importance of both health and early years practitioners' professional skillsets in working with families: maintaining a friendly and positive approach, active listening skills, and building a relationship and rapport with parents. Although neither study explored the impact on outcomes for children, feedback from parents, service leads and practitioners suggested beneficial impacts in terms of achieving a better and more holistic understanding of the child, the pooling of knowledge and services working together more effectively to support families.

Despite the identified benefits of joint working, future implementation of the Integrated Review remains dependent on policies and arrangements at a local level. Although the EYFS progress check at two years has statutory status and a review at two-and-a-half years is mandated in the Healthy Child Programme, the delivery of an integrated review is dependent on commissioning and implementation by local authorities. Implementation of the integrated review is patchy and Further research is needed to demonstrate the impact of an integrated child health and development review on improving school readiness.

Learning links

* The National Children's Bureau—'The Integrated Review: Experiences of Practice' resources: https://www.ncb.org.uk/integrated-review-resources
* E-learning for Healthcare module on the Ages and Stages Questionnaires: https://www.e-lfh.org.uk/programmes/ages-and-stages-questionnaires/.

Recommendations

* Invest in services for children under five years, ensuring provision at both a universal and targeted level. Funding streams should include inbuilt service evaluation and support for professional development. (*Evidence: strong.*)
* Promote partnership between services and parents in addition to joint working between health and early education services; for example, the implementation of an Integrated Review at age two- to two-and-a-half years. (*Evidence: emerging.*)
* Promote effective integration of the workforces by developing models of collaborative working, such as co-locating health, social care and early years workforces. (*Evidence: emerging.*)
* Work together through a process of shared decision-making, respecting each other's differing professional skills, experiences, and perspectives. (*Good practice.*)
* Consider developing the competencies and skills of health visiting teams and the early years workforce through shared education on new models of care. (*Good practice.*)

References

Allen, G. (2011). *Early Intervention: The Next Steps.* London: Cabinet Office.

All Party Parliamentary Group on Children's Centres (2016). *Family Hubs: The Future of Children's Centres.* London: 4Children.

Bedford, H., **Walton, A.**, and **Ahn, J.** (2013). *Review of Measures of Child Development.* London: Policy Research Unit in the Health of Children, Young People and Families.

Bronfenbrenner, U. (1979). *The Ecology of Human Development: Experiments by Nature and Design.* London: Harvard University Press.

Callanan, M., **Anderson M.**, **Haywood, S.**, **Hudson R.**, and **Speight S.** (2017). *Study of Early Education and Development: Good Practice in Early Education.* London: NatCen Social Research.

Cowley, S., **Whittaker, K.**, **Malone, M.**, **Donetto, S.**, **Grigulis, A.**, and **Maben, J.** (2015). Why health visiting? Examining the potential public health benefits from health visiting practice within a universal service: a narrative review of the literature. *International Journal of Nursing Studies*, **52**, 465–480.

Department for Education (DfE) (2013). *Sure Start Children's Centres Statutory Guidance.* London: DfE.

Department for Education (DfE) (2017). *Early Years Foundation Stage Statutory Framework (EYFS).* London: DfE.

Department for Education (DfE) and Department for Health (DH) (2011). *Supporting Families in the Foundation Years.* London: DfE and DH.

Department of Health (DH) (2011). Health Visitor Implementation Plan 2011–15: A Call to Action. [online] Available at: https://www.gov.uk/government/uploads/system/uploads/attachment_data/file/213759/dh_124208.pdf.

Field, F. (2010). *The Foundation Years: Preventing Poor Children Becoming Poor Adults.* London: The Cabinet Office.

Griggs, J. and **Bussard, L.** (2017). *Study of Early Education and Development (SEED): Meeting the Needs of Children with Special Educational Needs and Disabilities in the Early Years.* London: NatCen Social Research.

Kendall S., **Nash A.**, **Braun A.**, **Bastug G.**, **Rougeaux R.**, **Bedford H.** (2014). *Evaluating the Use of a Population Measure of Child Development in the Healthy Child Programme Two Year Review.* London: Policy Research Unit in the Health of Children, Young People and Families

Marmot, M. (2010). *Fair Society, Healthy Lives: Strategic Review of Health Inequalities in England post 2010.* London: The Marmot Review

Melhuish, E., **Gardiner, J.** and **Morris, S.** (2017). Study of early education and development (SEED): *Impact Study on Early Education Use and Child Outcomes up to Age Three.* NatCen Social Research: London.

Munro, E. (2009). Managing societal and institutional risk in child protection. *Risk Analysis*, **29**, 1015–1023.

Munro, E. (2011). *The Munro Review of Child Protection: Final Report. A Child-Centred System.* London: The Stationery Office.

National Audit Office (2016). *Entitlement to Free Early Education and Childcare.* London: National Audit Office.

National Children's Bureau (NCB) (2012). *A Know How Guide: The EYFS Progress Check at Two.* London: NCB.

National Children's Bureau (NCB) (2015a). *The Integrated Review: Bringing Together Health and Early Education Reviews at Age Two to Two-and-a-Half. Supporting Materials for Practitioners Working with Young Children.* London: NCB.

National Children's Bureau (NCB) (2015b). *The Integrated Review: Follow-up Report on Practice in Two Local Authority Areas.* London: NCB.

National Children's Bureau (NCB) and ICF GHK. (2014). *Review at 2-2½ Years: Integrating the Early Years Foundation Stage Progress Check and the Healthy Child Programme Health and Development Review.* London: NCB and ICF GHK.

Nutbrown, C. (2012). *Foundations for Quality: The Independent Review of early Education and Childcare Qualifications.* London: Department for Education.

Ofsted (2016). *The Annual Report of Her Majesty's Chief Inspector of Education, Children's Services and Skills 2015/16.* London: House of Commons.

Pia Otero, M. and Melhuish, E. (2015). *Study of early education and Development (SEED): Study of the Quality of Childminder Provision in England.* London: NatCen Social Research.

Public Accounts Committee (2016). *Report: Entitlement to Free Early Years Education and Childcare.* London: House of Commons.

Rutter, J. and Evans, B. (2012). *Improving our Understanding of Informal Childcare in the UK.* London: Daycare Trust.

Schonkoff, J. and Phillips, D. (Eds.) (2001). *From Neurons to Neighbourhoods: The Science of Early Child Development.* Washington, DC: National Academy Press.

Sammons, P., Sylva, K., Melhuish, E.C., Siraj, I., Taggart, B. and Elliot, K. (2002). *The EPPE Project: Technical Paper 8a – Measuring the Impact of Pre-School on Children's Cognitive Progress over the Pre-School Period.* London: DfES/Institute of Education, University of London.

Sammons, P., Sylva, K., Melhuish, E.C., Siraj-Blatchford, I., Taggart, B. and Elliot, K. (2003). *The EPPE Project: Technical Paper 8b – Measuring the Impact of Pre-School on Children's Social/Behavioural Development over the Pre-School Period.* London: DfES/Institute of Education, University of London.

Sammons, P., Sylva, K., Melhuish, E.C., Siraj, I., Taggart, B., Elliot, K. and Marsh A. (2004). *The EPPE Project: Technical Paper 11 – The Continuing Effects of Pre-school Education at Age 7 Years.* London: DfES/Institute of Education, University of London.

Sammons, P., Toth, K., and Sylva, K. (2015). *Pre-school and Early Home Learning Effects on A-Level Outcomes. Effective Pre-School, Primary and Secondary Education Project (EPPSE) Research Report.* Oxford: University of Oxford.

Save the Children (2016). *Lighting up Young Brains: How Parents, Carers and Nurseries Support Children's Brain Development in the First Five Years.* London: Save the Children.

Speight, S., Maisey, R., Chanfreau, J., Haywood, S., Lord, C., and Hussey, D. (2015). *Study of Early Education and Development (SEED): Baseline Survey of Families.* London: NatCen Social Research.

Sylva, K., Melhuish, E.C., Sammons, P., Siraj, I., and Taggart, B. (2004). *The EPPE Project: Technical Paper 12 – The Final Report: Effective Pre-School Education.* London: DfES/Institute of Education, University of London.

Sylva, K., Melhuish, E., Sammons, P., Siraj-Blatchford, I., and Taggart, B. (2008). *The EPPE 3–11 Project. Report from the Primary Phase: Pre-school, School and Family Influences on Children's Development during Key Stage 2 (Age 7–11).* London: DCSF.

Sylva, K., Sammons, P., Melhuish, E.C., Siraj-Blatchford, I. and Taggart, B. (1999). *The EPPE Project: Technical Paper 1 – An Introduction to the EPPE Project*. London: DfEE/Institute of Education, University of London.

Tickell, C. (2011). *The Early Years: Foundations for Life, Health and Learning: An Independent Report on the Early Years Foundation Stage to Her Majesty's Government*. London: Department for Education.

Chapter 31

School readiness and transition into school

Alan Emond and Jane Coad

Summary

This chapter:

- describes the concept of school readiness, its importance, and the debate about how to measure it
- discusses different ways of promoting children's readiness for school, and schools' readiness for children
- reviews the issue of the value of assessments at school entry, and the potential links with the early years foundation stage profile
- summarizes how children with medical needs can be helped in the transition into school.

Introduction

Starting school is one of life's major transitions, which for many children represents an exciting time where important formative positive relationships are formed and new learning is nurtured. However, for some it can be stressful for the child and parents or legal guardians, and may be a time when children with developmental difficulties or insecure attachments struggle.

The concept of school readiness

'Three qualities that are necessary for children to be ready for school are intellectual skills, motivation to learn, and ability to regulate emotion and make social relationships' (Robinson and Diamond, 2014). These qualities are partially genetically inherited, but also influenced by the health and well-being of the families of the children, and may be modifiable. In supporting such modifications, the Child Health Programme and early years services have an important role in identifying children with delays in developing these essential skills, and supporting their families.

School readiness is a complex construct which includes physical health and well-being, social competence, emotional maturity, language and cognitive development, and communication skills. UNICEF defines three dimensions of school readiness

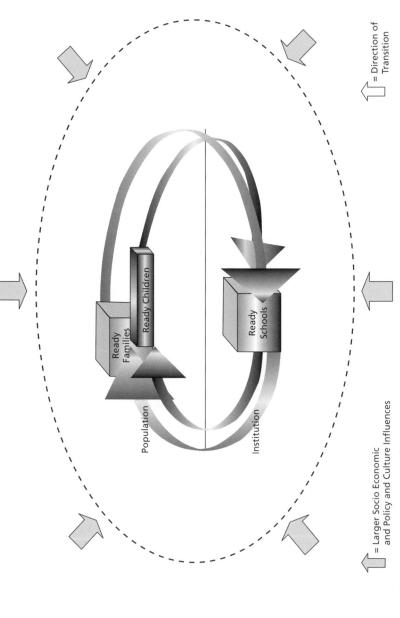

Fig. 31.1 Building Competency/Capacity for Transition to School.

as: '(1) *Ready children,* focusing on children's learning and development. (2) *Ready schools,* focusing on the school environment along with practices that foster and support a smooth transition for children into primary school and advance and promote the learning of all children. (3) *Ready families,* focusing on parental and caregiver attitudes and involvement in their children's early learning and development and transition to school' (see Figure 31.1).

The concept of school readiness has evolved from a development or maturational definition to a more socially constructed concept (UNICEF, 2012). It must be remembered that 'readiness' is a term relative to the culture and background of the family, and to the resources available to children in their homes and communities.

School readiness skills are cumulative in that there exists a hierarchy of achievement based on mastering earlier goals, that is, they build on earlier learned skills and behaviours. Readiness combines learning and development because achieving simpler skills allows for the acquisition of higher and more complex skills (Bowman et al., 2001).

Measuring school readiness

The checklist in Box 31.1 is an example of a comprehensive assessment of school readiness. There are a number of school readiness checklists, representing the many types of skills that children need to benefit from education. All are essentially normative, to allow comparisons of an individual with a 'typical' 5-year-old. However, they should not be considered as screening tests or as threshold measures, but should be viewed as guides to help parents to understand the complex developmental requirements for a child to succeed at school—it is not just a question of the child learning the alphabet or being able to count to 100!

Longitudinal studies have shown that children who were not mature in one of the key areas of school readiness when they started formal education have worse

---

Box 31.1 Topics to include in a school readiness checklist

- Social skills.
- Motor skills.
- Reasoning and concept development.
- Language skills—understanding and expression.
- Reading skills.
- Writing skills.
- Mathematics concepts.
- Science.
- Creative arts and music.

educational outcomes. In the cognitive area, a meta-analysis of six longitudinal studies (Duncan et al., 2007) showed that early mathematical skills had the greatest predictive power on subsequent educational attainment, followed by reading skills and then attention. Children's socio-emotional skills at school entry can affect peer relations, child–teacher relationships, individual learning, and the dynamics in the classroom. Poorly developed inter-personal skills lead to conflicts with teachers as well as peers, which can result in educational failure and social exclusion. Behaviour problems are associated with lower speech and language, motor, play, and peer-group skills, even after controlling for demographics. A study by Montes et al. (2012) found developmental delays of 0.6–1 standard deviations compared to children without behaviour problems, and that parents of children with behaviour problems were five times more likely to report their child was not ready for school.

The current situation in the UK is concerning: across England in 2018, only 70% of all children reached a good level of development by the age of 5 years (Gov.uk, 2018).

Children who are known to be eligible for free school meals lagged 19 percentage points behind their peers, and too few who start school behind their peers catch up by the time they leave education (Ofsted, 2014).

Promoting school readiness

Although the strongest predictor of school readiness is the family environment in which the child is raised, day care and preschool nursery settings can compensate for a lack of opportunity to learn and develop at home. Early education programmes enhance children's physical, intellectual, and social competencies, each contributing to a child's overall developmental competence and readiness for school. Many children start school with limitations in their social-emotional, physical, and cognitive development that might have been significantly modified by early recognition, support of the parents, and placement of the child in a good early years setting. A particularly important group is low birthweight and preterm infants (Roberts et al., 2011), for whom early interventions have been shown to prevent developmental delay and to improve grade retention (Brooks-Gunn et al., 1994). Nutritional support provided in preschool nursery settings can promote school readiness, by reducing iron deficiency and improving performance on standardized tests (Meyers et al., 1989). The effect of social deprivation and poverty on a young child's development is strongest during the earliest years. By the age of 3 years, there is a significant gap in cognitive test scores between children in the poorest fifth of the population compared with those from more affluent backgrounds (Carter-Wall and Whitfield, 2012) and evaluations suggest that at school entry, children from disadvantaged backgrounds could already be years behind their more economically advantaged peers (Ofsted, 2014).

Families' expectations of school readiness also impact a child's subsequent attainments. Parental beliefs and expectations are often cited as two explanations for the link between maternal education achievement and child learning outcomes (Haveman and Wolfe, 1995; Bornstein et al., 2003). Engaging with fathers is also important: Potter et al. (2012) reported a successful project in an area of multiple deprivation in the north of England which engaged fathers in their children's transition from an early years setting to formal schooling by using a highly individualized, strengths-based, empowerment-orientated approach, complemented by intensive follow-up contact via mobile phone.

In the US, the American Academy of Pediatrics recommends that paediatricians should promote the foundations of healthy child development in their contacts with families: reciprocal and nurturing relationships, routines, and regular times for meals, play, and sleeping, which help children know what they can expect and what is expected from them; praise as reward for everyday successes; reading together as a daily family activity; and rhyming, playing, and cuddling together often (High et al., 2008).

The teacher-completed Early Development Instrument (EDI) has been introduced in Canada as a measure of school readiness and shown to be useful at a population and an individual level. Janus and Duku (2010) showed that male gender, the child's suboptimal health, and coming from a family with low income contribute most strongly to the vulnerability at school entry.

In Australia, the Early Language in Victoria Study followed children from infancy to school entry, when teachers completed a school readiness assessment. 'The most influential factors in readiness for school were child language competencies and pre-literacy capacities, including phonemic awareness and letter knowledge' (Prior et al., 2010).

Preparation for school

The second aspect of school readiness is schools' readiness for children, also known as 'ready schools' or 'school ready'. The Professional Association for Childcare and Early Years (PACEY), a standard-setting professional association for everyone working in childcare and early years in England and Wales, published a comprehensive research report (PACEY, 2013) into what the term 'school ready' meant for childcare professionals, parents, and primary school teachers. Key findings are outlined in Box 31.2.

This report's key findings are helpful in listing what is important in preparation for school for the majority of children. However, there is limited robust international research on interventions to improve the preparation surrounding children from black and minority ethnic groups or with disabilities including speech and language needs. The extra needs, and the effectiveness of programmes for migrant, refugee, and travelling families to help their children achieve school readiness, are discussed in Chapter 26.

There is evidence from one review (Axford et al., 2013) that early preschool centre-based intervention programmes for disadvantaged children can improve a range of outcomes, including mother–infant interaction, home environment, child cognitive function, maternal employment and education, incidence of repeat pregnancies for teenage mothers, and maternal knowledge and attitudes about child-rearing. One small controlled study with deprived families in UK Sure Start areas (Ford et al., 2009) showed that 'scaffolded' educational activities delivered at home by mothers improved teachers' ratings at school entry of children's listening, writing, mathematics, and person-social skills.

Maintaining learning between early learning and primary school environments is a defining characteristic of ready schools. Ofsted (2014; Gov.uk, 2014) recommends 'institutional' preparation for the transition to school, with staff from the early years

---

Box 31.2 Key findings into what the term 'school ready' meant for childcare professionals, parents, and primary school teachers

1. Childcare professionals, parents, and teachers interpret the term 'school ready' in a way that is in stark contrast to that often stated by policymakers and regulators in England and more reflective of the approach taken by policymakers in Wales.

2. For a child to be considered school ready, professionals, parents, and teachers stated that cognitive and academic skills such as reading and writing were not as important as children being confident, independent, and curious. Teachers were the least likely to rate understanding of reading, arithmetic, and writing as of key importance to being school ready.

3. Both teachers and childcare professionals (58% and 40%, respectively) stated that they felt there needed to be greater emphasis on play which was felt to best support children's creativity, social, and emotional development.

4. Almost half of all respondents in the report (PACEY, 2013) identified a lack of communication and common expectation between each other as a barrier to preparing a child for school.

Adapted with permission from Professional Association for Childcare and Early Years (PACEY), *What does 'school ready' really mean? A research report from Professional Association for Childcare and Early Years,* Copyright © PACEY 2013, available from https://www.pacey.org.uk/Pacey/media/Website-files/school%20ready/School-Ready-Report.pdf.

---

setting and the school visiting each other's workplaces, and sharing learning materials and assessment approaches so that continuity is assured and a seamless transition achieved. The greater the gap between the early childhood care and the first primary school system, the greater the challenge for young children to transition from an early learning to a primary school environment. More recent research of largely US-based studies shows that preschool programmes can also enhance cognitive outcomes, social skills, and progress within school. Individualized teacher-directed instruction and small-group instruction produced the most positive gains. For example, the Getting Ready intervention in Head Start centres has been successful at promoting positive developmental outcomes and may also buffer the deleterious effects of parental depression on children's learning-related social behaviours (Sheridan et al., 2014).

Supporting families in school readiness

Carter-Wall and Whitfield (2012) reviewed the evidence on parental involvement in children's education and children's school readiness and subsequent attainment. A good example is the Family Literacy Initiative, an intervention involving several family literacy programmes in England and Wales for parents and their 3- to 6-year-old children. The initiative demonstrated evidence of impact on raising attainment: the children made gains in vocabulary, reading, and writing which were still evident 2 years later, and parents became better equipped to support children in reading and writing. Goodall et al. (2011) found robust evidence of the impact of family learning, literacy, and numeracy programmes on school readiness, which impact positively on disadvantaged families and bring benefits that outlast the duration of the intervention. Learning Wales have produced a collection of resources to help schools engage families and communities in children's learning (Learning Wales, 2016).

While there is some evidence on the effectiveness of language intervention practices that involve 'contingent language facilitation procedures', such as evidence that modelling and imitation are beneficial for young children with spoken language disorders who are entering school (i.e. at age 5 years), there are concerns about the methodological quality of studies. Roulstone et al. (2015) noted that there is limited robust international research on interventions to systematically improve the immediate environment surrounding children in order to improve language outcomes for children with or at risk of primary language impairment.

It is widely claimed that exposure to music in the preschool period can improve some aspects of cognitive development, especially in language and social and emotional skills, but the research base is limited. A controlled study of a music training programme on the auditory development of 6–7-year-old children showed that children in the music group had an enhanced ability to detect changes in tonal environment and an accelerated maturity of auditory processing (Habibi et al., 2016).

Health assessments at school entry

Although there is insufficient evidence to support a universal medical examination at school entry, starting school offers an opportunity to review the child's health and developmental status and access to primary health services. These reviews are recommended good practice (and are mandated in Scotland), and can be combined with weight measurement and screening for hearing and vision which have moderately strong evidence to support them. Child health programmes recommend that, soon after school entry, several reviews should be undertaken (usually by members of a school nursing team): a review of immunization status and to offer any missed immunizations, a review of access to primary care and dental care, and a review of any appropriate interventions for physical, emotional, or developmental problems that may have been missed or not addressed (see Chapter 23). Measuring height and weight is recommended for the National Child Measurement Programme (see Chapter 18), and two screening tests are justified: vision (by orthoptists or professional trained by and supported by orthoptists, see Chapter 21), and hearing using an agreed, quality-assured protocol in appropriate surroundings (see Chapter 20). Parental concern about hearing should always be noted and acted upon.

There is some moderate-quality evidence to support the use of the Strengths and Difficulties Questionnaire to aid the identification of emotional and behavioural difficulties prior to school entry. White et al. (2013) found that it was feasible to ask preschool education staff to assess children systematically for social and behavioural problems as part of the routine transition process at school entry, and this is being implemented in some districts in England, and in local authority areas in Scotland.

Further research is needed to determine how many children are newly identified, and how many receive an intervention as a result.

The early years foundation stage profile

In England, all schools have to complete the early years foundation stage (EYFS) profile (Gov.uk, 2017). This school entry profile is applied to all reception-year pupils in the summer term, summarizing and describing children's attainment. The EYFS profile, completed by early years practitioners based on observing a child's daily activities, describes the child's attainment in relation to the 17 early learning goals descriptors, and contains a short narrative describing the child's three characteristics of effective learning. The results are reported to local authorities, who use them to construct a baseline profile of the children entering each school, and allocate extra resources according extra needs identified.

The EYFS profile identifies the next learning steps and the support needed for each child and should be linked clearly to funding from the pupil premium. The EYFS profile is statutory for the academic year 2017–18 (Gov.uk, 2018), but the Test Standards Agency is reviewing the options for assessment in the reception year beyond 2019. The Scottish Government published their National Practice Guidance on Early Learning and Childcare: 'Building the Ambition' in 2014 (Gov.scot, 2014). Some sort of baseline assessment is regarded by early years educational experts as being essential to identify both children's potential and their needs. It would be efficient and cost-effective if the health and educational assessments in the early years could be coordinated, with information sharing about individual children, but few local authorities in the UK have achieved this.

Helping children with difficulties make a successful transition into school

For children who have special needs, who don't have English as a first language, or who live in difficult circumstances, a good transition from home or nursery to school is particularly important. The level of engagement by the child and family with the school from the start affects the child's subsequent attainment and social and emotional well-being. Good home-to-school transition programmes have been linked to better outcomes, particularly for at-risk groups. Research evidence (e.g. Bryan and Treanor, 2007) suggests that it is the children at greatest risk of poor transition experiences who benefit the most from good transitions and achieve better grades.

Children who are the youngest in their year may experience difficulties (Sanders et al., 2005). Preterm infants are especially vulnerable, especially if they are assigned according to their date of birth to a year group younger than they should have been if based on their due date (Odd et al., 2013). Children with medical conditions will need an individual healthcare plan drawn up with the school (see 'Supporting children with medical needs in primary school'), ideally before starting, to ensure that key school staff are trained and no lessons are missed because the necessary support is not in place. Children with special educational needs will require an Education, Health, and

Care plan before starting school (see Chapter 25). Looked after children and those from disadvantaged backgrounds will need targeted support.

Public Health England (2014a) published a useful guidance document 'Improving the home to school transition' written by the Institute of Health Equity, which clarifies good practice (Public Health England, 2014b). Many schools have open days, and encourage visits and familiarization lessons to help pupils adjust to the school environment, and have staggered part-time starts in the first term. Children at risk of difficult transition can be additionally helped by good communication and planning between preschool health staff, early years services, and school staff. Area special educational needs coordinators have a key role to play in planning transitions for vulnerable children. In school, special induction and orientation meetings, and one-to-one support during the transition period, can help the child settle in and participate in learning and social interaction.

Supporting children with medical needs in primary school

The responsibility for notifying the school when a child has been identified as having a medical condition which will require support in school rests with the school nurse, who should do this before the child starts at the school. Schools have a duty to provide for pupils with medical needs, and the Department for Education (2015) has issued helpful guidance for school governors and head teachers. A child with a medical condition cannot be denied admission or prevented from taking up a place in school because arrangements for their medical condition have not been made. Individual healthcare plans are recommended to facilitate these arrangements, to document the child's medical condition, the resulting health needs including medication, the specific support required for the pupil's educational, social, and emotional needs, and what to do in an emergency (see Box 31.3). Some children may have an emergency healthcare plan prepared by their lead clinician that could be used to inform development of their individual healthcare plan.

School nurses have an important coordinating role for implementing individual care plans, and can liaise with lead clinicians locally on specifying appropriate support for the child and the training needed for school staff. Community nursing teams are also a valuable source of advice, training and support in relation to children with a medical condition.

A senior nurse, in each area, should be identified to take responsibility for ensuring that adequate levels of suitably qualified staff, necessary equipment, and provision are available to allow children with complex healthcare needs to take full advantage of their education. There should be a named school nurse and doctor for each school and each school nurse should have access to a wider team of health support such as community children's nurses, paediatricians, and therapists.

Managing medicines in schools and early years settings

Disputes between health and education services over responsibilities to provide medication safely for children at school have been common, and sometimes a parent has to

Box 31.3 Components of an individual healthcare plan

- ◆ The medical condition, its triggers, signs, symptoms and treatments.

- ◆ The pupil's resulting needs, including medication (dose, side effects, and storage) and other treatments, time, facilities, equipment, testing, access to food and drink where this is used to manage their condition, dietary requirements, and environmental issues in school.

- ◆ Specific support for the pupil's educational, social, and emotional needs—for example, how absences will be managed, requirements for extra time to complete exams, use of rest periods or additional support in catching up with lessons, counselling sessions.

- ◆ The level of support needed (some children will be able to take responsibility for their own health needs) including in emergencies. If a child is self-managing their medication, this should be clearly stated with appropriate arrangements for monitoring.

- ◆ Who will provide this support, their training needs, expectations of their role, and confirmation of proficiency to provide support for the child's medical condition from a healthcare professional; and cover arrangements for when they are unavailable.

- ◆ Who in the school needs to be aware of the child's condition and the support required.

- ◆ Arrangements for written permission from parents and the head teacher for medication to be administered by a member of staff, or self-administered by the pupil during school hours.

- ◆ Separate arrangements or procedures required for school trips or other school activities outside of the normal school timetable that will ensure the child can participate (e.g. risk assessments).

- ◆ Where confidentiality issues are raised by the parent/child, the designated individuals to be entrusted with information about the child's condition.

- ◆ What to do in an emergency, including whom to contact, and contingency arrangements.

Adapted under the Open Government Licence v3.0 from Department of Education, *Supporting pupils at school with medical conditions: Statutory guidance for governing bodies of maintained schools and proprietors of academies in England*, © Crown Copyright 2014, available from https://www.gov.uk/government/uploads/system/uploads/attachment_data/file/306952/Statutory_guidance_on_supporting_pupils_at_school_with_medical_conditions.pdf.

become involved to give the medication in school, which is clearly not desirable for the parent or the child. The Department for Education and the Department of Health (2005) produced joint guidance 'Managing Medicines in Schools and Early Years Settings' to help all schools and all early years settings develop policies on managing medicines, and to put in place effective management systems to support individual children with medical needs.

Medicines should only be taken to school when it would be detrimental to a child's health if the medicine were not administered during the school or setting 'day'. Many medicines can be prescribed in dose frequencies which enable the drug to be taken outside school hours. If a medicine has to be taken during the school day, prescribers are encouraged to provide two prescriptions, one for home and one for use in the school or setting, avoiding the need for repackaging or relabelling of medicines by parents. Every school needs to have a medicines policy, and the child's individual healthcare plan should describe the arrangements for storing and giving the medicine safely.

Learning links

- There are several e-Learning for Health modules on the healthy school child such as Module 7, 'Speech Language and Communication Needs' and Module 13, 'Early Developmental Support': https://www.e-lfh.org.uk/programmes/healthy-school-child/.

Recommendations

- Use the school readiness concept as a framework to work with parents and ensure children have the necessary skills and maturity to benefit from formal education. (*Evidence: moderate.*)
- Use school readiness as an outcome measure for preschool child health programme and early years education services. (*Evidence: moderate.*)
- It is good practice for an integrated health and early years review at 24–30 months of age, involving the health visitor, the child's key worker at nursery or children's centre, the child, and the parent coming together to jointly review the child's health, development and learning, to provide early intervention and support for families in deprived areas. (*Good practice.*)
- Appoint a named school nurse and doctor for each school, with each school nurse having access to a wider team of health support such as community children's nurses, paediatricians, and therapists. (*Evidence: moderate.*)
- Children with medical needs may require individual healthcare plans to support their transition into reception class. (*Good practice.*)

Acknowledgement

Text extracts from UNICEF, *School Readiness: A Conceptual Framework*, Copyright © 2012 United Nations Children's Fund, New York, USA reproduced with permission from UNICEF, available from https://www.unicef.org/earlychildhood/files/Child2Child_ConceptualFramework_FINAL(1).pdf.

References

Axford, N. and Morpeth, L. (2013). Evidence-based programs in children's services: a critical appraisal. *Children and Youth Services Review*, **35**, 268–277.

Blair, C. (2002). School readiness as propensity for engagement: integrating cognition and emotion in a neurobiological conceptualization of child functioning at school entry. *American Psychologist*, **57**, 111–127.

Bornstein, M.H., Hendricks, C., Hahn, C.-S., et al. (2003). Contributors to self-perceived competence, satisfaction, investment, and role balance in maternal parenting: a multivariate ecological analysis. *Parenting: Science and Practice*, **3**, 285–326.

Bowman, B.T., Donovan, S., and Burns, M.S. (Eds.) (2001). *Eager to Learn: Educating Our Preschoolers*. Washington, DC: National Research Council, National Academy of Sciences.

Brooks-Gunn, J., McCarton, C.M., Casey, P.H., et al. (1994). Early intervention in low-birth-weight premature infants: results through age 5 years from the Infant Health and Development Program. *JAMA*, **272**, 1257–1262.

Bryan, R. and Treanor, M. (2007). *Evaluation of Pilots to Improve Primary and Secondary School Transitions*. Edinburgh: Scottish Executive.

Carter-Wall, C, and Whitfield, G. (2012). The Role of Aspirations, Attitudes and Behaviour in Closing The Educational Attainment Gap. [online] The Joseph Rowntree Foundation. Available at: https://www.nationalnumeracy.org.uk/research-role-aspirations-attitudes-and-behaviour-closing-educational-attainment-gap-2012.

Department for Education (2015). *Supporting Pupils at School with Medical Conditions: Statutory Guidance for Governing Bodies of Maintained Schools and Proprietors of Academies in England*. London: Department for Education.

Department for Education and Skills/Department of Health (2005). *Managing Medicines in Schools and Early Years Settings*. London: Department for Education.

Duncan, G.J., Dowsett, C.J., Claessens, A., et al. (2007). School readiness and later achievement. *Developmental Psychology*, **43**, 1428.

Ford, R.M., McDougall, S.J.P., and Evans, D. (2009). Parent-delivered compensatory education for children at risk of educational failure: improving the academic and self-regulatory skills of a Sure Start preschool sample. *British Journal of Psychology*, **100**, 773–797.

Goodall, J., Vorhaus, J., Carpentieri, J., Brooks, G., Akerman, A., and Harris, A. (2011). *Review of Best Practice in Parental Engagement*. Research Report DFE-RR156. London: Department for Education. Available at: https://www.education.gov.uk/publications/RSG/publicationDetail/Page1/DFE-RR156.

Gov.scot (2014). National Practice Guidance on Early Learning and Childcare. [online] Available at: http://www.gov.scot/Publications/2014/08/6262 [Accessed 26 Sep. 2017].

Gov.uk (2014). Helping disadvantaged children start school. [online] Available at: https://www.gov.uk/government/publications/are-you-ready-good-practice-in-school-readiness [Accessed 26 Sep. 2017].

Gov.uk (2017). Early years foundation stage profile: 2017 handbook. [online] Available at: https://www.gov.uk/government/publications/early-years-foundation-stage-profile-handbook [Accessed 28 Sep. 2017].

Gov.uk (2018). Early years foundation stage profile 2017–18. [online] Available at: https://www.gov.uk/government/statistics/early-years-foundation-stage-profile-results-2017-to-2018 [Accessed 12 Nov. 2018].

Habibi, A., **Cahn Damasio, A.**, and **Damasio, H.** (2016). Neural correlates of accelerated auditory processing in children engaged in music training. *Developmental Cognitive Neuroscience*, **21**, 1–14.

Haveman, R. and **Wolfe, B.** (1995). The determinants of children's attainments: a review of methods and findings. *Journal of Economic Literature*, **33**, 1829–1878.

High, P.C., **American Academy of Pediatrics Committee on Early Childhood, Adoption, and Dependent Care, and Council on School Health** (2008). School readiness. *Pediatrics*, **121**, e1008–e1015.

Janus, M. and **Duku, E.** (2010). The school entry gap: socioeconomic, family, and health factors associated with children's school readiness to learn. *Early Education and Development*, **18**, 373–403.

Learning Wales (2016). Family and community engagement toolkit for schools. [online]. Available from: http://learning.gov.wales/resources/browse-all/family-and-community-engagement-toolkit/?lang=en [Accessed 12 Nov. 18].

Meyers, A.F., **Sampson, A.E., Weitzman, M., Rogers, B.L.**, and **Kayne, H.** (1989). School Breakfast Program and school performance. *American Journal of Diseases of Children*, **143**, 1234–1239.

Montes, G., **Lotyczewski, B.S., Halterman, J.S.**, and **Hightower, A.D.** (2012). School readiness among children with behavior problems at entrance into kindergarten: results from a US national study. *European Journal of Pediatrics*, **171**, 541–548.

Odd, D., **Evans, D.**, and **Emond, A.** (2013). Preterm birth, age at school entry and educational performance. *PLoS One*, **8**, e76615.

Ofsted (2014). Are you ready? Good practice in school readiness. [online] Available at: www.ofsted.gov.uk/resources/140074.

Potter, C., **Walker, G.**, and **Keen, B.** (2012). Engaging fathers from disadvantaged areas in children's early educational transitions: a UK perspective. *Journal of Early Childhood Research*, **10**, 209–225.

Prior, M., **Bavin, E.**, and **Ong, B.** (2011). Predictors of school readiness in five-to six-year-old children from an Australian longitudinal community sample. *Educational Psychology*, **31**, 3–16.

Professional Association for Childcare and Early Years (PACEY) (2013). What does school ready really mean? A research report from Professional Association for Childcare and Early Years. [online] Available at: https://www.pacey.org.uk/Pacey/media/Website-files/school%20ready/School-Ready-Report.pdf.

Public Health England (2014a). Good quality parenting programmes and home to school transition. [online] Available at: https://fingertips.phe.org.uk/documents/Early_intervention_health_inequalities.pdf [Accessed 26 Sep. 2017].

Public Health England (2014b). *Improving the Home to School Transition*. Health Equity Briefing 1b. Publications Gateway Number: 2014334. London: Public Health England.

Robinson, C.D. and **Diamond, K.E.** (2014). A quantitative study of head start children's strengths, families' perspectives, and teachers' ratings in the transition to kindergarten. *Early Childhood Education Journal*, **42**, 77.

Roberts, G., **Lim, J., Doyle, L.W.**, and **Anderson, P.J.** (2011). High rates of school readiness difficulties at 5 years of age in very preterm infants compared with term controls. *Journal of Developmental & Behavioral Pediatrics*, **32**, 117–124.

Roulstone, S.E., **Marshall, J.E., Powell, G.G.**, et al. (2015). *Evidence-Based Intervention for Preschool Children with Primary Speech and Language Impairments: Child Talk–An*

Exploratory Mixed-Methods Study. Southampton: NIHR Journals Library. Available at: https://www.ncbi.nlm.nih.gov/books/NBK311174/.

Sanders, D., White, G., Burge, B., et al. (2005). *A Study of the Transition from the Foundation Stage to Key Stage 1*. London: Department for Education and Skills.

Scottish Government (2014). Building the Ambition: National Practice Guidance on Early Learning and Childcare Children and Young People (Scotland) Act 2014. [online] Available at: http://www.gov.scot/Resource/0045/00458455.pdf.

Sheridan, S., Knoche, L., Edwards, C., et al. (2014). Efficacy of the Getting Ready Intervention. *Early Education and Development*, **25**, 746–769.

UNICEF (2012). *School Readiness: A Conceptual Framework*. New York: United Nations Children's Fund.

White, J., Connelly, G., Thompson, L. and Wilson, P. (2013). Assessing wellbeing at school entry using the strengths and difficulties questionnaire: professional perspectives. *Educational Research*, **55**, 87–98.

Chapter 32

Enhancements to child health programmes in the UK

Alan Emond and Alice Haynes

Summary

This chapter reviews the evidence supporting five enhancements to the child health programmes in the UK currently being evaluated:

- Flying Start
- Family Nurse Partnership (FNP)
- A Better Start
- Maternal Early Childhood Sustained Home-visiting (MECSH)
- Trial of Healthy Relationship Initiatives for the Very Early-years (THRIVE).

Flying Start

Flying Start (Children in Wales, 2014) is the Welsh Government's targeted early years programme aimed at families with children below 4 years of age living in some of the most deprived areas in Wales. Flying Start started in 2007 and was initially administered as a grant to local authorities, targeted on the catchment areas of schools in deprived areas. The expansion of the scheme from 2011 resulted in changed criteria where funding was allocated according to the estimated number of 0–3-year-olds living in income benefit households in local authority areas. In 2016–2017, 37,628 children were in receipt of Flying Start services in Wales. Flying Start is one of the Welsh Government's top priorities in policies to reduce the impact of poverty.

Key components of Flying Start are:

- quality, part-time childcare for 2–3-year-olds (2.5 hours a day, 5 days a week)
- an enhanced health visiting service (one full-time equivalent health visitor per 110 children under 4 years)
- access to parenting support (positive parenting groups or one-to-one home visits)
- support for children's speech, language, and communication (language and play groups).

In addition to the four core elements, an element of outreach work is included, allowing local authorities to deliver all elements of Flying Start to a small percentage of their population who live outside of designated Flying Start areas.

Several evaluations of Flying Start have been undertaken since 2009, using a variety of different methodologies. The Welsh Government's national evaluation of the programme was published in December 2013—'National Evaluation of Flying Start: Impact Report'. More recent evaluations published in 2017 include educational outcomes and qualitative research with Flying Start families. These reports are available from http://gov.wales/statistics-and-research/national-evaluation-flying-start/?lang=en.

The evaluations showed that families in Flying Start areas did have more health visitor contacts and a higher take-up of parenting programmes, language and play, and other early years services. Respondents felt more positive about the services and the support provided to parents, and users reported positive impacts on themselves as parents and on their children. However, the analysis showed no differences between parents in Flying Start areas and parents in comparison areas on parenting self-confidence, mental health, or home environment measures. There were also no differences between Flying Start and non-Flying Start areas in terms of children's cognitive and language skills, their social and emotional development, and their independence/self-regulation. Living in a Flying Start area after it was introduced was related to better school attendance and an increased chance of children with special educational needs being identified early.

The evaluations have recognized that families in Flying Start areas were more deprived than those in comparison areas, and therefore started in a lower baseline position, so the programme 'brought about parity' with less disadvantaged comparison areas. It has also been difficult to be certain what level of support each individual child received from Flying Start, so it has not been possible to show that being in receipt of Flying Start improved child development, school readiness, or educational attainment.

Further evaluations of Flying Start are planned—what is needed is to have data on families' engagement with Flying Start at the individual level, and to link these data with educational outcomes.

A Better Start

A Better Start (Abetterstart.org.uk, 2017) is a 10-year strategic investment by the Big Lottery Fund in England, focused on developing and testing new approaches to promoting good Early Childhood Development (ECD). The programme is made up of five local partnerships, working in wards with high levels of economic deprivation in Blackpool, Bradford, Lambeth, Nottingham, and Southend-on-Sea. Each partnership has developed a locally tailored strategy which draws on their analysis of strengths of the community and the specific challenges they face. Implementation of the local strategies began in 2015.

The partnerships are each led by a voluntary sector organization and comprise a range of partners including parents, members of the community, statutory agencies (such as senior representation from the local authority, clinical commissioning groups, hospital trusts, and the police), and the community sector. The programme is provided for all families living in the target wards, from pregnancy until their child turns four.

The strategies are aimed at achieving four interlinked outcomes:

- Improving children's diet and nutrition, for example, through healthy diet and be-haviours in pregnancy, breastfeeding, and physical activity.
- Improving speech, language, and communication skills, for example, through parent–child relationships and interaction, such as talking, reading, and playing.
- Enhancing social and emotional development, for example, through parent–child relationships and good parental mental health.
- Bringing about systems change to embed a shift towards prevention-focused, re-sponsive, co-produced, and evidence-based support for children and families.

Intrinsic to A Better Start is a belief in the importance of co-production (Alakeson et al., 2013), a partnership between professionals, the wider community and parents through which support for children and families is designed, planned, and delivered. Decision-making is shared and inclusive, and all partners are seen as equal and valued for their distinct strengths and assets. The expected benefits of this approach include more effective service provision and the embedding of reciprocal and enduring rela-tionships between all partners to build and sustain local communities.

A Better Start is a 'test and learn' programme. Reviews of the evidence were conducted to support the initial development of the A Better Start programme (Dartington Social Research Centre, 2013a, 2013b). The long-term investment provides the opportunity for partnerships to rigorously design, implement, evaluate, and adapt approaches to promoting ECD on a small scale to learn what works and what does not. A national, independent evaluation of A Better Start is being led by the Warwick Consortium over the 10 years of the programme. It will evaluate the set-up, implementation, and effectiveness of the programme within and across the areas. The impact evaluation comprises a longitudinal cohort study of families in the 5 funded and 15 external com-parison areas (Warwick Consortium, 2015). The partnerships are also evaluating their programmes and services locally, providing further detailed analysis of individual services and service configurations, and building evaluation capabilities.

A Common Outcomes Framework for A Better Start was developed by the Personal Social Services Research Unit (2016) at the London School of Economics in collabor-ation with the five A Better Start partnerships and a range of experts in ECD. Available for use in any local area, it sets out key population-level outcomes and indicators to help local areas track ECD outcomes, and to compare trends to national level data where these are available. It is based on critical milestones in the early years—birth outcome, school readiness, and key stage attainment. It is underpinned by a review of the evidence base and driven by availability of routinely collected data.

The London School of Economics has developed a model of 'preventomics' which includes a number of practice tools to assist local areas understand the potential down-stream public sector cost savings from investing in prevention in the early years.

Learning, tools, and resources from the A Better Start national evaluation, partner-ships, and development support programme are being made freely available to sup-port other local areas to improve ECD outcomes. Further information about A Better

Start, the partnerships, and available resources and tools can be found at http://www.abetterstart.org.uk and https://www.biglotteryfund.org.uk/abs.

The establishment of a core outcome set, and the philosophy of sharing learning both between partnerships and to support early child development more widely, are to be commended. The results of the evaluations of specific programmes within A Better Start are awaited with interest.

Family Nurse Partnership (FNP)

The FNP is a preventative programme targeted at young mothers, which was developed in the US as the Nurse-Family Partnership Programme by David Olds (Olds, 2006) and since 2007 has been implemented in the NHS in England (Fnp.nhs.uk, 2015) and since 2010 in Scotland (Gov.scot, 2017). The FNP is a licensed, intensive home-visiting intervention that involves up to 64 structured home visits from early pregnancy until the child's second birthday by specially recruited and trained family nurses. It has been offered to first-time mothers under 19 years of age recruited in pregnancy. The goals of the FNP are to:

♦ improve maternal health during pregnancy

♦ better child development

♦ increase maternal economic self-sufficiency.

The FNP aims to affect risks and protective factors within prenatal health-related behaviours, develop sensitive and competent care giving, and modify the parental life course. Core specialist training for nurses includes motivational interviewing and the adoption of a guiding autonomy-supportive communication style with clients.

Three evaluations of the FNP in the US (Olds et al., 1986, 2002; Kitzman et al., 1997) and one in the Netherlands (Mejdoubi et al., 2014) have shown positive results for mothers and babies. Benefits for mothers include improved pregnancy health and behaviours (e.g. reduced smoking in pregnancy), a reduction in short inter-pregnancy intervals, and an increase in maternal employment and economic self-sufficiency. Childhood outcomes include reductions in child abuse and neglect, improved school readiness, and a reduction in behavioural and emotional problems at age 6 years.

In 2006, the UK Government announced its intention to test the FNP programme, and it was adapted under licence for delivery in England from early pregnancy until children were 2 years old. Initial implementation in England in 2007–2008 involved ten sites and focused on feasibility and acceptability of the manualized programme adapted for the English setting. The FNP was delivered well in England with fidelity to the programme model; young mothers and fathers liked the programme and valued the materials that were used, engaged well, and there was a good potential for positive outcomes and longer-term cost savings. In 2009–2010, a pragmatic individually randomized controlled trial (RCT) 'Building Blocks' was carried out in 18 NHS sites in England, comparing usual care with usual care plus FNP (Robling et al., 2016). The English RCT was not able to replicate the benefits shown in the American evaluations, as the FNP did not have an impact across the study's four main short-term outcomes—prenatal tobacco use, birth weight, subsequent pregnancy by 24 months, and emergency department attendances and hospital admissions in first 2 years of life. A wide range of secondary outcomes assessed also didn't show significant benefits for the FNP, but weak effects were seen on intention-to-breastfeed, maternally reported child cognitive development, and language development. Although this trial did not provide sufficient evidence to recommend wider roll-out of the FNP across the NHS, more research is needed. A longer-term follow-up to age 6 years is being funded by the National Institute for Health Research and is due to report in 2018. One of the strengths of the FNP is that all sites are required to demonstrate fidelity to the programme by measuring how core model elements are being achieved ('Fidelity Goals'), resulting in continuous quality improvement (see Chapter 37).

Following the publication of the Building Blocks trial, the FNP in the UK has been extended to include 20–24-year-old mothers and adapted to be more flexible for individual family's needs and better integrated with local service provision. 'FNP Next Steps' aims to achieve broader and greater outcomes for families, with clear evidence of cost-effectiveness. The A Better Start partnerships are trialling adaptations to the FNP, to the way in which the programme is delivered (termed 'personalization') and in the clinical content of the programme. Personalization includes changes to the eligibility criteria, greater flexibility in the content of sessions, increasing or decreasing the amount of support women receive, and early graduation from the programme. The partnerships are developing and testing clinical adaptations on breastfeeding, attachment, domestic abuse and healthy re-lationships, and perinatal mental health. These adaptations may increase the ef-fectiveness of the FNP in the British context, but evaluations are awaited. Learning will be made available from the FNP national website (http://fnp.nhs.uk/evidence/fnp-next-steps).

Maternal Early Childhood Sustained Home-visiting (MECSH)

The MECSH programme (Earlychildhoodconnect.edu.au, 2014) is a structured pro-gramme of sustained home visiting delivered by health visitors for families at risk of poorer maternal and child health and development outcomes. There are MECSH-licensed sites in Australia, South Korea, and the US and at several sites in the UK and the Channel Islands (Kemp et al., 2017). The MECSH programme components are outlined in Box 32.1 (Kemp et al., 2017; Earlychildhoodconnect.edu.au, 2014; Kemp 2018).

The MECSH programme is delivered through at least 25 home visits by the same health visitor during pregnancy and the first 2 years post birth, group activ-ities, and engagement with community, services, and supports, delivered as part of a comprehensive, integrated approach to services for young children and their families.

The first RCT of MECSH conducted in Sydney, Australia (Kemp et al., 2011) showed that intervention mothers were more likely to experience a normal, unassisted vaginal

Box 32.1 MECSH programme components

1. Supporting mother and child health and well-being, including observation and support of child, maternal and family health and development, parent–infant interaction, and provision of primary healthcare and health education.

2. Supporting mothers to be future oriented and aspirational for themselves, their child, and family.

3. Supporting family and social relationships within the extended family, with the family's communities, and with other health and social services.

4. Delivery of a structured programme of parent education about child development using the 'Learning to Communicate' programme.

5. Additional support in response to need including interventions by the health visitor and accessing additional services.

6. Integration into health visitor professional development and practice and child and family service systems, so that the effects of the programme 'spill over' to the whole population.

Adapted with permission from Kemp L., *MECSH: Maternal Early Childhood Sustained Home-visiting At a Glance*, Western Sydney University, School of Nursing and Midwifery, Translational Research and Social Innovation, Liverpool, NSW, Australia, 2018.
Source: data from MECSH, earlychildhoodconnect.edu.au; and Kemp L *et al.* Maternal Early Childhood Sustained Home-visiting (MECSH): a UK update. *Journal of Health Visiting*, Volume 5, Issue 8, pp. 392–397. Copyright © 2017 MA Healthcare Limited.

birth than the general Australian population, had better self-rated perinatal health, and felt more enabled and confident to care for themselves and their baby. The mothers showed improved verbal and emotional responsiveness, used more developmentally appropriate play materials, and generally had more involvement with their children. The intervention children were breastfed for longer, and children of mothers who were distressed in pregnancy showed improved in cognitive development (scores on the Bayley Mental Developmental Index). Interestingly, the programme benefitted their parenting of older and subsequent children, and population-level data showed that the children living in the trial community had fewer developmental vulnerabilities at school entry.

A large, 'arms-length', multisite randomized trial in Australia based on MECSH, the right@home trial (Goldfeld et al., 2017) has recently completed. The intervention included additional modules focusing on parent care, responsivity, and the home learning environment. The trial demonstrated benefits for mothers (warmer parenting and more facilitation of their child's learning) and infants (safer family homes and more regular bedtimes) (Goldfeld et al., 2018).

In the UK, MECSH is being piloted in Essex (Plastow, 2013), and a UK update has recently been published (Kemp et al., 2017), but more evidence is needed of its sustained impact and cost-effectiveness of the intensive programme of home visits before it can be more widely implemented in the NHS.

Trial of Healthy Relationship Initiatives for the Very Early-years (THRIVE)

The effectiveness of two parenting support programmes targeted at pregnant women with additional health and social care needs (mental health difficulties, addiction, domestic abuse, or been in care) is being evaluated in a large trial in the west of Scotland (THRIVE) (Thrive.sphsu.mrc.ac.uk, 2013). The programmes Enhanced Triple P for Baby (Sanders, 2012) and Mellow Bumps (MacBeth et al., 2015) are being compared with usual NHS care, with the outcomes of anxiety and depression and parenting self-efficacy in the mothers, the quality of parent–child interaction, and the language development of the child at 18 months. The interventions are being compared in a large, well-funded RCT with a cost-effectiveness evaluation, and the results should be relevant to the wider NHS.

Learning links

+ A Better Start: https://www.abetterstart.org.uk/content/expert-presentations
+ Family Nurse Partnership: http://fnp.nhs.uk/fnp-next-steps/kse/
+ Flying Start: http://www.childreninwales.org.uk/resources/
+ MECSH: http://www.earlychildhoodconnect.edu.au/home-visiting-programs/mecsh-public/about-mecsh
+ THRIVE: http://thrive.sphsu.mrc.ac.uk/practitioners.

Recommendations

+ Evaluate through the life course of the child health programme, from programme initiation, data linkage, to educational outcomes. (*Evidence: strong.*)
+ Develop process measures in the enhanced child health programme to ensure that all families received similar input. (*Evidence: strong.*)
+ Assess the added value of the enhanced targeted programme by comparison with families receiving usual care who are living in similar areas of social deprivation. (*Evidence: strong.*)
+ Consider a cost-effectiveness analysis as part of every impact assessment of a new enhancement to the child health programme. (*Evidence: moderate.*)

Acknowledgement

Thanks to Lynn Kemp (MECSH) for providing material to write the chapter.

References

Abetterstart.org.uk (2017). A Better Start – Evaluation & Learning. [online] Available at: https://www.abetterstart.org.uk/ [Accessed 20 Sep. 2017].

Alakeson, V., Bunnin, A., and **Miller, C.** (2013). *Coproduction of Health and Wellbeing Outcomes: The New Paradigm for Effective Health and Social Care.* London: OPM Connects.

Children in Wales (2014). The Flying Start Network. [online] Available at: http://www.childreninwales.org.uk/our-work/early-years/flying-start-network/ [Accessed 19 Sep. 2017].

Dartington Social Research Centre (2013a). *The Science Within: What Matters for Child Outcomes in the Early Years.* Dartington: The Social Research Unit.

Dartington Social Research Centre (2013b). *What Works: An Overview of the Best Available Evidence on Giving Children a Better Start.* Dartington: The Social Research Unit

Earlychildhoodconnect.edu.au (2014). About MECSH. [online] Available at: http://www.earlychildhoodconnect.edu.au/home-visiting-programs/mecsh-public/about-mecsh [Accessed 28 Sep. 2017].

Fnp.nhs.uk (2015). The Family Nurse Partnership. [online] Available at: http://fnp.nhs.uk/ [Accessed 28 Sep. 2017].

Goldfeld, S., Price, A., Bryson, H., et al. (2017). 'right@home': a randomised controlled trial of sustained nurse home visiting from pregnancy to child age 2 years, versus usual care, to improve parent care, parent responsivity and the home learning environment at 2 years *BMJ Open*, **7**, e013307.

Gov.scot (2017). Family Nurse Partnership Programme. [online] Available at: http://www.gov.scot/Topics/People/Young-People/early-years/parenting-early-learning/family-nurse-partnership [Accessed 28 Sep. 2017].

Goldfeld, S., Price, A., and **Kemp, L.** (2018). Designing, testing, and implementing a sustainable nurse home visiting program: right@ home. *Annals of the New York Academy of Sciences*, **1419**, 141–159.

Kemp L. (2018). *MECSH: Maternal Early Childhood Sustained Home-Visiting At a Glance.* Liverpool, NSW: Western Sydney University, School of Nursing and Midwifery, Translational Research and Social Innovation.

Kemp, L., Cowley, S., and **Byrne, F.** (2017). Maternal Early Childhood Sustained Home-visiting (MECSH): a UK update. *Journal of Health Visiting*, **5**, 392–397.

Kemp, L., Harris, E., McMahon, C., et al. (2011). Child and family outcomes of a long-term nurse home visitation programme: a randomised controlled trial. *Archives of Disease in Childhood*, **96**, 533–540.

Kitzman, H., Olds, D.L., and **Henderson, C.R.** (1997). Effect of prenatal and infancy home visitation by nurses on pregnancy outcomes, childhood injuries, and repeated childbearing. A randomized controlled trial. *JAMA*, **278**, 644–652.

MacBeth, A., Law, J., McGowan, I., Norrie, J., Thompson, L., and **Wilson, P.** (2015). Mellow Parenting: systematic review and meta-analysis of an intervention to promote sensitive parenting. *Developmental Medicine and Child Neurology*, **57**, 1119–1128.

Mejdoubi, J., van den Heijkant, S.C., van Leerdam, F.J., et al. (2014). Effects of nurse home visitation on cigarette smoking, pregnancy outcomes and breastfeeding: a randomized controlled trial. *Midwifery*, **30**, 688–695.

Olds, D.L. (2006). The nurse-family partnership: an evidence-based preventive intervention. *Infant Mental Health Journal*, **27**, 5–25.

Olds, D.L., Henderson, C.R., Jr., Tatelbaum, R., and **Chamberlin, R.** (1986). Improving the delivery of prenatal care and outcomes of pregnancy: a randomized trial of nurse home visitation. *Pediatrics*, **77**, 16–28.

Olds, D.L., Robinson, J., and O'Brien, R. (2002). Home-visiting by paraprofessionals and by nurses: a randomized, controlled trial. *Pediatrics*, **110**, 486–496.

Personal Social Services Research Unit (2016). *A Better Start: Developing an Early Years Outcomes Framework using Area-Level Routine Data*. London: London School of Economics.

Plastow, L. (2013). Implementing maternal early childhood sustained home visiting in Essex. *Journal of Health Visiting*, **1**, 96–103.

Robling, M., Bekkers, M.-J., Bell, K., et al. (2016). Effectiveness of a nurse-led intensive home-visitation programme for first-time teenage mothers (Building Blocks): a pragmatic randomised controlled trial. *The Lancet*, **387**, 146–155.

Sanders, M.R. (2012). Development, evaluation, and multinational dissemination of the Triple P-Positive Parenting Program. *Annual Review of Clinical Psychology*, **8**, 345–379

Thrive.sphsu.mrc.ac.uk (2013). Trial of Health Relationships Initiatives for the Very Early years (THRIVE). [online] Available at: http://thrive.sphsu.mrc.ac.uk/ [Accessed 28 Sep. 2017].

Warwick Consortium (2015). The impact and economic evaluation of A Better Start. [online] Available at: https://www.abetterstart.org.uk

Section 7

Implementation of a healthy child programme

Chapter 33

Delivering and managing an effective child health programme across the UK

Mitch Blair

Summary

This chapter:

♦ describes the necessary steps required to deliver and manage a child health programme (CHP), using the principles of implementation and improvement science in order to embed learning within the programme

♦ discusses a number of prerequisites for high-quality provision, including workforce capacity and competence

♦ reviews the evidence for accredited training, the use of learning sets, and data feedback loops

♦ emphasizes that the establishment of a local CHP steering group is a key organizational mechanism to bring stakeholders together

♦ outlines variations in different UK country programmes.

Introduction

Most of the preceding chapters of this book have reviewed the scientific evidence base for different interventions or topics which come within the umbrella term the 'child health programme' (CHP). The core components of the CHP or the equivalent well-child programmes in other countries are:

1. screening and case finding through surveillance

2. health promotion and health education including specific programmes (e.g. injury prevention and smoking cessation)

3. parenting support

4. immunization.

This chapter describes how the whole clinical public health programme is delivered, managed, and improved. The practical aspect of the implementation of such a programme also has an evidence base in its own right (Blair, 2014). This is what some refer to as translational science, and more recently, improvement science. Two forms of translational research exist, T1—that is bench to bedside; from the discovery of a particular phenomenon to its use at the bedside, and T2—which is the systematic review of randomized controlled trials and the development of clinical guidelines for use in practice. A third possible form is emerging which is the translation of such guidance in practice through health services research and improvement science which we might class as T3. This chapter is concerned primarily with the last of these forms of translational research.

Why a programme?

The first issue here is the recognition that a programme is more than the sum of its parts and has a number of advantages in terms of its 'brand recognition' both for policymakers and professionals, including development of a coherent set of knowledge, skills, and attitudes of those professionals who are implementing it on the ground, and for commissioners to appreciate that this is a holistic public health programme with its own distinct identity and content. Who the programme is delivered by becomes less important than the capacity, skills, and competencies of the workforce responsible for its delivery. Whether the CHP is delivered in a home setting, community centres, GP surgeries, or indeed preschool and school settings is a matter for local decision-makers. The principal issue is to ensure that it is implemented with the highest possible quality within the resources available.

The Council of Europe guidelines on child friendly health services reinforces this approach with the guiding philosophy to 'place children's rights, needs and resources at the centre of health care activities, taking into account children's opinions and evolving capacities'. This implies the adoption of an integrated and multidisciplinary approach, sometimes referred to as a 'continuum of care'. They were ratified by all European Health Ministers in 2011 and by all three major European Paediatric Associations (Lenton et al., 2016).

This allows us to think about the delivery of interventions (e.g. immunization) in terms of doing the right things (evidence), to the right children (need), with the right workforce (competencies), at the right time, and in the right location. Evidence and competencies required are well defined but workforce and location may well differ between areas. This is explored in more detail in Chapter 34 in relation to quality assurance and improvement of the programme.

Another dimension to be considered here is the reach of the programme; that is, who the recipients are of the interventions contained within it. It is tempting in times of austerity to focus on those in most need of services, but this must not be at the expense of delivering a high-quality universal service to all. This is the essence of a proportionate universal approach, and the appropriate combination of both approaches is needed to ensure a shift in the population curve (e.g. improving mental health or language skills for all as well as a focus on those at particularly high risk). The analogy often used in adult medicine is to reduce the levels of blood pressure for all through reduction in salt content of foods overall or to screen for those at high risk and treat.

Implementation of the child health programme

A number of theoretical frameworks have been developed to help us to understand how such scientific innovations are implemented. Laura Damschroeder and colleagues' (2009) 'Comprehensive Implementation Research Framework' (CIRF) is a review of reviews which identifies five major domains which are necessary to consider for implementation. These are the intervention, inner and outer settings, the individuals involved, and the process by which implementation is accomplished (see Figure 33.1—major domains of the CIRF).

Without adaptation, interventions usually come to a setting as a poor fit resisted by those who will be affected by them and requiring an active process to engage individuals in order to accomplish implementation. The left side of Figure 33.1 shows how the intervention has not been adapted to the setting with the puzzle not fitting well with the other pieces. Interventions can be conceptualized as having core components (as was described earlier) and an 'adaptable periphery'; that is, those elements, structures, and systems related to the intervention and the organization into which it is being implemented. Examples of this in the context of the CHP might be utilizing the practice nurse who is carrying out immunizations to opportunistically give breastfeeding support and advice to a mother attending with her infant, or the use of on screen pop-ups and reminders during a consultation with the general practitioner to enquire about postnatal depression during the 6–8-week review.

The inner setting in Figure 33.1 refers to the features of structural, political, and cultural context through which the implementation process will proceed, that is, aspects *within* the organizational boundaries. The outer setting includes the economic, political, and social context *outside* the organization. It is clear that the line between the inner and outer setting is often blurred and the interface is dynamic and sometimes quite precarious. The textured hash lines in the diagram convey some of the issues, such as networks, communications and readiness, that all interrelate and influence implementation.

The next major domain includes the individuals involved with delivery of the intervention and/or implementation process. Those individuals have the ability to make choices, wield power, and influence others with predictable or unpredictable consequences. They are the carriers of cultural, organizational, professional, and individual mind-sets, norms, interests, and affiliations. They are not passive recipients of innovations but will want to seek them out, experiment with them and evaluate them, develop feelings about them, challenge them, worry about them, complain about them, etc.

From the above description, one can see that implementation is very much a human process. In a number of these theoretical frameworks there are particular individuals who actively promote the implementation process and may come from either the inner or outer setting (e.g. local champions or external change agents) and are thus overlapping two domains (inner and outer settings). The fifth and last major domain is the implementation process itself, which usually requires an active change process aimed to achieve use of the intervention, as designed, at individual and organizational levels. The multiple series of cycles and shadowed arrows represent multiple simultaneous activities taking place within the organization. These subprocesses may be formally planned or spontaneous, linear or non-linear, but are all aimed in the same

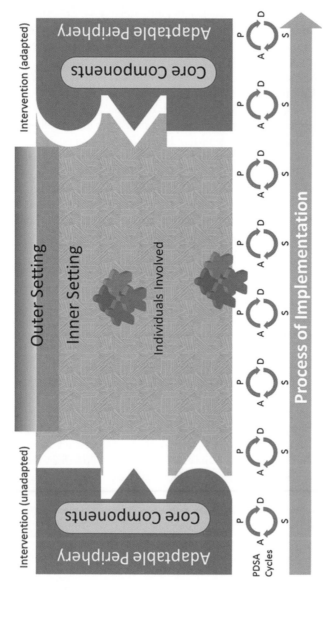

Fig. 33.1 People and processes in implementation of an innovation.

Adapted with permission from Damschroder, L.J. et al., Fostering implementation of health services research findings into practice: a consolidated framework for advancing implementation science. *Implementation Science*, Volume 4, Issue 50. pp.40–55, Copyright © 2009 under the Creative Commons Attribution License 4.0.

general direction, that is, of effective implementation. The CIRF provides a very useful framework on which to measure the success or otherwise of the implementation of the CHP in a particular setting.

There is much to learn from the implementation of other specific programmes, for example, the Family Nurse Partnership (FNP; http://fnp.nhs.uk/), an intensive preventive care programme for the most vulnerable families (under 19 years age) in our society. The programme was developed by David Olds in the US after many years of experimentation and development of randomized controlled trials in the US (Olds et al., 1997). It is a highly specified programme with mentalization, strict training and quality assurance, and enhanced support and clinical supervision of practitioners (see Chapter 32 for more details of this and other enhanced programmes). Practitioners who go through the rigorous training programme are 'accredited' by the leading organization. Olds has developed a licensing scheme which ensures that no practitioners can use the FNP without strict adherence to the core components of the intervention using standardized tools. The largest randomized controlled trial of this programme has taken place in England, Scotland, and Northern Ireland (Wales does not use FNP) and although the results were disappointing for some of the key outcomes (prenatal tobacco use, birthweight, emergency department attendances and emergency hospital admissions within 24 months of birth of the mother's first child, and subsequent pregnancies within 24 months of birth of mother's first child), it may be too early to establish whether there are longer-term benefits to families many years later—so-called sleeper effects (Robling et al., 2016).

The FNP uses regular data feedback loops to practitioners and parents and there is a sense that a close community of practitioners has developed over the years through the development of a number of 'learning sets'. Participants have quoted many benefits which they have gained from action learning (Weinstein, 1995)—see Box 33.1

Many of the disciplines and behaviours that are seen to characterize a learning organization are within action learning sets: team learning, dialogue, suspending assumptions, personal mastery, taking risks, converting mistakes into learning, asking questions, and building in time for reflection. Action learning can be seen as a step towards promoting organizational learning—although these behaviours are not enough on their own. Similarly, there have been a number of small-scale studies exploring the use of learning sets in relation to child and maternal health programmes (World Health Organization, 2014).

There is also good evidence from a number of different types of organization within industry and elsewhere that points to better outcomes when the organization is said to

---

Box 33.1 Benefits of 'action learning sets'

- Learning a more 'evidenced' way of working.
- Learning to network.
- Learning to relate to, and communicate with, others more effectively.
- Gaining increased self-confidence; (increased competence?)
- Gaining increased awareness; (of what?)
- Gaining increased readiness to take responsibility and initiative.

be a 'learning organization'; that is, they are skilled at five main activities: systematic problem-solving, experimentation with new approaches, learning from past experience, learning from best practices of others, and transferring knowledge quickly and efficiently throughout the organization (Garvin, 1993).

There is good evidence that the use of accredited programmes (i.e. those that have been officially recognized in order to maintain standards) improves health outcomes. A systematic review of 26 studies evaluating the impact of accreditation showed benefits for those patients with acute myocardial infarction, trauma, ambulatory surgical care, infection control, and pain management with subspecialty accreditation improving both the process's structure and organization of healthcare (Nicklin, 2011). The authors conclude that 'accreditation programme should be supported as a tool to improve the quality of healthcare services'.

The delivery of an effective CHP requires sufficient capacity, competence, and confidence of the workforce. In turn, this should translate to increased parental competency and confidence. Aristotle described three key forms of knowledge: *episteme* (facts), *techne* (skill), and *phronesis* (practical wisdom). In other words, sufficient numbers of health and other professionals are required with the appropriate competencies for the programme activities to be delivered as intended by policymakers.

In England, the Ofsted inspection process in early years settings has identified that close inter-professional and parent–professional partnership working enhances the chances of 'school readiness' (Ofsted, 2014). Despite there not being a standard definition of this concept, the notion encompasses sufficient maturation of physical, social, and emotional as well as communication development (see Chapter 31). This is a good example of increasing the capabilities of the total workforce concerned with child health and development.

However, having said this, there is much argument about the ideal health visitor caseload required to deliver the programme in its various forms and ensuring a focus on 'proportionate universalism'. This phrase refers to Michael Marmot's concept of providing services according to need in a graded way so that those most in need receive the greatest input (Marmot and Bell, 2012). Unfortunately, often the converse applies; that is, there is an inverse relationship so that those at most in need in fact receive lower-quality services in many parts of the country—the 'inverse care law'. For those parents who experience multiple disadvantages who are least likely to access group or centre-based programmes, the purposeful linking of these families to key services is a critical function of relationship-based practice through home visiting (Daro and Dodge, 2010). A survey by the Institute of Health Visiting, however, has shown that only 55% of health visitors are able to offer continuity of care to families most of the time and the universality of population cover is less than parents would prefer and diminishes the confidence in effective recognition and response to need. In the UK, 63% of health visitors have caseloads of 300 families, or more, 20% over 400, and 16% with caseloads of 500–1000 children under 5 years. The recommended caseload average of 250 children is believed to be the maximum for safe and effective practice (Institute of Health Visiting, 2012). As with most professional recommendations on average caseload, it is recognized that there will be variations in interpretation based on case mix and local needs assessments as well as the competencies and skill mix within the local workforce in the different UK countries and regions. Only high-quality scientific evidence relating workload and child health outcomes can further refine these estimates.

In recent years, it has become quite clear that the CHP workforce is now considerably extended beyond traditional health visiting and midwifery and school nursing to include nursery and children's centre professionals and school-based teaching and welfare staff. Despite the access to books such as this one and a considerable number of high quality e-learning resources (see 'Learning links'), there is a variable commitment to how much of the CHP content should be included in different professionals' formal undergraduate and postgraduate learning. The 'A Better Start' UK programme is currently experimenting with different forms of staffing and delivery of the Healthy Child Programme and components (abetterstart.org.uk, 2017) (see Chapter 35 for more details of this and other enhanced programmes). The teams are brought together from around the country through the development of communities of practice, learning and development events, and a number of cross-site development projects focusing on diet and nutrition in pregnancy and the early years, social and emotional development, and speech and language development (Institute of Health Visiting, 2012). The involvement of the wider health visiting team and community nursery nurses in early identification and management of behaviour problems in children has been described (Nathan et al., 2007). An important characteristic of ensuring high-quality delivery of such programmes is close clinical supervision, preceptorship, and support of both medical and nursing teams. In work-based clinical practice, the evidence base for being exposed to a wide patient mix is strong in terms of learning in these settings (de Jong et al., 2013); that is, extensive experience is important to develop competence and confidence in practice.

With such a diverse group of individuals working towards a common aim, it is necessary to develop a management system which can help coordinate the activities, hold individuals to account, and drive improvement. This is discussed in the next section.

The role of the child health programme coordinator

When one scrutinizes the number of different professionals involved in the delivery of the CHP and the various organizations that employ them, it soon becomes very clear that the coordination and management of such a programme requires some purposeful overarching structure in all areas. This is a public health programme and it is expected that the health professional lead for the programme is a senior clinician with public health expertise (e.g. health visitor, public health nurse, or doctor). This coordinator needs to be supported by a steering group, with leads from key professional groups. Commissioners of the programme where they exist would also be members of such a group.

The six functions of such a steering group have been well described and include the following:

1. Set goals (expectations) to share ownership of the programme and to develop agreed written aims, objectives, referral guidelines, administrative processes, and training standards.

2. Set standards to develop quality standards for the provision of the CHP in primary care and school and methods for monitoring these (see Chapter 34).

3. Promote coverage to ensure equitable delivery of the programme and that hard-to-reach children and those looked after are not missed by the universal programme (proportionate universalism).

4. To introduce and coordinate new programmes and alterations to the existing programme.

5. To establish, develop, and maintain information systems to support the monitoring and feedback of the programme (see Chapter 34).

6. To facilitate consultation with parents, children, and voluntary groups in the planning and implementation of the programme.

7. Be transparent and accountable through the production and dissemination of regular reports on quality and learning through improvement.

The composition of the steering group is shown in Figure 33.2, with the option that other individuals would join as required for key specialist areas of interest (Blair, 2001).

A major advantage of such a group would be the harnessing of expertise and skills to provide maximum 'collective impact' on children's health and well-being in the early years up to and including school entry. The evidence base for such groups is well described in a variety of fields (Kania and Kramer, 2008) (see Chapter 34). At a recent workforce census of the Royal College of Paediatrics and Child Health, only 25 individual paediatricians had CHP activities as part of their consultant job plans. There is a diminishing number of paediatricians with this as an area of responsibility. Currently we do not have data which informs us of the public health workforce roles in this area.

Variations exist in each of the four UK country programmes (see Table 33.1) with Wales and Scotland having a more frequent review regimen. The evidence base for all the programmes is drawn from Hall and Elliman (2006). The degree to which they

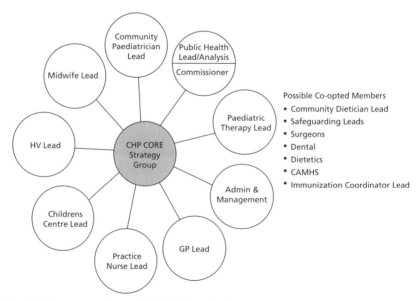

Fig. 33.2 The composition of the CHP local strategy group.

Table 33.1 CHP in UK countries

	England	Wales	Scotland	Northern Ireland
Name of programme	Healthy Child Programme	Healthy Child Wales Programme	Scottish Child Health Programme	Healthy Child, Healthy Future Programme
Date of Publication	2009	2016	2015	2010
Delivery types	Universal/ Progressive	Universal/ Enhanced/ Intensive	Universal/ non-universal	Thresholds of need model (4 levels)
Ages of reviews				
Early antenatal	✔	✔	✔	✔
Late antenatal	✔	✔	✔	✔
Birth–72 hours	✔	✔	✔	✔
10–14 days	✔	✔	✔	✔
3–5 weeks			✔	
6–8 weeks	✔	✔	✔	✔
2 months		✔		
3 months		✔	✔	
4 months		✔	✔	
6 months		✔	✔	
9–12 months	✔			✔
13–15 months		✔	✔	
27–30 months	✔	✔	✔	✔
42 months		✔		
School entry (4–7 years)	✔	✔	✔	✔

Source: data from Llywodraeth Cymru Welsh Government, *An overview of the Healthy Child Wales Programme*, © Crown Copyright 2016, available from http://gov.wales/docs/dhss/publications/ 160926healthy-childrenen.pdf; Sustain, *Healthy Child Programme 0–5: Integrated Commissioning and Delivery Toolkit*, Copyright Sustain 2015, available from http://www.sustain-improvement.com/downloads/ 2/6/no/all; and DHSSPS-Northern Ireland, *Healthy Child, Healthy Future A Framework for the Universal Child Health Promotion Programme in Northern Ireland*, © Crown Copyright 2010, available from https://www. health-ni.gov.uk/sites/default/files/publications/dhssps/healthychildhealthyfuture.pdf.

vary the intensity of the programme according to the needs of the population is referred to formally in all but the Scottish programme. Each of the countries offers a set of resources to support practitioners.

A very well-developed and comprehensive set of materials for both practitioners and commissioners has been developed in the East of England which includes detailed descriptions of practitioner expectations and also commissioning support for key performance indicators (Healthy Child Programme 0–5: Integrated Commissioning & Delivery Toolkit (Sustain, 2015)).

Others have attempted to develop a suite of measures to support international comparison of well-child programmes (see Table 33.2). Regular reporting against these measures over time would allow appraisal of how well we are achieving our objectives.

Table 33.2 Suggested reporting measures for core items of the child health programme

Element of the core CHP	Suggested measure
Child health reviews (growth and developmental surveillance and health promotion)	*Nutrition/growth*: % initiation rates for breastfeeding % infants breastfed at 6 months (exclusive) % children of healthy weight at school entry *Development*: % of children at school entry with previously unidentified emotional or behavioural problems % of children at school entry with a good level of development as measured by and internationally comparable tool much as the Early Development Instrument (Offord Centre for Child Studies) *Injury*: Rate of hospital admission for scalds and burns in children 0–4 years Rate of admission for fracture of the long bones in children 0–4 years Rate of admission for poisonings in children 0–4 years *Exposure to second-hand smoke*: % maternal smoking at postnatal review *Dental health*: % of children at school entry with no dental caries
Immunization	% coverage of completed immunization at 1, 2, and 5 years
Screening	% coverage of neonatal hearing screening by 28 days Median and range of age at fitting of hearing aids for bilateral congenital deafness % coverage of bloodspot testing by 10 days Median and range of age at orchidopexy for undescended testes Median and range of age at operative intervention for congenital hip dysplasia Median and range of age at removal of congenital cataract

Chapter 34 will expand on the topic of quality assurance of the various programmes and how this has been achieved by a number of countries.

Learning links

- ◆ E-Learning for Healthy Child Programme:
  - • 'Leadership, Monitoring and Quality: Part 1: Principles': https://portal.e-lfh. org.uk/Component/Details/12693
  - • 'Leadership, Monitoring and Quality: Part 2: In Practice': https://portal.e-lfh. org.uk/Component/Details/31222.

Recommendations

- ◆ Consider use of a formal implementation framework, for example, CIRF could be used to identify and control facilitating and impeding factors in the implementation of the CHP in each locality. (*Evidence: moderate.*)
- ◆ Use an accreditation system to ensure CHP integrity and sustainability and that the workforce is appropriately trained. (*Evidence: strong.*)
- ◆ Learning sets should be used to support the implementation of the CHP and adaptation to local circumstances. (*Evidence: strong.*)
- ◆ Nominate a senior clinical professional with public health expertise as coordinator in each locality; consider developing a local CHP strategy and implementation group accountable to local commissioners and the national public health body. (*Good practice.*)
- ◆ Quality of the CHP should be assessed by such a steering group. (*Good practice.*)

References

abetterstart.org.uk (2017). A Better Start: Evaluation and Learning. [online] Available at: https://www.abetterstart.org.uk/ [Accessed 28 Sep. 2017].

Blair, M. (2001). The need for and the role of a coordinator in child health surveillance/promotion. *Archives of Disease in Childhood*, **84**, 1–5.

Blair, M. (2014). Getting evidence into practice – implementation science for paediatricians. *Archives of Disease in Childhood*, **99**, 307–309.

Damschroder, L.J., Aron, D.C., Keith, R.E., et al. (2009). Fostering implementation of health services research findings into practice: a consolidated framework for advancing implementation science. *Implementation Science*, **4**, 40–55.

Daro, D. and Dodge, K.A. (2010). Strengthening home-visiting intervention policy: expanding reach, building knowledge. In: Haskins, R. and Barnett, W.S. (Eds.), *Investing in Young Children: New Directions in Federal Preschool and Early Childhood Policy*, pp. 79–86.

Washington, DC: National Institution for Early Education Research and Brookings Institution. Available at: https://www.brookings.edu/wp-content/uploads/2016/07/1013_ investing_in_young_children_haskins_ch7.pdf [Accessed 1 May 2017].

de Jong, J., Visser, M., Van Dijk, N., et al. (2013). A systematic review of the relationship between patient mix and learning in work-based clinical settings. A BEME systematic review: BEME Guide No. 24. *Medical Teacher*, **35**, e1181–e1196.

Garvin, D.A. (1993). Building a learning organization. *Harvard Business Review*, **71**, 78–91.

Hall, D. and Elliman, D. (2006). *Health for all Children* (4th edn. rev.). Oxford: Oxford University Press.

Institute of Health Visiting (2012). Results of the State of Health Visiting Survey 2016. [online] Available at: www.ihv.org.uk [Accessed 1 May 2017].

Kania, J. and Kramer, M. (2008). Collective impact. *Stanford Social Innovation Review*, **1**, 36–41.

Lenton, S., Wettergren, B., Huss, G., et al. (2016). A consensus on the improvement of community and primary care services for children, adolescents and their families in Europe. European Academy of Paediatrics (EAP) European Confederation of Primary Care Paediatricians (ECPCP) European Paediatric Association (EPA). [online] Available at: http://www.epa-unepsa.org/.

Marmot, M., Allen, J., Goldblatt, P., et al. (2010). *Fair Society, Healthy Lives: The Strategic Review of Health Inequalities in England post-2010*. London: Institute of Health Equity.

Nathan, D., Smedley, A., Griffiths, H., Shepherd, L., and Stark, W. (2007). Learning sets ... the way forward? *Community Practitioner*, **80**, 28–31.

Nicklin, W. (2011). The value and impact of health care accreditation: a literature review. Available at: https://accreditation.ca/sites/default/files/value-and-impact-en.pdf [Accessed 20 April 2017].

Ofsted (2014). Are you ready? Good practice in school readiness. [online] Available at: https:// www.gov.uk/government/uploads/system/uploads/attachment_data/file/418819/Are_you_ ready_Good_practice_in_school_readiness.pdf [Accessed 26 July 2017].

Olds, D.L., Eckenrode, J., Henderson, C.R., Jr., et al. (1997). Long-term effects of home visitation on maternal life course and child abuse and neglect. Fifteen-year follow-up of a randomized trial. *JAMA*, **278**, 637–643.

Robling, M., Bekkers, M.J., Bell, K., et al. (2016). Effectiveness of a nurse-led intensive home-visitation programme for first-time teenage mothers (Building Blocks): a pragmatic randomised controlled trial. *The Lancet*, **387**, 146–155.

Sustain (2015). Healthy Child Programme 0–5: Integrated Commissioning and Delivery Toolkit. [online] Available at: http://www.sustain-improvement.com/downloads/2/6/no/all.

Weinstein, K. (1995). *Action Learning: A Journey in Discovery and Development*. London: Harper Collins.

Wood, R. and Blair, M. (2014). A comparison of child health programmes recommended for preschool children in selected high-income countries. *Child: Care, Health and Development*, **40**, 640–653.

World Health Organization (2014). WHO recommendation on community mobilization through facilitated participatory learning and action cycles with women's groups for maternal and newborn health. [online] Available at: http://apps.who.int/iris/bitstream/ 10665/127939/1/9789241507271_eng.pdf?ua=1 [Accessed 30 Apr. 2017].

Chapter 34

Quality assurance and data requirements of the child health programme

Mitch Blair and Andy Spencer

Summary

This chapter:

- describes the desired outcomes of a child health programme
- argues that appraisal of programme quality and continuous monitoring are essential to ensure confidence in its safety and effectiveness
- discusses a number of quality improvement methods
- provides some international examples of quality dashboards, and how they are used to feedback information to parents, health professionals, and policymakers in the pursuit of continuous quality improvement.

Introduction

'It is clear that only what can be measured can be improved.' ◊

Lord Ara Darzi (2008)

In Chapter 33, we considered the role of the child health programme (CHP) coordinator and steering group; one of their functions is to ensure that the quality of the programme is monitored and continuously improved.

....

◊ Reprinted from *The Lancet*, Volume 371, Issue 9624, Darzi A, Quality and the NHS Next Stage Review, pp. 1663–1564, Copyright © 2008, with permission from Elsevier, https://www.sciencedirect.com/journal/the-lancet.

What is meant by quality in relation to the child health programme?

The effective implementation of the CHP should lead to strong parent–child attachment and positive parenting, resulting in:

- better social and emotional well-being among children
- care that helps to keep children safe
- healthy eating and increased physical activity leading to a reduction in obesity
- prevention of some serious and communicable diseases through immunization
- increased rates of initiation and continuation of breastfeeding
- readiness for school and improved learning
- early recognition of growth disorders and recognition of obesity
- early detection of and action to address developmental delay, abnormalities and ill health, and concerns about safety through screening and surveillance
- identification of factors that could influence health and well-being in families
- better short- and long-term outcomes for children who are at risk of social exclusion.

All four UK countries have very similar if not identical objectives. Scotland specifically emphasizes strong parent–child attachment and positive parenting in its desired outcomes (Gov.scot, 2015).

According to the US Institute of Medicine, health services need to be safe, timely, equitable, effective, efficient, and person centred (Institute of Medicine, Committee on Quality of Health Care in America, 2001). The Organisation for Economic Co-operation and Development published a quality framework for Europe (Arah et al., 2006) with many similarities; for example, both call for improvements to patient safety and stress the importance of learning lessons from adverse events. Inherent in these approaches is a need to appreciate how the 'whole health system' works to support high-quality delivery (see Figure 34.1).

Practical issues in the measurement of quality

A quality indicator is defined as a periodic measurement of an aspect of clinical practice, benchmarked against a standard, which can be used to drive an improvement and will normally relate to infrastructure, process, or outcome (Donabedian, 1997). Assessment of the quality of the immunization or screening activities requires a pathway approach where each of the structure, process, and outcome are clearly defined and linked. Optimum outcome is defined by all the parts working together. Inherent in this approach is a need to appreciate how the 'whole health system' works to support high-quality delivery (Alliance for Health Policy and Systems Research and World Health Organization, 2009). Let us take immunization as an example.

Immunization of a defined population requires the following structural measures: a register of new births and those eligible for immunization, an invitation system, vaccine supply, equipment, and people to give the vaccine. Process measures would

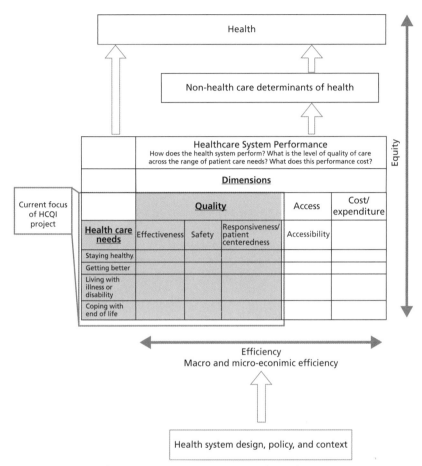

Fig. 34.1 Framework for Health Care Quality Indicators (HCQIs).

Adapted from Arah O.A. *et al.*, A conceptual framework for the OECD Health Care Quality Indicators Project, *International Journal for Quality in Health Care*, Volume 18 Supplement 1, pp. 5–13, Copyright © 2006, with permission from Oxford University Press.

include an invitation delivered in a timely way, a process for identifying those non-attenders and arrangements for re- invitation, and a recording process for collecting completed/missed vaccinations. Output measures might include recorded percentage immunized and outcome, reduction of new cases of vaccine-preventable disease, the number suffering complications from the immunization (patient safety), and the level of satisfaction with the experience of care. The latter may relate to perceptions of waiting times, child-friendly facilities, or attitude and competence of staff.

Similarly when we look at all the components required of a screening programme, we would need to define the following: the target population to be covered, the invitation for screening, whether the primary screening has been completed, repeat test if needed, completion of secondary screening and outputs, diagnostic tests carried out, intervention put in place, initial outcomes to individual and population, and sustained impact (value). Let us apply this framework to the example of phenylketonuria (PKU)/congenital hypothyroidism (CHT) care pathways, standards, and quality assurance.

In the UK, about 1 in 3000 babies will be born with CHT and about 1 in 13,000 will be born with PKU (Simpson et al., 1997). Without timely identification and treatment these conditions will cause irreversible severe learning difficulties. Both these conditions can be easily and reliably detected in the neonatal period, by bloodspot screening.

Analyses of samples are carried out in centralized laboratories on blood collected by heel prick. Ideally, the screening programme should ensure that all infants are tested, and that those with either PKU or CHT commence treatment within the first 3 weeks of life.

Because the conditions being screened for are rare and the consequences of missing them are so significant, it is vital to ensure that the service is running in the most effective, efficient, equitable, and acceptable way possible.

A number of standards have been developed to represent key stages in the pathway (see Table 34.1).

Table 34.1 The acceptable standards of heel prick blood screening programme

Standard 1a. Identify the population and coverage: coverage (CCG responsibility at birth)	≥ 95.0% of eligible babies have a result for each of the 9 conditions recorded on the CHIS at less than or equal to 17 days of age
Standard 1b. Identify the population and coverage: coverage (movers in)	≥ 95.0% of eligible babies have a result for each of the 9 conditions (or 5 conditions if not eligible for expanded screening) recorded on the CHIS at less than or equal to 21 calendar days of notifying the CHRD of movement in
Standard 2. Coverage: timely identification of babies with a null or incomplete result recorded on the CHIS	CHRD performs regular checks (ideally daily, minimum weekly) to identify babies ≥ 17 days and ≤ 364 days with a null or incomplete result
Standard 3. Test: barcoded NHS number label is included on the blood spot card	≥ 90.0% of blood spot cards are received by the laboratory with the baby's NHS number on a barcoded label
Standard 4. Test and intervention/treatment: timely sample collection	≥ 90.0% of first blood spot samples are taken on day 5
Standard 5. Test and intervention/treatment: timely receipt of a sample in the newborn screening laboratory	≥ 95.0% of all samples received less than or equal to 3 working days of sample collection

(continued)

Table 34.1 Continued

Standard 6. Test and intervention/treatment: quality of the blood spot sample	Avoidable repeat rate is ≤ 2.0%		
Standard 7a. Test and intervention/treatment: timely taking of a second blood spot sample for CF screening	≥ 95% of second blood spot samples taken on day 21 to day 24 (this allows for day 21 to fall on a weekend when a special visit is not warranted)		
Standard 7b. Test and intervention/treatment: timely taking of a second blood spot sample following a borderline CHT screening	≥ 95.0% of second blood spot samples taken as defined		
Standard 7c. Test and intervention/treatment: timely taking of a second blood spot sample for CHT screening for preterm infant	≥ 95.0% of second blood spot samples taken as defined		
Standard 9. Intervention/ treatment: timely processing of CHT and IMD (excluding HCU) screen positive samples	100% of babies with a positive screening result (excluding HCU) have a clinical referral initiated within 3 working days of sample receipt by screening laboratory		
Standard 11. Intervention/ treatment: timely entry into clinical care	Condition	Intervention/ treatment	Thresholds
	IMDs (excluding HCU) and CHT (suspected on first sample)	Attend first clinical appointment by 14 days of age	Acceptable: 100%
	CHT (suspected on repeat following borderline TSH)	Attend first clinical appointment by 21 days of age	Acceptable: 100%
	CF (2 CFTR mutations detected) and HCU	Attend first clinical appointment by 28 days of age	Acceptable: ≥ 95.0% Achievable: 100%
	SCD	Attend first clinical appointment by 90 days of age	Acceptable: ≥ 90.0% Achievable: ≥ 95%
Standard 12a. Minimizing harm: timeliness of results to parents (CCG responsibility at birth)	100% of babies with a not suspected result for each of the conditions for whom a not suspected results letter was despatched directly to parents by the CHRD within 6 weeks of birth		

(*continued*)

Table 34.1 Continued

Standard 12b. Minimizing harm: timeliness of results to parents (movers in)	100% of babies with a not suspected result for each of the conditions for whom a not suspected results letter was despatched directly to parents by the CHRD within 6 weeks of notification of moving in
(NB: standards 8 and 10 are lab standards for specialist accreditation)	

CF, cystic fibrosis; CHIS, Child Health Information System; CHRD, Child Health Record Departments; CHT, congenital hypothyroidism; HCU, homocystinuria; IMD, inherited metabolic disease; SCD, sickle cell disease; TSH, thyroid-stimulating hormone.

Adapted under the Open Government Licence v3.0 from Public Health England, *NHS Newborn Blood Spot Screening Programme Standards*, © Crown Copyright 2017, available from https://www.gov.uk/government/uploads/system/uploads/attachment_data/file/585415/Newborn_Blood_Spot_Screening_Programme_Standards.pdf.

The standards can be further elaborated in terms of acceptable and achievable parameters:

1. The *acceptable* threshold is the lowest level of performance which programmes are expected to attain to ensure patient safety and programme effectiveness.
2. The *achievable* threshold represents the level at which the programme is likely to be running optimally.

A recent study from Scotland has reported on 30 years of testing for hypothyroidism and demonstrated clear improvements over time in a number of parameters such as timeliness of testing and repeats as well as age at start of replacement treatment (Mansour et al., 2017). The researchers recommended a number of improvements including reducing the age at initial capillary sampling to as close to 96 hours as possible, the introduction of 6-day laboratory reporting, and electronic messaging for repeat samples and notification of midwives. This is a good example of continuous quality improvement.

Other measures of the child health programme

Screening and immunization are relatively easy measures to collect. The reason that many outcomes are difficult to measure is because they are often dependent on the recording of a clinical diagnosis; for example, in the case of a condition such as speech and language delay, there is a need to agree on clear diagnostic criteria so that the target population can be identified. An example of an outcome from the CHP that is easier to measure might be the proportion of children with healthy weight for age. The problem in using outcome measures in both of these examples is that the attribution of interventions from specific health services to an improvement in outcome is often difficult and imprecise due to a myriad of confounding factors such as child co-morbidities, parental mental health issues and family social environment—all of which may be unrelated to the particular intervention.

Further work is always required to elucidate the cause of poor (or good) perform-ance; 'the ability to identify specific elements of the service that are working well or not, is fundamental to driving up quality' (Hanafin and Cowley, 2006). Using time series analyses of accurate measurements, such as these, can be helpful in attrib-uting specific interventions to outcome especially if there is a plausible mechanism postulated.

Quality improvement methodology provides a number of tools which would allow for the identification of issues and modifications to be made to the programme through process mapping, the use of action effect diagrams, statistical process control charts, and root cause analysis, among others. Often less sophisticated methods can be used.

A good example of using this type of methodology has been in the investigation of adverse events such as late diagnosis or adverse reactions to immunization. The fol-lowing case scenario (Box 34.1) illustrates the issue.

This is what is often referred to as a 'sentinel' case—a failure of the screening/sur-veillance system—which has many learning points: recording of screening, orientation of parents to PCHR, appointment and recall systems, and referral guidance (was not marked as an urgent referral by the referring GP) among them. Many of these factors can be improved through improved professional education and adherence to standard operating procedures.

It demonstrates the importance of ensuring that there is a quality assurance process with clear accountabilities in the delivery of the CHP. From the above, it is clear that

---

Box 34.1 The 'missed hip'

Dinesh is a 16-month-old boy who is seen by the paediatrician in his general clinic, referred by the general practitioner (GP) at 14 months because of concerns that the toddler's gait appears to be unusual. Parents are well-educated profes-sionals both working full-time with grandparent support for child care of Dinesh and his 3-year-old sister, Rekha. On closer questioning, the parents had noticed a difference in the appearance between the buttock creases but had been reassured by the nursery nurse at the baby clinic that this was nothing to worry about: 'not all babies look the same'. They had a parent-held Personal Child Health Record (PCHR) but had not read the insert about hip surveillance. Hip examination at birth was recorded as normal, the 6–8-week review was completed by the GP but the PCHR recording for the physical examination was only partially completed (blank section for hip examination and head circumference measurement), with a missed 1-year review (no appointment had been received). On examination, the baby's general appearance and neurodevelopment was normal other than an antalgic gait and a 2 cm leg length difference with limited external abduction of the right hip. X-ray confirmed the clinical findings of subluxation of that hip and underdeveloped acetabulum. He is referred urgently to orthopaedics for assess-ment and surgical intervention.

understanding data and data management is a prerequisite to high-quality information in order to support quality assurance.

Data and data management to support the child health programme

We are in the midst of a digital revolution and the NHS is awash with data. Sadly, many health professionals see data collection as someone else's responsibility and are so convinced that NHS data is unreliable that they take little interest in analysing results or thinking about new and innovative ways to convert data into meaningful information. It is now a professional responsibility to ensure that clinical data is as accurate as it can be, and we need to advise collectively on which key data items and analyses are required to make sound judgements for the future.

Using data to drive up quality is becoming embedded into the NHS through online resources for patients such as NHS Choices, 'I want great care ', and the 'My Hospital Guide'. Much of the approach has been developed from pioneering work in cardiac surgery where outcomes published by surgeons has led to a situation where all cardiac surgeons are forced to scrutinize every aspect of their practice. Although there might be some unwanted consequences, such as surgeons turning down high-risk cases even though it offers the best outcome for the patient, evidence shows that the results in the UK have dramatically improved and are now acknowledged to be among the best in the world. Patients facing surgery can access mortality data for their surgeon on NHS Choices.

As more data are published and made available to the public and policymakers, clinicians are becoming more aware of how data pertaining to their patients are being collected, coded, and interpreted. One aspect that requires good clinician scrutiny and involvement is in classification and coding of healthcare processes and outcomes. The subsequent section describes how this has developed to date.

Classification and coding systems

Information pertaining to patient symptoms and diagnosis is coded using Read Codes in general practice, whereas hospital data are coded using the tenth revision of the International Statistical Classification of Diseases (ICD-10). ICD-10 is a disease classification owned and used by the World Health Organization. In the ICD-10, similar diseases are clustered together and assigned to the same code, even though the outcomes might be very different. This leads to problems when attempting to use the ICD-10 for monitoring quality and consequently it has been much criticized by clinicians who often view the collection of hospital data with disdain (Spencer and Davies, 2012). However, these data are extremely important in the NHS as they are used to develop Health Resource Groups, which are used to support costing, commissioning, and contract negotiations. Hospital Episode Statistics (HES) are used for multiple purposes including monitoring patient outcomes. This is important when looking at the outcomes of the CHP newborn screening and immunization programmes; for example, in terms of ear, eye, hip, heart, and testes operative interventions or admissions with vaccine-preventable disease.

Primary care systems are migrating from Read Codes to SNOMED CT so that the coding systems used in both primary and secondary care will be the same. Every newly acquired hospital electronic health record has to provide access to SNOMED CT for clinical coding. New administrative datasets such as the Maternity Services Data Set and the Children and Young People's Health Services Data Set (CYPHS) are also SNOMED CT compatible. This is a significant step towards developing interoperable solutions across the NHS.

Data sources to support preventive child health services

So what measurements are available to examine the impact of public health initiatives around pregnancy, childbirth, screening programmes in the very young, nutritional health of the child population, and accident prevention? The Children and Young CYPHS Data Set (Content.digital.nhs.uk, 2017) requires that all community services funded by the NHS are required to submit these data monthly. The CYPHS Data Set describes national definitions for the extraction of data in relation to the following key areas:

- Personal and demographic.
- Social and personal circumstances.
- Breastfeeding and nutrition.
- Care event and screening activity.
- Diagnoses, including long-term conditions and childhood disabilities.
- Scored assessments.

Statistics arising from this data collection are published by NHS digital in summary form and as an interactive Excel spreadsheet where different health providers can be compared. It is the stated intention that information from the data set will be made widely available to commissioners, providers, clinicians, service users and the general public to inform choice through monthly and annual statistical publications. Reference to the denominator population is required to allow coverage and timeliness to be derived. Recent audits in England have shown a 90% reliability rate and this is likely to improve over time.

A key aim of most preventive child healthcare programmes is the early detection and proactive management of children who have significant neurodevelopmental impairments. Certainly inclusion of diagnoses and scored assessments within this data set should lead to the possibility of monitoring outcomes. This has been tested with a neurodisability service in Northern England.

A subset of SNOMED CT terms has been developed to describe technology dependency, family-reported issues, and functional disability as well as the underlying diagnoses. Collecting data using the paediatric subset in neurodevelopment clinics in Sunderland led to the first description of the complexity of work undertaken by the department, leading to additional resourcing of the service (Horridge et al., 2016).

The Sunderland experience illustrates three important points:

1. It is essential for the interpretation of electronic records that professionals work together to update the terminology and ensure that everyone is using the same terms in the same way.

2. As patients and parents are to have access to their notes, terminology should be designed to be as understandable as possible.

3. As funding for health services becomes more and more dependent on data, outcomes and not just activity data are going to be increasingly important.

The Maternity Services Data Set (Content.digital.nhs.uk, 2017b) provides important data about fetal anomaly and neonatal screening and much else besides. Data pertaining to immunization rates are very comprehensively covered and include an interactive dashboard to allow comparisons between local authorities. Similarly, there are good demographic data from the National Child Measurement Programme which shows the prevalence of overweight and obesity in children. HES data may also provide useful outcome data in recording the causes of admission to hospital. Geographical variations in healthcare by local authority or Clinical Commissioning Group are published online in the 'Atlas of Variation' (https://fingertips.phe.org.uk/profile/atlas-of-variation). The indicators used cover the care of mothers, babies, children, and young people including mental health and childhood accidents. Hospital admission rates are used as a metric for a range of chronic and acute diseases. Examples of indicators used include the percentage of mothers who are smoking at the time of delivery and the rate of children aged 0–17 years who were the subject of a child protection plan. Despite these developments, there is a need to bring these elements together into a comprehensive dashboard system specifically focused on the CHP or its equivalents in the other countries.

Improving the integration of care through information systems

Another important aspect of information management is the ability to retrieve all the pertinent information relevant to the care of the individual child. Unfortunately, this can be exceedingly difficult because children are seen by multiple different health and non-health professionals and in multiple different settings. Consequently information about children's health is held in a plethora of different systems including Maternity Systems, GP systems, local authority databases, and hospital electronic health records which are not interoperable (see Figure 34.2).

This means that a health professional seeing a child in an emergency may be deprived of vital information which could have life-limiting consequences in the most extreme cases. National digital strategies are aiding integration through the development of a standard for electronic community child health and the Personal Child Health Record.

There are many different stakeholders involved in data collection and usage but they fall primarily into three large groups: patients and carers, providers of care, and public health as illustrated in Figure 34.3.

The seamless flow of information with appropriate access and security arrangements is the goal of a well-functioning child health information infrastructure fit to support twenty-first-century care.

The use of quality dashboards

A number of attempts have been made to identify a standardized set of measures, outcomes, and indicators for the CHP. Hampshire et al. (1999) carried out a detailed study of 25 general practices and their quality measures. Regular feedback of data on

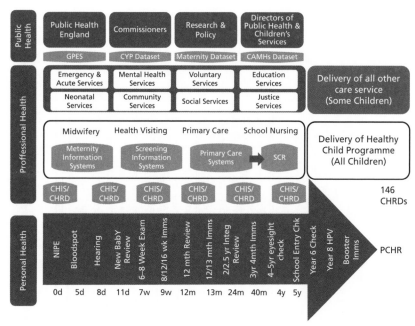

Fig. 34.2 Child health information sources to support preventive care in England.

Reproduced under the Open Government Licence v3.0 from National Information Board, *Healthy Children: Transforming Child Health Information*, NHS England Publication Gateway Reference 05454, © Crown Copyright 2016, available from https://www.england.nhs.uk/wp-content/uploads/2016/11/healthy-children-transforming-child-health-info.pdf.

these measures led to gradual improvement of quality, highlighting the importance of data feedback loops and the need for regular collaboration with stakeholders to ensure a continuous improvement cycle as described in Chapter 33.

The Welsh Government and its partners (Healthy Child Wales Programme (HCWP)) have developed shared outcome frameworks to help us understand the impact their policies, programmes, services, and behaviours are having on health and well-being in Wales (Welsh Government, 2016). The HCWP will contribute to improving outcomes across the early years and public health outcomes frameworks, specifically by defining key indicators:

◆ Percentage of 0–7-year-old Welsh residents presenting at emergency departments having had accidental injuries in the home.

◆ Percentage of children reaching or exceeding their developmental milestones between ages 2 and 3 years (also applicable under 'learn and develop')

◆ Percentage of 4-year-olds up to date with immunizations.

◆ Percentage of 4–5-year-olds who are a healthy weight.

◆ Dental caries at age 5.

◆ Also, the HCWP will contribute to the Child Poverty Strategy outcome indicator:

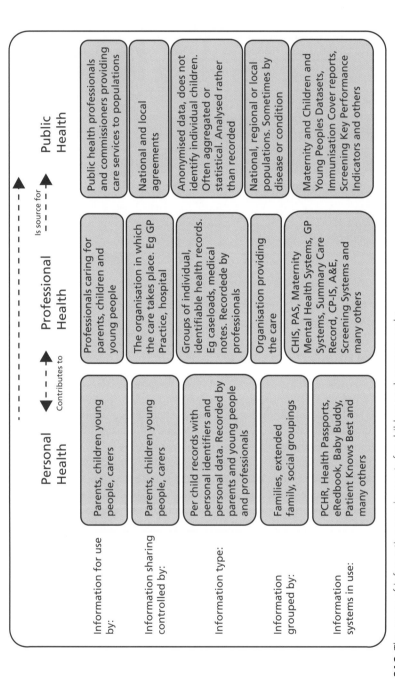

Fig. 34.3 The scope of information requirements for children and young people.

♦ Percentage of children living in low-income households who are reaching health, social, and cognitive development milestones when entering formal education (Public Health Wales Observatory and Aneurin Bevan University Health Board, 2013).

A promising development in England is the work of CHIMAT, the health intelligence network for children, which produces an area-wide graph benchmarking key measures of interest in relation to the aims of the CHP—a compilation of these is shown in Figure 34.4.

In Scotland, there are high-quality reliable data on coverage of the key reviews and this has the additional advantage of indicating a breakdown by socio-economic status (in this

| Compared with benchmark | Better | Similar | Worse | | Lower | Similar | Higher | | Not compared |

Indicator	Period	◁▷	England	East Midlands region	Derby	Derbyshire	Leicester	Leicestershire	Lincolnshire	Northamptonshire	Nottingham	Nottinghamshire	Rutland
Under 18 conceptions	2016	◁▷	18.8	19.4	26.0	16.9	24.0	13.7	20.5	20.9	26.9	18.3	4.7*
Smoking status at time of delivery (current method)	2016/17	◁▷	10.7	13.3	14.5	14.1	10.2	8.6*	13.3*	14.4	17.6	14.8	*
Low birth weight of term babies	2016	◁▷	2.79	2.77	2.90	2.20	5.22	2.43	2.37	2.44	3.99	2.17	2.67
Infant mortality	2014–16	◁▷	3.9	4.3	6.0	3.7	5.1	3.9	3.0	4.3	5.9	4.4	4.9
Breastfeeding prevalence at 6–8 weeks after birth - current method	2016/17	◁▷	44.4*	*	43.8	40.3	57.7	*	*	*	48.4	*	*
Reception: Prevalence of overweight (including obese)	2016/17	◁▷	22.6	22.7	23.5	23.7	21.2	20.3	24.6	22.1	26.0	21.8	24.0
A&E attendances (0–4 years)	2016/17	◁▷	601.8	*	679.9	508.2	627.1	586.7	625.3	390.6	*	*	607.6
Emergency admissions (aged 0–4)	2015/16	◁▷	155.0	134.2	84.8	150.0	83.8	93.2	157.4	184.0	109.5	140.0	141.6
Hospital admissions for accidental and deliberate injuries in children (aged 0–4)	2016/17	◁▷	126.3	98.2*	62.7	105.4	67.9	80.6	109.2	122.3	*	*	103.5
Children with one or more decayed, missing or filled teeth	2016/17	◁▷	23.3	25.1	24.0	20.4	38.7	22.3	24.0	24.3	25.9	20.1	15.6
Population vaccination coverage - MMR for two doses (5 years old) <90% 90% to 95% ≥95%	2016/17	◁▷	87.6	88.8	85.2	93.1	89.9	93.8*	86.3	86.5	82.5	88.2	*
Proportion of children aged 2–2½ offered ASQ-3 as part of the Healthy Child Programme or integrated review	2016/17	◁▷	89.4*	78.5	95.9	72.0	*	41.6	83.7	96.7	99.9	93.3	*
Children achieving a good level of development at the end of reception	2016/17	◁▷	70.7	68.9	68.0	70.4	64.4	70.1	69.6	69.8	66.2	68.1	75.7

Fig. 34.4 CHIMAT benchmarking indicators.

Adapted from The National Child and Maternal Health Network (CHIMAT), *Public Health and NHS Outcomes Frameworks for Children,* Crown Copyright © available from https://fingertips.phe.org.uk/profile-group/child-health/profile/cyphof, under the Open Government Licence v3.0.

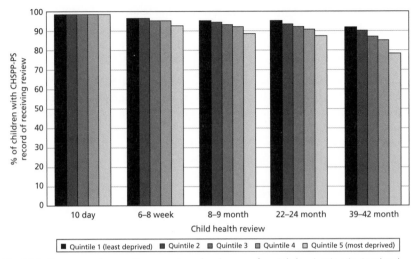

Fig. 34.5 Coverage of surveillance reviews by degree of social deprivation in Scotland.

Reproduced with permission from Wood R. *et al.*, Trends in the coverage of 'universal' child health reviews: observational study using routinely available data, *BMJ Open*, Volume 2, Issue 2, pp. 759–759, Copyright © 2012, Published by the BMJ Publishing Group Limited.

case, the index of multiple deprivation). Figure 34.5 indicates a drop off in the coverage of the most deprived part of the population as the child becomes older, suggesting some disengagement of families themselves or services with families (Wood et al., 2012).

A natural corollary of this would be further investigation with parents about the acceptability and perceived value of such reviews. It is quite possible that there are real issues about convenience of appointments or indeed the possibility that certain families might be better targeted for home visiting to reduce the effects of stigma and to also maximize the value of a holistic assessment, taking into account the full set of socio-demographic factors affecting the child's life. In the UK, there are very few studies which have explored parental attitude to the CHP in detail.

Importance of feedback to local child health programme steering group and practitioners

Feedback loops are an essential method of assuring quality by making parts of the system more visible to change and to ensure that both practitioners and parents are kept informed of progress against desired outcomes. The rationale for all of these is if you show people where they can improve, they will take steps to improve. However, there is no doubt that people react in different ways when they are made aware of these sorts of data output and these can be summarized as follows:

1. The data are wrong.

2. Ok, the data are correct enough but there is not a problem (e.g. different case mix, more deprivation, etc.).

3. Ok, the data are correct enough and there is a problem, but it is not my problem (ascribed to John Wennberg, 2010).

Only when there has been some degree of iteration, do clinicians and others start to take the need to change seriously. We know this is true because we have all done it. Add to this the fact that before the process starts clinicians have to be aware of the data that are out there now, be prepared to look at it, and take some ownership. Care must be taken that decisions are not made on a single snapshot view of red, amber, and green indicators alone without sufficient detail of trend data over time (Anhøj and Hellesøe, 2016).

Despite the limitations described above, there is much to learn from looking at examples from elsewhere in the world. Colleagues in Carolina in the US have used a system to provide continuous improvement for their Bright Futures well child programme. The Child and Adolescent Health Measurement Initiative (CAHMI) is a national initiative based out of the Bloomberg School of Public Health at Johns Hopkins University in Baltimore, Maryland (http://www.cahmi.org/). Originally housed at FACCT (Foundation for Accountability), the CAHMI was established in 1998. The mission of the CAHMI is to advance patient-centred innovations and improvements in children's health and healthcare quality. They have achieved this through using the Online Promoting Healthy Development Survey (PHDS) for practice improvement and maintenance of certification.

The Online PHDS is designed to support paediatric providers and practices in their efforts to improve well-child care, and the tool can be used to fulfil the American Board of Pediatrics Maintenance of Certification Part 4 requirement. In order to maintain certification with the American Board of Pediatrics, paediatricians are required to demonstrate competence in systematic measurement and improvement in patient care by participating in an American Board of Pediatrics-approved quality improvement project. This is known as 'Performance in Practice' or 'Maintenance of Certification (MOC) Part 4'. Since 2013, this system is available to paediatricians as an option to fulfil the quality improvement MOC requirement.

The PHDS was designed to measure the communication-dependent aspects of care—what providers and parents discuss at the visit. The PHDS not only assesses whether recommended care is provided, but also the degree to which parents have their informational needs met and whether the care provided is family-centred. These are the aspects of quality care that are best measured by asking parents directly.

The PHDS collects data in the following domains:

- *Anticipatory guidance and education for parents*: measures whether parents' information needs were met with regard to age-specific topics based on American Academy of Pediatrics Guidelines.
- *Developmental surveillance*: assesses whether the provider asked about and addressed parents' concerns about their child's learning, development, and behaviour.
- *Developmental screening*: determines whether standardized screening tools for developmental and behavioural delays were used.
- *Follow-up for children at risk*: measures whether children at risk were referred and received follow-up services.
- *Assessment of psychosocial well-being and safety in the family*: assesses whether providers asked about parents' emotional and mental well-being, as well as smoking, alcohol and drug abuse, and physical safety in the home.

◆ *Family-centred care*: measures whether providers interact with the family in a respectful manner, engage the parent as a partner in care, and listen to and address parents' concerns.

The PHDS also gathers information useful for describing the population served and determining their healthcare needs. This includes measures of the following:

◆ *Children's healthcare utilization*: to determine rates of routine or emergency room visits.

◆ *Children's health status*: to assess rates of children at risk for developmental and behavioural delays, special healthcare needs, and overall health status.

◆ *Parenting to optimize development*: to assess the proportion of parents reading to young children, applying injury prevention measures, or experiencing depression.

◆ *Access and care coordination*: to monitor problems with access to paediatric care and coordination among providers.

Table 34.2 show some examples of the types of output produced.

Our Australian colleagues have also looked at other measures to help inform their preventive child health programmes, such as the Australian Early Development Census (https://www.aedc.gov.au/). This index provides a number of dimensions, which have been measured in Australian localities for many years now and give some indication to local policy makers and the public about the vulnerabilities of children in their area. This allows for a very highly visible map to be produced and year-on-year improvements with modification of interventions and programmes put in place to support improved outcomes (see Figure 34.5).

Table 34.2 CAHMI PHDS

Preventive health care					
Measure % (CI)	**Nationwide**	**Special healthcare needs**	**Non-special healthcare needs**	**Public**	**Private**
Well visits: child had one or more preventive medical care visits during past 12 months (children age 0 to 17 years)	**88.5** (88.0–89.0) 64,575,112	**91.4** (90.2–92.6) 12,802,108	**87.8** (87.2–88.4) 51,773,003	**91.4** (90.6–92.3) 19,056,563	**89.5** (88.9–90.1) 40,129,169
Dental visits: child had one or more preventive dental care visits during past 12 months (children age 1 to 17 years)	**78.4** (77.6–79.1) 54,293,506	**84.1** (82.8–85.5) 11,636,399	**76.9** (76.1–77.8) 42,657,107	**76.2** (74.7–77.7) 14,827,895	**82.4** (81.6–83.2) 35,178,486

(continued)

Table 34.2 Continued

Preventive health care					
Surveillance: parent reports that a doctor or other healthcare provider asked basic questions about parent's concerns (children with healthcare visit in past 12 months, age 0 to 5 years)	**48.0** (46.5–49.5) 11,267,674	**55.4** (51.3–59.4) 1,563,476	**47.0** (45.3–48.6) 9,704,198	**42.6** (39.7–45.4) 3,447,002	**53.1** (51.3–54.9) 7,154,997
Screening: standardized developmental and behavioural screening (SDBS) was conducted during a healthcare visit (children who had at least one health care visit in past 12 months, age 10 months to 5 years)	**19.5** (18.3–20.8) 3,880,957	**23.9** (20.8–27.1) 626,385	**18.9** (17.5–20.2) 3,254,572	**23.6** (21.2–26.1) 1,590,401	**17.8** (16.3–19.2) 2,042,796

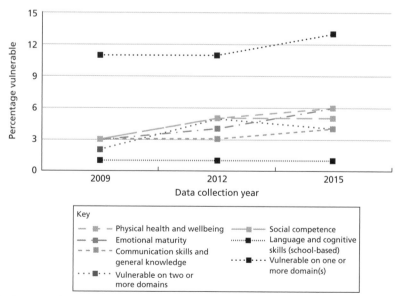

Fig. 34.6 Trends in developmental vulnerability for children in the North Sydney area (2009–2015) using the Australian version of the Early Development Instrument (AvEDI).

Table 34.3 Key performance indicators—a dashboard from New Zealand

DHB	WCTO referral by 28 days	WCTO core contact 1 before 50 days	All WCTO core contacts received by age 1	Breastfed at 2 weeks	Breastfed at LMC discharge at 6 weeks	Breastfed at 3 months	Smoke-free household at 6 weeks	Screened for family violence	SUDI prevention information provided
National target									
National target	90%	90%	90%	85%	75%	70%		90%	90%
All ethnicities									
Auckland	92%	82%		77%	75%	65%		47%	100%
Bay of Plenty	89%	78%		81%	76%	61%		52%	99%
Canterbury	85%	77%		75%	72%	61%		59%	100%
Capital and Coast	87%	59%		77%	74%	65%		45%	100%
Counties Manukau	81%	81%		73%	68%	50%		47%	99%
Hawkes Bay	93%	71%		78%	70%	54%		74%	100%
Hutt	76%	66%		73%	68%	55%		61%	99%
Lakes	93%	80%		78%	71%	53%		42%	100%
MidCentral	89%	75%		74%	69%	57%		62%	100%
Nelson Marlborough	95%	84%		79%	71%	61%		69%	100%
Northland	80%	47%		81%	78%	63%		40%	97%
South Canterbury	90%	81%		78%	73%	60%		76%	100%
Southern	89%	78%		80%	75%	62%		60%	100%
Tairawhiti	92%	79%		79%	71%	51%		78%	98%
Taranaki	80%	80%		76%	70%	57%		61%	100%
Waikato	80%	82%		77%	70%	56%		53%	100%
Wairarapa	91%	67%		70%	64%	52%		60%	100%
Waitemata	88%	84%		80%	76%	65%		43%	100%
West Coast	93%	86%		89%	78%	61%		66%	99%
Whanganui	88%	72%		77%	70%	55%		56%	100%

DHB	Newborn enrolled with GP	Children 0-4 enrolled with oral health service	Reduce dmft in 5-year-old children	Fully immunized at age 5	B4SC started before 4½	Children with healthy weight at age 4	Children with BMI > 98th percentile are referred	Children have low SDQ-P scores	Children with high SDQ-P scores are referred
National target									
National target	90%	95%	4.00	95%	95%	75%	95%	N/A	N/A
All ethnicities									
Auckland	74%	85%	4.62	87%	90%	92%	100%	98%	100%
Bay of Plenty	74%	93%	4.80	81%	88%	93%	76%	94%	98%
Canterbury	80%	62%	4.11	93%	96%	93%	93%	96%	100%
Capital and Coast	77%	97%	3.93	90%	78%	92%	82%	97%	100%
Counties Manukau	73%	84%	4.80	92%	89%	88%	99%	95%	100%
Hawkes Bay	83%	89%	3.79	93%	92%	90%	87%	94%	99%
Hutt	81%	97%	3.72	92%	88%	90%	85%	99%	93%
Lakes	82%	105%	4.68	85%	85%	90%	93%	93%	97%
MidCentral	72%	95%	4.62	93%	79%	91%	93%	94%	100%
Nelson Marlborough	72%	83%	4.06	88%	80%	94%	76%	95%	100%
Northland	82%	72%	5.78	84%	70%	92%	95%	95%	97%
South Canterbury	81%	85%	3.67	95%	96%	91%	86%	96%	100%
Southern	69%	80%	3.64	92%	90%	92%	91%	96%	97%
Tairawhiti	77%	101%	4.96	88%	85%	90%	69%	92%	100%
Taranaki	79%	95%	4.14	94%	53%	92%	86%	92%	100%
Waikato	72%	72%	4.92	87%	94%	90%	78%	96%	99%
Wairarapa	84%	83%	3.81	96%	80%	89%	77%	95%	100%
Waitemata	70%	92%	4.22	84%	86%	93%	100%	98%	100%
West Coast	77%	97%	4.55	80%	71%	88%	86%	96%	100%
Whanganui	88%	104%	4.88	90%	88%	92%	81%	91%	100%

B4SC, B4 School Check; BMI, body mass index; DHB, district health board; LMC, lead maternity carer; SUDI, sudden unexpected death in infancy; WCTO, Well Child/Tamariki Ora.

Adapted from Nationwide Service Framework Library, Well Child / Tamariki Ora Quality Improvement Framework, *WCTO Quality Indicator Report - September 2017*, Copyright © Ministry of Health–Manatū Hauora, 2018, available from https://nsfl.health.govt.nz/dhb-planning-package/well-child-tamariki-ora-quality-improvement-framework, under a Creative Commons Attribution 4.0 International Licence.

New Zealand has produced a standardized dashboard which should be developed at local level with robust and available measures focusing on three key aspects—access, outcome, and quality—which can be collected continuously to help inform real-time quality improvements. The discs below show how close to the individual target each measure is (see Table 34.3).

In the East of England, a comprehensive integrated commissioning and delivery toolkit has been developed which very clearly describes the CHP, its aims, professional responsibilities, and key performance indicators which could act as a useful model for others as a policy document for multiple stakeholders to integrate their data (Sustain, 2015).

It is clear that if we are to take the endeavour of well child care provision seriously as a society then we need to ensure there are credible systems of quality assurance in place with appropriate reporting mechanisms, providing feedback to practitioners, public health, and users of the service alike.

Learning links

◆ National Screening Committee: https://cpdscreening.phe.org.uk/elearning

◆ E-Learning for health leadership, monitoring, and quality: https://www.e-lfh.org.uk/programmes/healthy-child-programme/.

Recommendations

◆ Each country should agree a core set of indicators for their CHP which localities would be expected to report to on a periodic basis. Additional local measures may be collected as necessary to support continuous quality improvement of the well child programme and support benchmarking across areas and between countries over time. (*Evidence: strong.*)

◆ Integration of existing information systems with the aim of unifying the child health record should be prioritized, to optimize patient safety, efficiency, and effectiveness in the delivery of the CHP. (*Evidence: strong.*)

◆ Integrate existing information systems to unify the child health record and optimize patient safety, efficiency and effectiveness in the delivery of the CHP. (*Evidence: strong.*)

◆ Regular feedback of performance measures to practitioners should be a function of all local CHP steering groups and could be linked to professional certification. (*Evidence: strong.*)

◆ Develop a national measure to capture parent experience as part of child health programme. (*Evidence: strong.*)

References

Alliance for Health Policy and Systems Research and World Health Organization (2009). *Systems Thinking for Health Systems Strengthening*. Geneva: World Health Organization. Available at: http://apps.who.int/iris/bitstream/10665/44204/1/9789241563895_eng. pdf?ua=1 [Accessed July 17, 2017].

Anhøj, J. and Hellesøe, A.-M.B. (2016). The problem with red, amber, green: the need to avoid distraction by random variation in organisational performance measures. *BMJ Quality and Safety*, **26**, 81–84.

Arah, O.A., Westert, G.P., Hurst, J., and Klazinga, N.S. (2006). A conceptual framework for the OECD Health Care Quality Indicators Project. *International Journal for Quality in Health Care*, **18**(Suppl. 1), 5–13.

Content.digital.nhs.uk (2017). Children and Young People's Health Services Data Set. [online] Available at: http://content.digital.nhs.uk/maternityandchildren/CYPHS [Accessed 28 Sep. 2017].

Content.digital.nhs.uk (2017)b. Maternity Services Data Set. [online] Available at: http:// content.digital.nhs.uk/maternityandchildren/maternity [Accessed 28 Sep. 2017].

Donabedian, A. (1997). The quality of care. How can it be assessed? *JAMA*, **260**, 1743–1748.

Gov.scot (2015). Universal Health Visiting Pathway in Scotland: Pre-Birth to Pre-School. [online] Available at: http://www.gov.scot/Resource/0048/00487884.pdf [Accessed April 25, 2017].

Hampshire, A.J., Blair, M.E., Crown, N.S., et al. (1999). Is pre-school child health surveillance an effective means of detecting key physical abnormalities? *British Journal of General Practice*, **49**, 630–633.

Hanafin, S. and Cowley, S. (2006). Quality in preventive and health-promoting services: constructing an understanding through process. *Journal of Nursing Management*, **14**, 472–482.

Horridge, K., Harvey, C., McGarry K., et al. (2016). Quantifying multi-faceted needs captured at the point of care. Development of a Disabilities Terminology Set and Disabilities Complexity Scale. *Developmental Medicine and Child Neurology*, **58**, 570–580.

Institute of Medicine, Committee on Quality of Health Care in America (2001). *Crossing the Quality Chasm : A New Health System for the 21st Century*. Washington, DC: National Academy Press.

Mansour, C., Ouarezki, Y., Jones, J., et al. (2017). Trends in Scottish newborn screening programme for congenital hypothyroidism 1980–2014: strategies for reducing age at notification after initial and repeat sampling. *Archives of Disease in Childhood*, **102**, 936–941.

Public Health Wales Observatory and Aneurin Bevan University Health Board (2013). Plentyn Gwent Child Early Years Surveillance Tool. [online] Available at: http://www2. nphs.wales.nhs.uk:8080/PubHObservatoryProjDocs.nsf/3653c00e7bb6259d80256f2700 4900db/2e87bb1fb95c6ed680257d5100447247/$FILE/PlentynGwentChild_pdf_v1.pdf [Accessed April 25, 2017].

Simpson, N., Randall, R., Lenton, S., and Walker, S. (1997). Audit of neonatal screening programme for phenylketonuria and congenital hypothyroidism. *Archives of Disease in Childhood. Fetal and Neonatal Edition*, **77**, F228–F234.

Spencer, S.A. and Davies, M.P. (2012). Hospital episode statistics: improving the quality and value of hospital data: a national internet e-survey of hospital consultants. *BMJ Open*, **2**, e001651.

Sustain (2015). Healthy Child Programme 0–5: Integrated Commissioning and Delivery Toolkit. [online] Available at: http://www.sustain-improvement.com/downloads/2/6/no/all.

Wennberg, J. (2010). *Tracking Medicine- A Researcher's Quest to Understand Health Care.* Oxford: Oxford University Press.

Welsh Government (2016). An overview of the Healthy Child Wales Programme. [online] Available at: http://gov.wales/docs/dhss/publications/160926healthy-childrenen.pdf [Accessed April 25, 2017].

Wood, R., Stirling, A., Nolan, C., Chalmers, J., and Blair, M. (2012). Trends in the coverage of 'universal' child health reviews: observational study using routinely available data. *BMJ Open*, **2**, e000759.

Chapter 35

Conclusions and recommendations

Alan Emond

Conclusions

The research evidence base supporting the child health programme (CHP) has enlarged in the last 15 years, and there is a lot of support to promote health for all children based on a framework of proportionate universalism. This approach appears to be the best investment, as it aims to reduce inequalities in children's health and development, which should reduce inequalities in their educational attainments, their life chances, and their economic potential. How to obtain best value (return on investment for commissioners) still needs further evaluation— buy enhanced services for some families based on assessed need, or target services based on risk factors for a subgroup of the population? Both are certainly needed, but more evidence of impact and cost-effectiveness is required. Conclusions about the long-term benefits of investing in early child development are often based on the associations of adverse child experiences with poor outcomes—not enough research has been done on how to promote resilience, that is, positive outcomes as an adaptation to adversity.

To show the effectiveness of complex CHPs requires a different approach to evaluating effectiveness of drug treatments. It is often not possible to randomize children to receive a preventative intervention, and 'gold standard' level 4 randomized controlled trial-based evidence was rarely found in this review. However, valid comparison groups are essential when assessing effectiveness of interventions, and follow-up is needed to measure the 'washout' of the effects over time. To obtain medium-term outcomes of interventions in the first 1000 days, improved data linkage is required. Better data linkage between preschool CHPs and school entry assessments would be a big step forward, making a school readiness assessment both an outcome for the CHP as well as a baseline for future educational progress. More studies are needed which are able to track impact through childhood and into adulthood.

Across the four nations of the UK, the commissioning environment for the CHP and supporting specialist services for children are becoming more complex, and all countries are trying to do more with reducing resources. In this changing landscape, there is an even greater need for quality evidence to help make rational choices over resource allocation. The good news is that there are quality reviews to help, for example, 'Foundations for Life' from the Early Intervention Foundation (Asmussen et al., 2016), with accompanying commissioner guides.

The provider landscape in the early years is also becoming more diverse, with more varied organizations contributing to the CHP from the health, education, and independent sectors. Although local provision to suit local needs must be good, there is widespread concern about the effect of professional skill mix on both the quality and quantity of CHP provision, and the impact of skill mix on families. There is rightly an emphasis on evaluation with new programmes and enhancements to the existing CHP, but evidence is also needed for the benefit of 'usual care' in the new multi-provider environment—testing what works in the practices of health visitors for example, or evaluating the integrated 2-year check in different settings.

For practitioners working to deliver the CHP, the evidence is clear that families must be engaged as partners in a philosophy of empowerment to give their children the best start in life: to effect this, professionals need to be culturally competent, have a developmental approach to children's health and well-being, and have a good understanding of the signals of risk in families which warrant further assessment for enhanced support.

Above all, to ensure continuous quality improvement, the CHP has to be commissioned, managed, and delivered as a *programme*—with commissioners ensuring that a senior clinician is in charge, that the workforce is well trained, well managed, and given enough time to undertake the multiple level tasks required, and that key measures of process and outcome are routinely collected and reported annually.

Suggestions for further research needed

1. *Cost-effectiveness*. More cost–benefit studies are needed to show return on investment for early intervention. The Early Intervention Foundation has developed a database of studies that have sufficient reliability to form the basis of analysis of impact. Analyses of these impacts are planned, leading to further reports on cost-effectiveness of early intervention.

2. *UK studies*. Too many interventions operating in the UK are based on evidence from other locations, without appropriate adaptation for the diverse British population or for the NHS and educational services in the different countries of the UK. More evaluation needs to be built in, to assess the relevance of findings from one location for another. Learning from innovation needs to be shared, as is happening with A Better Start and the Family Nurse Partnership.

3. *Exposures in pregnancy*. The review identified many gaps in knowledge of the current exposure to harm; for example, research is needed on blood levels of heavy metals in pregnant women in the UK, and on quantifying exposure to phthalates in pregnancy. Research is needed to determine the normal ranges for vitamin D levels in black African and Asian women living in the UK to inform better identification of infants at risk, and rational prescribing of vitamin D supplements. The benefits of iodine supplementation in pregnancy need to be evaluated in a well-designed and adequately powered trial.

4. *Perinatal mental health*. Evaluation is urgently needed of computer and web-based interventions in NHS services to support pregnant women with anxiety and

depression. Also, the effectiveness of mindfulness-based interventions to support pregnant women with anxiety and depression need to be evaluated.

5. *Transition to parenthood.* More research is needed on how to effectively engage grandparents during pregnancy to improve preparation for parenthood for first-time parents. Evaluations are needed of the use of social media to reach digital native young parents to provide evidence-based guidance on infancy and childhood using a developmental approach.

6. *Early child development.* More evaluation is required of the benefits and harms of tablets and smartphones on young children's development, to give evidence-based guidance to parents and grandparents on how to control screen time for children.

7. *Promoting physical activity.* More research evidence is needed on the impact of healthy eating and exercise programmes for young children in preventing obesity and improving well-being.

8. *Injury prevention.* Evaluation is needed of the effectiveness of provision of safety equipment for families living in deprived areas.

9. *Sudden infant death syndrome (SIDS).* More evaluation of the effectiveness of baby boxes in preventing SIDS in low-risk populations is required. If a scoring system can be derived to identify a relatively small group of mothers at higher risk of SIDS, these could be targeted for enhanced messaging.

10. *Children with special needs.* Further research is needed to determine how many children are newly identified by the use of the Strengths and Difficulties Questionnaire at school entry, and how many receive an intervention as a result.

    More evidence is needed on the effectiveness of the joint health and education plans in meeting the needs of children with special educational needs.

    Assistive devices may promote some children's social and cognitive development, but more evidence on the effect of the assistive devices is needed.

11. *Vulnerable children.* More research is needed on how to promote resilience in looked after children, how to promote healthy attachments, and the best ways to encourage children to develop self-regulation.

12. *Programme development.* The introduction of the electronic Personal Child Health Record needs to be carefully evaluated. More evidence is required of the effectiveness of the enhancements and adaptations to the CHP currently being implemented.

Finally, the authors and editor hope that the fifth edition of *Health for all Children* will help to support an effective evidence-based CHP relevant to the needs of children and families across the UK. The evidence base is growing fast, and fewer years should pass until the next edition: at least the revisions based on new evidence will be easier with the online book. A culture of embedded learning is growing, but the approach needed is summarized in the conclusion of the 'Foundations for Life' review: 'The challenge of improving the evidence base is the responsibility of everyone involved in early intervention, of commissioners, providers and practitioners, all must contribute' (Asmussen et al., 2016).

Reference

Asmussen, K., Feinstein, L., Martin, J., and Chowdry, H. (2016). Foundations for Life: What Works to Support Parent Child Interaction in the Early Years. [online] Early Intervention Foundation. Available at: http://www.eif.org.uk/publication/foundations-for-life-what-works-to-support-parent-child-interaction-in-the-early-years.

Index

Tables, figures, and boxes are indicated by an italic *t, f,* and *b* following the page number.